Breastfeeding For Dummies®

Cheat Sheet

Ten Reasons to Breastfeed

1. Breast milk is individually formulated for *your* baby — not the kid on the formula can!
2. Breastfeeding helps shrink your uterus after delivery.
3. Breast milk tastes different depending on what you eat, so maybe your baby will be a gourmet eater later in life!
4. Breastfed babies spend less time at the pediatrician's office, because they're sick less often.
5. You'll have bigger breasts while you're breastfeeding. (No, it won't last forever!)
6. You can take breast milk anywhere without needing a bigger diaper bag.
7. Breastfeeding burns as many calories per day as a trip to the gym.
8. If you have older kids, breastfeeding can help you teach them about the facts of life.
9. Breastfeeding may raise your baby's IQ 5 to 10 points.
10. You never run out of breast milk at 2 a.m. and need to run to the all-night convenience store for more.

Essential Vocabulary

Alveoli: The cells where milk is produced.

Areola: The brownish area surrounding the nipple. For proper *latch-on* to occur (see the definition later in this list), the baby must take both the nipple and a good portion of the areola into his mouth.

Breast pump: A mechanical device for removing milk from your breast. Breast pumps can be as simple as a manual, bicycle-horn type or as complicated as an electrical pump that removes milk from both breasts at the same time (see Chapter 5).

Colostrum: A thick, creamy fluid containing high amounts of antibodies and protein. This is the first milk your body produces in the days immediately following delivery.

Engorgement: The congestion of the blood vessels in the breast that occurs when your milk production begins to change from colostrum to mature milk. The increased volume of milk can cause your breasts to become hot, swollen, and tender (see Chapter 6).

Foremilk: The first milk produced in a feeding.

Hindmilk: The milk produced at the end of a feeding. It has a higher amount of fat than foremilk and has a sleep-inducing effect on the baby.

Inverted nipples: Nipples that invert rather than protruding from the breast tissue, which can cause challenges during early breastfeeding (see Chapter 4).

Lactation consultant: A specialist in the field of breastfeeding (see Chapter 4).

Latch-on: The attachment of the baby to the breast. If latch-on is poor, your baby may not get enough milk and/or your nipples may become very sore (see Chapter 6).

Let-down reflex: Your body's release of milk in response to nipple stimulation (see Chapter 6).

Mastitis: An infection in the breast (see Chapter 8).

Milk ducts: The conduits that carry breast milk from the alveoli to the nipple.

Postpartum: The time period from the day you deliver the baby to six weeks after delivery.

Rooming in: Keeping the baby in your room the entire time you're in the hospital, rather than sending him to the nursery (see Chapter 6).

Tandem nursing: Breastfeeding two babies of different ages, such as a newborn and a toddler (see Chapter 16).

Weaning: The process of ending breastfeeding (see Chapter 12).

For Dummies: Bestselling Book Series for Beginners

Breastfeeding For Dummies®

Cheat Sheet

Breastfeeding Month by Month

Sleeping and eating: 1 month

In the first month, your baby may:

- Sleep most of the time.
- Nurse every two to three hours.
- Perfect his rooting reflex.
- Have a strong sucking reflex.
- Love being held close.
- Start focusing on your face (by the end of the month).

Smiling away: 2 months

This month, your baby may:

- Recognize your face and associate you with feeding.
- Start to smile!
- Possibly develop colic — watch what you eat (see Chapter 8).

"Hey, I'm here!": 3 months

This month, your baby may:

- Become a social butterfly.
- Develop a schedule of sorts (but don't get too used to it!).
- Respond to your voice.
- Prefer one breast side or a certain breastfeeding position over another.

"Is that my voice?": 4 months

This month, your baby may:

- Find his voice — he may vocalize and sometimes squawk!
- Love being touched. Try massaging his back or legs during nursing. Massaging may help him gain weight faster.
- Start getting teeth — look for them before you discover them with an "ouch!"

Wiggle worm: 5 months

This month, your baby may:

- Start moving parts of his body — and realizing that they belong to him. He'll often play with his hands and feet while nursing.
- Be more distracted by voices or outside events while nursing.

"I'm ready for more": 6 months

This month, your baby may:

- Be ready to start solid foods (see Chapter 10).
- Start drinking a little from a sippy cup.
- Possibly have one or more teeth.

"Can't slow me down": 7 months

This month, your baby may:

- Start to crawl or roll across the floor. Expect lots more wiggling during nursing as well!
- Want to nurse for shorter times so he can get moving again.

Anxious: 8 months

This month, your baby may:

- Develop stranger anxiety, wanting to be close only to you.
- Show an attachment to a certain blanket or stuffed animal.

Growing up: 9 months

This month, your baby may:

- Seem less interested in nursing.
- Nurse for comfort more than for nutrition.
- Nurse more at night than during the day.

"Where's my baby?": 10 to 12 months

During these months, your baby may:

- Cruise alongside furniture or start to take a few tentative steps.
- Still be interested in nursing. Keep going if you're both interested. Your baby is little for such a short time; hold on tight, but also give him wings to fly.

Item 4481-0.

For more information about Wiley Publishing, call 1-800-762-2974.

For Dummies: Bestselling Book Series for Beginners

Breastfeeding FOR DUMMIES®

Breastfeeding FOR DUMMIES®

by Sharon Perkins, RN,
and Carol Vannais, RN

WILEY

Wiley Publishing, Inc.

Breastfeeding For Dummies®

Published by
Wiley Publishing, Inc.
111 River St.
Hoboken, NJ 07030-5774
www.wiley.com

Published by Wiley Publishing, Inc., Indianapolis, Indiana

Published simultaneously in Canada

For general information on our other products and services or to obtain technical support, please contact our Customer Care Department within the U.S. at 800-762-2974, outside the U.S. at 317-572-3993, or fax 317-572-4002.

Wiley also publishes its books in a variety of electronic formats. Some content that appears in print may not be available in electronic books.

Library of Congress Control Number: 2004100678

ISBN: 0-7645-4481-0

Manufactured in the United States of America

10 9 8 7 6 5 4 3 2 1

About the Authors

Sharon Perkins, RN: Sharon Perkins is an RN with 17 years experience, all in some area of maternal–child health. She's currently the RN coordinator for in vitro fertilization at Cooper Center in Marlton, New Jersey, but has also worked in labor and delivery, home health, and neonatal intensive care. Sharon is the coauthor of *Fertility For Dummies*, published in 2003. She lives in Medford, New Jersey, with her husband John, a soon-to-be-retired Air Force pilot, and wonders what she's going to do when he's hanging around the house all the time! She has five children, none of whom (amazingly enough) are living at home at the moment, two wonderful daughters-in-law, and the smartest grandchild in the world.

Carol Vannais, RN: Carol Vannais has been an RN for 33 years. She is currently a staff nurse at Cooper Center for In Vitro Fertilization in Marlton, New Jersey, a very large infertility center where she's worked for six years. Prior to Cooper Center, she worked in labor and delivery for 18 years as an RN and a Certified Childbirth Instructor. She summarizes her maternal–child health experience as taking care of babies from the very, very beginning (as embryos) to the very end (delivery). Prior to working in maternal– child health, she worked in critical care. She lives in New Jersey with her husband Leon. She has four sons who are a constant reminder of her title of "mother"!

Dedication

From Sharon: To my children and grandson, who provided the raw material for this book.

From Carol: This book is dedicated to my children. If it weren't for them, I would not know how a nursing mother truly feels. And to my husband, Leon; without his support, my climb to become an author would have been insurmountable. And last, but far from least, to my Dad. Remembering your creative ability with your hands, your heart, and your mind helped me to accept this challenge without fear.

Authors' Acknowledgments

From Sharon: When I wrote *Fertility For Dummies,* I used up all my good acknowledgments! For this book, I thank everyone in my family again, including my children and husband John. You're all still wonderful and supportive.

Much of what I know about breastfeeding came from my own experiences; much I learned from patients. In 11 years as a labor and delivery nurse, and 3 years working the neonatal intensive care unit, I had the privilege of helping many new moms learn to breastfeed, under many different conditions. As we go through life, we gain much from the people we meet and care for, and often they aren't aware of how they've shaped us. To all I've cared for, I thank you for what you've taught me. I thank God for the ability to care for others, as well as the ability to write about my experiences.

To my coauthor from *Fertility For Dummies,* Jackie Thompson, a million thanks for everything, from being a constant cheerleader to refusing to ever let me get discouraged — about anything! You're a true friend.

To Carol, who had the guts to sign on to write this book, even though she didn't think she'd live through it — you did it! And you did a great job. Your name moved from the acknowledgments section of *Fertility For Dummies* to the front cover of this one, and you deserve to be there!

Both Carol and I want to thank Kathy Cox, our acquisitions editor, for trusting us to write this book; Joan Friedman, our project editor, for being a great support from beginning to end, as well as a great editor; Kathryn Born, for her (once again) wonderful illustrations; and lactation consultant Shirley Donato, our friend as well as our technical advisor, who kept us accurate and up-to-date on the latest in breastfeeding. And, of course, our agent, Jessica Faust, for her help in bringing this book to life.

And to all the people whose names we never hear, but who were instrumental in creating this book, we thank you all. We may not know you, but we appreciate you!

From Carol: It's kind of funny that after months and months of writing words, I find myself "speechless"! I feel like the people at the Academy Awards. How do you acknowledge so many people who are a part of your life?

I undertook this challenge because I truly felt that it would be a life experience that I would never forget. Thirty-two years of being a nurse helped prepare me for my introduction to authorship by teaching me "to learn, to teach, and to live." My wish is that this book will help all mothers not only to breastfeed their children but also to learn and to live!

I would like to personally thank my children: Ryan, Jonathan, Rebecca, Joshua, and Rory. If I were writing a book about my personal breastfeeding experiences, it would be titled *The Good, The Bad, and The Ugly*! There were many ups and downs, but we all persevered because breastfeeding is a family affair. Their support during the last few months meant so much to me. Of course, they were probably being nice mostly to avoid being immortalized in print. Only kidding, guys!

My grandmother was an important person in my early breastfeeding days. She nursed her children, so she could relate to my early problems. I'll never forget the day she showed up at my house with boxes and boxes of tea bags. Apparently, way back then, it was thought that drinking tea helped with your milk supply. She was hell-bent on making sure that my supply would not diminish!

My mother has been so supportive. She knew that I had a full load with writing the book, working full-time, preparing for my oldest son's wedding, and maintaining a big house. She was always there to say, "Keep up the good work — you'll never regret it, and the dirt will still be there when it's done!" It's funny, because those are words for every breastfeeding mom to live by too!

A special thanks to two special breastfeeding friends. It seems like only yesterday that I was commiserating with you about my breastfeeding problems, yet it was over 16 years ago. My friendships remain strong with Denise and Chris. You both were my "bosom buddies" for quite a few years. As in our nursing days, we've struggled and succeeded in some hardships in our lives. Our breastfeeding bonding has cemented a lifetime friendship, for which I am eternally grateful.

And lastly, I'd like to thank Sharon. As a friend and coauthor, she's often gone above and beyond the call of duty. She has listened to my ideas. She encouraged me when I felt overwhelmed. And she did it all with a smile! I know that we have a true friendship, because it has only grown with this experience.

Publisher's Acknowledgments

We're proud of this book; please send us your comments through our Dummies online registration form located at www.dummies.com/register/.

Some of the people who helped bring this book to market include the following:

Acquisitions, Editorial, and Media Development

Project Editor: Joan Friedman

Acquisitions Editor: Kathy Cox

Technical Editor: Shirley Donato

Editorial Manager: Michelle Hacker

Editorial Assistant: Elizabeth Rea

Cover Photos: A9LWA-Dann Tardif/CORBIS

Cartoons: Rich Tennant, www.the5thwave.com

Production

Project Coordinator: Courtney MacIntyre

Layout and Graphics: Andrea Dahl, Stephanie D. Jumper, Kristin McMullan, Barry Offringa, Jacque Schneider

Special Art: Kathryn Born

Proofreaders: Dwight Ramsey, Charles Spencer, TECHBOOKS Production Services

Indexer: TECHBOOKS Production Services

Special Help: Mary Yeary

Publishing and Editorial for Consumer Dummies

Diane Graves Steele, Vice President and Publisher, Consumer Dummies

Joyce Pepple, Acquisitions Director, Consumer Dummies

Kristin A. Cocks, Product Development Director, Consumer Dummies

Michael Spring, Vice President and Publisher, Travel

Brice Gosnell, Associate Publisher, Travel

Kelly Regan, Editorial Director, Travel

Publishing for Technology Dummies

Andy Cummings, Vice President and Publisher, Dummies Technology/General User

Composition Services

Gerry Fahey, Vice President of Production Services

Debbie Stailey, Director of Composition Services

Contents at a Glance

Table of Contents

Introduction

It's probably safe to assume that if you're reading these words, you're either considering having a baby or you're already pregnant. Either way, congratulations — you're embarking on an incredible journey!

One of the most important decisions you make when you're pregnant is whether to breastfeed or bottle feed. Believe it or not, this decision is even more important than whether to buy the $300 Peg Perego stroller or stick with a more basic model! Your baby can be happy and healthy no matter which approach to feeding you choose; this book helps you make an informed decision by showing you the pros and cons of each. More importantly, it can help you make the right decision for you and your baby.

About This Book

Just because women have been breastfeeding without the aid of books for thousands of years doesn't mean that it always goes smoothly. Every breastfeeding mom has questions and concerns about whether breastfeeding is the right choice.

Back in the days when we were breastfeeding, information on breastfeeding was sparse, and lactation consultants — professionals who provide nursing moms with information and support — were almost nonexistent. Times have certainly changed; many hospitals today make a visit from the lactation consultant mandatory before you are discharged, and breastfeeding books and support groups are everywhere.

Yet, of the more than 60 percent of new moms who start breastfeeding in the hospital, almost a third stop breastfeeding before six months — the length of time that the American Academy of Pediatrics (AAP) recommends breastfeeding exclusively. And even fewer are still breastfeeding when their babies reach 1 year of age, despite the AAP's counsel that a full year of breastfeeding is best for the child. With all the information and support available, why do so few moms continue breastfeeding for the recommended length of time?

Many new moms stop breastfeeding because it isn't as easy as they thought it would be. After being told how natural and instinctive breastfeeding is, you may expect it to be intuitive. For many women, it just isn't. Most new moms experience at least one breastfeeding problem difficult enough to cause them to consider giving up nursing. Others never begin because of misinformation or apathy on the part of their doctors, families, or hospital staff.

We didn't write this book to try to cure all breastfeeding problems or to force everyone to try it. Breastfeeding for a full year is not for everyone. Breastfeeding for even a month isn't for everyone. We wrote this book to encourage women to give breastfeeding a try and to give them the information they need to succeed even if they run into problems — and they probably will!

Neither of us were militant breastfeeders, and this book is not written from the viewpoint that breastfeeding for only a short time, or choosing not to breastfeed at all, makes you less of a mother. We don't believe that to be true. What we do believe is that breastfeeding is beneficial for you and your baby, that it brings you both benefits beyond convenience, and that it's worth the effort it takes to learn. Our goal is to make the learning effort fun — or at least as painless as possible — for both of you!

How to Use This Book

We'd like every new mom who tries breastfeeding to succeed for six months to a year, and we'd like more new moms to give it a try. We wrote this book to encourage you to seriously consider breastfeeding your new baby and to at least try it in the hospital. We hope this book helps you through the sometimes difficult first days of breastfeeding, as well as through challenges you may face throughout the first year of the baby's life, especially if you return to work.

This book is meant as a resource, which means you can flip to the table of contents or index, find what you're looking for, read about it, and put the book away. Or you can read it from front to back, memorize it, and recite it to all your friends.

We try to give you all the information you need in an easy-to-read, humorous way, without overloading you with details. The book is broken into five parts, which take you from the planning stages as you prepare for delivery all the way to breastfeeding as you plan for your next baby.

We include personal stories about our own breastfeeding experiences throughout the book because sometimes just knowing that someone else has been through problems and survived can help you keep breastfeeding on the not-so-good days. Our experiences weren't all wonderful, and most likely yours won't be either. But we kept breastfeeding — over and over! — because we thought it was worth the effort. We hope you will, too!

How This Book Is Organized

Breastfeeding For Dummies is divided into five parts. If you're still in the planning stages of breastfeeding, you may want to start with Part I. If you're in the hospital and need to know how to get started breastfeeding today, definitely jump directly to Part II! The following sections explain how the book is organized.

Part I: Getting Ready to Breastfeed

If you're just beginning to think about breastfeeding, we suggest you start with Part I. First, we give you the pros and cons of breastfeeding, including who should *not* breastfeed. We also help you set up your nursery and tell you how to get yourself physically ready for breastfeeding. (Don't worry — we don't demand any strenuous exercise!)

Part II: Putting Breastfeeding into Action

Now that you've got the new baby, as well as breasts filled with milk, what's next? These chapters show you how to start breastfeeding in the hospital. They help you through the first sleep-deprived and sometimes difficult weeks of breastfeeding, and they describe how to breastfeed under special circumstances, such as when you adopt a baby or have a baby with a physical handicap.

Part III: Growing with Your Baby

How does breastfeeding change month by month? How do you keep your partner happy and involved as a new parent? When's the best time to wean, and how do you go about it? All these questions and more are addressed in Part III.

Part IV: Breastfeeding in the Real World

Everyone has to leave the house sometime. In this part we discuss breastfeeding as a working mom, breastfeeding in public (from Disney World to the diner), and knowing the legal issues related to breastfeeding. We also take a peek ahead to planning your next pregnancy, nursing during pregnancy, and tackling the task of nursing two children at a time.

Part V: The Part of Tens

This section is a perfect read when you don't feel like being so serious about breastfeeding. Want to know the ten most common wives' tales about breastfeeding and the truths behind them? Looking for great underwear — or great bumper stickers? Want to know where to look for breastfeeding answers in the middle of the night (besides in this book)? Look no further than the chapters in Part V.

Icons Used in This Book

Throughout this book, you'll encounter icons in the margins. Icons give you hints about the type of information you'll find in a given paragraph. We use the following four icons:

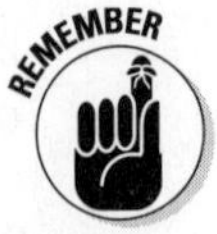

Paragraphs with this icon contain information you want to store in your mental filing cabinet. These reminders can help you get through even the roughest days of early breastfeeding.

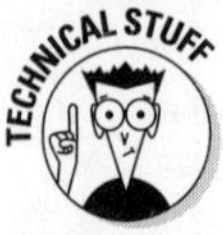

If you're the curious sort who needs to know the *why* of everything, be sure to read the paragraphs marked by this icon. If you're content knowing the *how* of breastfeeding, feel free to skip these paragraphs; your nursing experience will be just as good without them.

Paragraphs marked by this icon offer special bits of advice and information that can make your breastfeeding experience more successful and enjoyable.

This symbol alerts you to potential health issues or other problems you may encounter during your pregnancy or your breastfeeding experience.

Part I
Getting Ready to Breastfeed

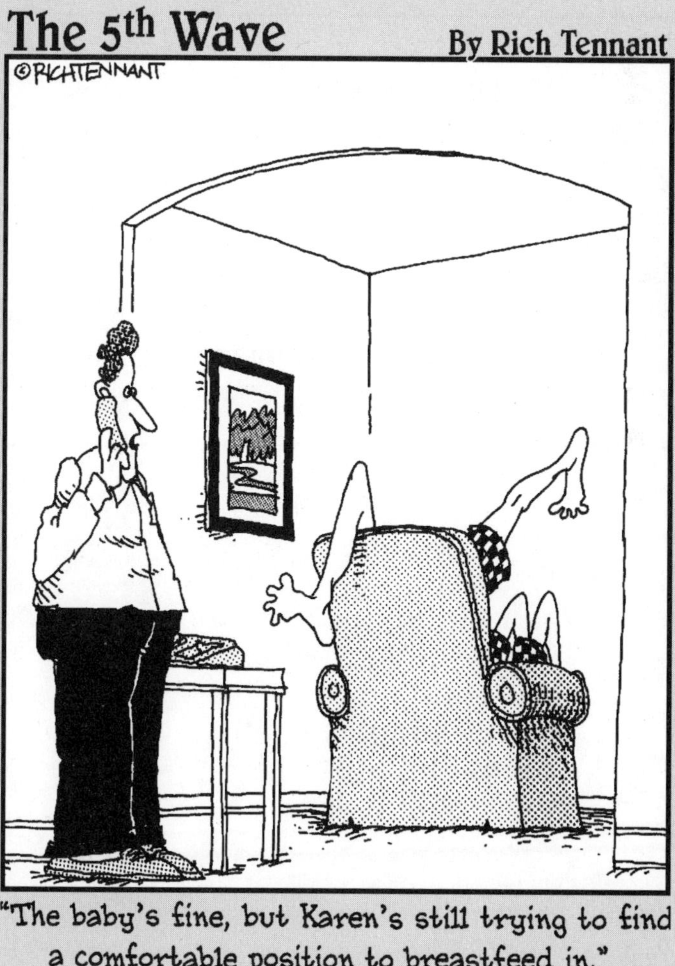
The 5th Wave
By Rich Tennant
©RICHTENNANT

"The baby's fine, but Karen's still trying to find a comfortable position to breastfeed in."

In this part . . .

Having a baby involves lots of decision making, from picking out a name to picking out a bigger house! Choosing whether to breastfeed or bottle feed can be one of the most important decisions, as well as one of the hardest. Friends and family all have opinions about breastfeeding, and some information you read and hear may seem contradictory. In this part, we discuss the pros and cons of breastfeeding, what breastfeeding really involves, and how to stock your nursery to make your new job easy (and fun!).

Chapter 1

Deciding to Breastfeed

In This Chapter

- Distinguishing between formula and breast milk
- Understanding how your breasts produce milk
- Weighing your feeding options

If this were the year 2000 BC rather than 2000+ AD, this book wouldn't be necessary. If you wanted your baby to survive more than a week or two, you'd have to breastfeed, unless you had a friend who was willing to do the job for you.

Somewhere in the last 4,000 years, however, the idea took root that breastfeeding a baby was a distasteful task, better left either to a hired nurse or to anyone willing to wield a rubber nipple. Chances are that your great-grandmother breastfed her children, but your mom and grandma probably didn't. That's because in the early twentieth century, most doctors told their patients that baby formula was a more modern and better way to feed a baby.

Now the pendulum is swinging back to breastfeeding as the best feeding method. You may have friends who are fervent — and vocal — proponents of either breast or bottle. But your friends can't make your decision for you; only *you* can determine if breastfeeding is the right choice for you and your child. This book can help you make that decision.

In this chapter, we offer an overview of breastfeeding, including a look at some differences between breast milk and formula, a lesson in how your breasts make milk, and a brief discussion of some of the advantages and disadvantages of breastfeeding (which we discuss in detail in Chapters 2 and 3). We hope the information here is food for thought, whether you may be planning to breastfeed for three days or three years.

Comparing Formula and Breast Milk

One of the first issues to consider when deciding how to feed your baby is the quality of the food itself. Perhaps you've heard that breastfed babies get hungry sooner than bottle-fed babies. Does that mean formula sustains babies better than breast milk? Maybe you've read that formula contains more protein than breast milk. Does that mean your milk is somehow deficient?

In this section, we soothe concerns you may have about the quality of milk your body produces, and we address misconceptions about the differences between breast milk and formula.

A lesson from Little Miss Muffet

You may remember the old nursery rhyme about Little Miss Muffet, sitting on a tuffet, eating her curds and whey. Looking at curds and whey is a good place to start as we examine the differences between breast milk and formula.

Most baby formulas are derived from cow's milk (although dairy-free formulas are also available). When milk — from the breast or from a cow — is digested, it breaks down into two byproducts: curds and whey. The *curd* is white and rubbery, and the *whey* is liquid.

REMEMBER

When cow's milk breaks down, the curd that forms is hard for human babies to digest. Breast milk, on the other hand, forms more whey than curd, and the curd is softer and more easily digested. Because the baby can digest breast milk more easily than cow's milk, he's less likely to decorate your favorite sweater with spit-up.

Formula makers are striving to make their formulas contain more whey and less curd, so they can be digested more like breast milk. Some formulas, like Nutramigen and Alimentum, are made of *hydrolyzed* protein, which is already broken down, so they are more easily digested than standard cow's milk or soy formulas. In all cases, breast milk is still the gold standard that formula companies are continually trying to match!

Custom-made nutrition

Formula and breast milk look very different; formula is creamier and looks richer than breast milk. This may lead you to believe that formula is more nutritious for your baby, but that's not the case.

One of the most amazing things about breast milk is that *your* milk is specially formulated to have the right composition for *your* baby, and to contain exactly the right amounts of nutrients. Bottle-fed babies receive the exact same nutrients every time they eat. Breast milk, on the other hand, continually changes in composition so that your baby gets what he or she needs at any age.

Considering colostrum

The first liquid the breasts produce (starting a few months before the baby is born) actually doesn't even look like milk. *Colostrum,* which is yellow and thicker than breast milk, is a great example of how your body custom-makes the right nutrition for your baby. Here are some of its benefits:

- Colostrum has a high concentration of antibodies, especially *IgA,* an antibody that helps protect the lungs, throat, and intestines.
- Colostrum helps "seal" the permeable newborn intestines to prevent harmful substances from penetrating the gut.
- Colostrum is very high in concentrated nutrition.
- Colostrum has a laxative effect, which helps the baby pass the first bowel movements (and prevents newborn jaundice).
- Colostrum is low in fat, high in proteins and carbohydrates, and very easy to digest.

Within a few days after delivery, your body begins to produce mature milk that takes over the work of giving your baby the necessary ingredients for healthy growth. Colostrum is still present for around two weeks; the milk produced during this time is called *transitional* milk.

Comparing ingredients

Breast milk contains more than 100 ingredients that the formula industry simply can't duplicate. For example, breast milk is full of antibodies that protect babies from illness and help them develop their own immune systems. Some other key differences between the ingredients in breast milk and formula include the following:

- Formula has a higher protein content than human milk. However, the protein in breast milk is more easily and completely digested by babies.
- Breast milk has a higher carbohydrate content than formula and has large amounts of *lactose,* a sugar found in lower amounts in cow's milk. Research shows that animals whose milk contains higher amounts of lactose experience larger brain development.

- Minerals such as iron are present in lower quantities in breast milk than in formula. However, the minerals in breast milk are more completely absorbed by the baby. In formula-fed babies, the unabsorbed portions of minerals can change the balance of bacteria in the gut, which gives harmful bacteria a chance to grow. This is one reason why bottle-fed babies generally have harder and more odorous stools than breastfed babies.

Table 1-1 summarizes these and other significant differences between breast milk and formula.

Table 1-1 Breast Milk and Formula at a Glance

Breast Milk	***Formula***
Contains proteins that don't cause allergies	Contains dairy-based proteins, which some babies are allergic to or may have difficulty digesting
Forms a softer curd and more whey	Forms larger, harder-to-digest curd
Contains growth-promoting hormones	Contains less-easily digested growth-promoting hormones (or sometimes none at all)
Contains lactose as its main sugar	May contain less lactose than breast milk
Gives baby more carbohydrates	Gives baby fewer carbohydrates
Contains oligosaccharides, good for a healthy gut	Deficient in oligosaccharides
Has a higher fat content	Has a lower fat content
Contains *lipase* (which helps to break down fats) and *cholesterol* (which is important for brain and nerve development)	Does not contain lipase or cholesterol
Is broken down and absorbed more easily than formula	Is more difficult to digest than breast milk, which means more is excreted
Contains DHA for nervous system development	May or may not contain DHA
Offers babies antibodies that protect them from disease	Does not contain antibodies
Contains lower amounts of vitamins and minerals, because they are easily absorbed	Contains higher amounts of vitamins andminerals to offset poor absorption

Who is breastfeeding today?

More women are choosing to breastfeed today than at any time in the last 70 years. Who is most likely to breastfeed in the United States today? One study conducted by Abbot Laboratories yielded the following statistics about women who breastfeed while they are in the hospital.

Maternal age:

- Less than 20 years old: 54%
- 20–24 years old: 62%
- 25–29 years old: 70%
- 30–34 years old: 73%
- Over 34 years old: 74%

Employment status:

- Women working full-time: 65%
- Women working part-time: 69%
- Stay-at-home moms: 66%

A year after delivery, these numbers change dramatically.

- Women working full-time: 10%
- Women working part-time: 16%
- Stay-at-home moms: 21%

We discuss the difficulties of working and breastfeeding in detail in Chapter 13.

Overall, 67 percent of all new moms breastfeed in the hospital, and 31 percent are still breastfeeding six months later. A year after delivery, only 17 percent are breastfeeding.

Feeding frequencies

Breastfed babies often want to eat again sooner after a feeding than bottle-fed babies, which may lead you (or an outspoken relative) to conclude that you aren't producing enough milk, or your milk isn't rich enough. We're happy to clear up this misconception!

REMEMBER

Breastfed babies eat more often than bottle-fed babies because the fats and proteins in breast milk are more easily broken down than the fats and proteins in formula, so they are absorbed and used more quickly. This means that breastfed babies often have fewer digestive troubles than bottle-fed babies. (Fats in formula aren't as well absorbed, which is one reason why bottle-fed babies have more unpleasant smelling bowel movements.) However, it also means that if you choose to breastfeed, you can expect to be on call for feedings every few hours. (A bottle-fed baby, by contrast, may be able to sleep longer between feedings.)

An important consideration for breastfeeding mothers is the length of time your baby spends nursing on each breast. As we discuss in Chapter 8, a baby receives thinner breast milk known as *foremilk* (with a lower fat content) at the beginning of a feeding, and thicker milk (with a higher fat content) after he has been nursing for several minutes. This thicker milk is called *hindmilk.* Allowing the baby to completely empty the breast ensures that he gets an adequate amount of hindmilk. Hindmilk has a sleep-inducing effect, resulting in the relaxed look your baby may have at the end of a meal.

Getting to Know Your Breasts

If you're thinking about breastfeeding, you may be curious about how this whole process works. Your breasts have been with you a long time, but outside of puberty, you probably haven't paid much attention to their functioning.

Everything changes with pregnancy. The breasts you thought you knew start to seem like someone else's. To help you understand the changes, in this section we explain what breasts are, what's inside them, and what makes them work.

Labeling your parts

Your breasts began to develop a very long time ago — about seven weeks after you were conceived, in fact. By the time you were born, all the components of adult breasts were already in place. In fact, both boy and girl babies often produce a small amount of fluid right after delivery (sometimes called *witch's milk*).

When you experienced puberty, your body released estrogen that started the process of your breasts becoming mature. From the first time you noticed puffiness of the *areola* (the darker area around the nipple), it probably took around three or four years for fully functioning breasts to develop.

Breast tissue is made up of glandular (or *lobular*) tissue, fatty tissue, milk ducts, and connective tissue (see Figure 1-1). Glandular tissue is firm, while fatty tissue is softer. (The upper, outer part of the breast has a higher percentage of glandular tissue than other areas of the breast.) Glandular tissue contains the milk ducts and lobules that produce milk. This tissue starts to grow in preparation for pregnancy after you ovulate, and it is responsible for the breast tenderness you may experience just before your period.

Around 15 to 20 lobes are distributed around each breast. Each lobe is further divided into lobules that contain *alveoli,* saclike structures that produce milk. The lobes are attached to mammary ducts that carry milk to little openings in the nipple. The nipple is surrounded by pinkish tissue that turns darker during pregnancy and remains darker after you've delivered. This is the *areola.* Milk is stored in small cavities called *lactiferous sinuses* beneath the areola. Small bumps on the areola are called *Montgomery's glands;* they produce secretions to lubricate and cleanse the areola.

Touring the milk factory

Starting with the delivery of your baby, this is how your body makes milk, beginning with colostrum:

1. **The levels of *estrogen* and *progesterone* (hormones that increase during pregnancy) in your body drop after you deliver your placenta.** This process usually occurs very shortly after you deliver — within hours, if not minutes. For more information about what occurs during and after delivery, see *Pregnancy For Dummies, 2nd Edition,* by Joanne Stone, M.D., Keith Eddleman, M.D., and Mary Duenwald (Wiley).

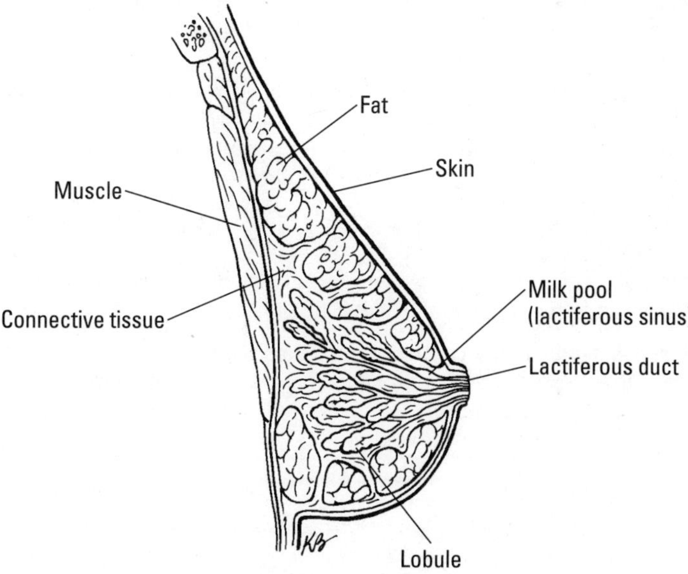

Figure 1-1: A look at your breasts from the outside in.

2. **The level of *prolactin* (another hormone that increases during pregnancy) stays high and actually increases after delivery.** This prompts your body to begin producing milk.
3. **Milk forms in the small cluster of cells called the *alveoli* and travels down your milk ducts.** It then pools in the lactiferous sinuses behind your nipple.
4. **Your baby begins nursing and empties the lactiferous sinuses.** Ideally, this occurs immediately after delivery (see Chapter 6).
5. ***Oxytocin,* a hormone that causes muscle contractions, is released as the baby sucks.** Oxytocin stimulates the muscles around your milk glands and ducts to contract, which moves your milk toward the nipple. This is known as your *let-down reflex.*
6. **Milk is continually squeezed through your milk ducts to the nipple as your baby sucks.**
7. **When the baby removes milk from the breast, your body is stimulated to produce more.** If you're not nursing, after three or four days your milk supply dries up. The more milk your baby takes, the more your breast makes.

A brief history of breastfeeding

Back in caveman days, moms were the sole providers of milk for their babies; if you couldn't nurse your baby, your baby didn't survive long. But around 600 or 500 BC, the Egyptians, Romans, and Greeks started something new with their royal babies: Royal moms began hiring other women, called *wet nurses,* to breastfeed their babies. A wet nurse was a woman who had recently had a child of her own, thereby making her capable of producing milk. Wet nurses sometimes nursed several children at a time.

Wet nursing continued as an upper-middle-class custom for centuries in many parts of the world, interspersed with attempts to give babies milk from various animals. Some rather odd sources (like pigs) were attempted, but eventually cows and goats won out as the best animal substitutes for human milk.

In the eighteenth century, some women tried *dry nursing* (or *pap feeding*), which involved giving babies flour, bread, or cereal mixed with broth or water. These mixtures didn't sit well with most babies' digestive systems. Many babies in orphanages, where pap was used extensively, died.

The formulation of useable breast milk substitutes really became popular in the 1930s. When women were needed in the workplace during World War II, bottle-feeding became the norm in the United States. Formula companies continued to tout their products after World War II ended. Doctors jumped on the formula band wagon, and breastfeeding in the United States dropped to an all-time low of around 20 percent between 1956 and 1966.

The "back to nature" movement in the 1970s that brought us natural childbirth also brought a new interest in breastfeeding. Every decade since has seen an increase in the percentage of moms who start breastfeeding in the hospital.

Making an Informed Choice

In this chapter, we've discussed the nutritional advantages of breastfeeding, and we discuss the physical, financial, and other benefits in detail in Chapter 2. You may already be wondering why, given all the plusses of breastfeeding, everyone isn't doing it.

Are there disadvantages to breastfeeding? Nothing in this world comes without some sort of price, so of course there are. From our perspective, the main disadvantages to breastfeeding are:

- **You're always on call.** You'll be the only meal ticket in town for your baby, which means you'll be on call for every feeding.
- **You may have to watch what you eat.** Some things you eat (like chocolate) may not agree with the baby (see Chapter 7).
- **If you're extremely modest, breastfeeding may be hard.** Keep in mind that you can manage to breastfeed without ever going public. We discuss breastfeeding in public in Chapter 14.
- **Breastfeeding can be difficult to establish.** Breastfeeding isn't always simple at first; both you and your baby have to learn how to do it. Putting a bottle in the baby's mouth is simpler than teaching some babies how to nurse efficiently.

Interestingly, these disadvantages aren't at the top of the list of reasons why women choose not to breastfeed, according to the American Academy of Pediatrics (AAP). An AAP study found that some of the most common reasons women did not breastfeed were:

- Apathy on the part of physicians
- Disruptive schedules in the hospital
- Early discharge from the hospital
- Lack of societal support
- The need to go back to work
- Free handouts of formula and other gift packs in the hospital

This certainly isn't an exhaustive list. Some women have personal reasons for not feeling comfortable with breastfeeding, and others have health issues that make breastfeeding difficult, if not impossible. We devote Chapter 3 to a detailed discussion of some reasons why breastfeeding isn't the best choice for everyone.

But with the AAP study in mind, we encourage you to take steps early to ensure that you have a good breastfeeding support network in place. In Chapter 4, we tell you how to pick a supportive doctor, and in Chapter 6, we discuss dealing with an uncooperative hospital. Chapter 13 shows you how to breastfeed when you go back to work, and Chapter 14 helps you deal with family and friends. As for the gift pack, we hope that you give your feeding decision serious enough consideration that it won't be swayed by a few free cans of formula and a baby bib!

Chapter 2

The Advantages of Breastfeeding

In This Chapter

- Decreasing childhood illnesses
- Helping yourself physically and emotionally
- Reducing the money and time spent on feeding

Studies have shown that breastfeeding is good for both you and your baby. In this chapter, we review the physical, emotional, and other benefits of breastfeeding, from the well-known to those still being studied.

As you discover in this chapter, breastfeeding for even a short time has benefits. Even if you aren't certain whether you want to breastfeed for months (or years), the information here can help you decide whether to give breastfeeding a try.

Benefiting Your Baby

In addition to being a tailor-made food for your baby (see Chapter 1), breast milk has benefits for infants that formula can't duplicate. The closer science looks at breast milk, the more benefits it uncovers.

Building the immune system

Breast milk contains large numbers of cells called *macrophages,* which are white blood cells that attack and destroy harmful bacteria in a baby's body. The presence of macrophages helps keep breastfed babies healthier overall than those who drink formula.

Your breast milk contains antibodies that protect your baby from illnesses that you've been exposed to in the past, as well as from the bacteria and viruses you're exposed to every day — germs that could make your baby ill. In addition, breastfed babies' own immune systems tend to mature faster than those of bottle-fed babies, so breastfed babies can fight off bacteria and viruses at a younger age.

Breastfed babies also have a higher antibody level after receiving the common infant vaccinations, meaning their protection level is higher.

Decreasing ear infections

Ear infections (called *otitis media*) are very common in infancy; two out of three children under the age of 3 have had at least one. Any parent who has spent a sleepless night rocking a wailing, ear-tugging baby can confirm that ear infections are no fun at all.

Breastfed babies suffer from fewer ear infections than bottle-fed babies. Bottle-fed babies who are fed lying down experience the highest number of ear infections. Previously, many doctors thought that the difference in positioning of the breastfed baby lowered the rate of ear infections. While feeding position may play a part, new studies have shown that even if breast milk is bottle-fed, babies have a lower rate of ear infections. This suggests that antibodies in breast milk are also responsible for the lower incidence of infection.

TECHNICAL STUFF

Another possible reason for increased ear infections in bottle-fed infants is that because milk from a bottle flows even when the baby isn't sucking, milk can pool in the baby's mouth and enter the Eustachian tubes. Breast milk flows only as the baby sucks and is swallowed without pooling in the mouth. Even if breast milk does enter the Eustachian tubes, its anti-inflammatory properties make it less likely to cause infection.

TIP

The frequency of ear infections seems to be directly related to the length of time a baby is breastfed and whether or not the baby is given breast milk exclusively. Giving breast milk exclusively for the first six months is the best protection against your baby developing ear infections even after he stops breastfeeding.

Aiding jaw and teeth development

TIP

Breastfeeding results in better jaw alignment and aids in shaping the hard palate. (This may be a big money saver down the road if your children inherit your less-than-perfect receding chin!) Many breastfed babies' teeth also come in straighter and stronger than those of their bottle-fed friends. Keep in mind, though, that there are some hereditary jaw lines even breastfeeding can't overcome!

Babies use different jaw muscles to get milk from the breast than from the bottle. The effort gives a baby's jaw a good workout, which may result in a straight, braces-free smile down the road. All that jaw action also helps encourages proper speech patterns.

Breastfeeding may also help your baby avoid the dentist's drill in the future, because breast milk is deposited at the back of the throat and immediately swallowed. When you bottle-feed, by contrast, milk pools in the mouth, so the baby's teeth are bathed in milk.

Lessening the chance of SIDS

Sudden Infant Death Syndrome, or SIDS, is every parent's nightmare. The first time your baby sleeps through the night, you'll probably wake up in a panic, scared to death that SIDS has struck.

Ever since doctors began recommending that babies sleep on their backs rather than their stomachs, the incidence of SIDS has decreased 40 percent. But 3,000 babies in the United States still die every year from SIDS, and the devastating death of a healthy, normal infant literally overnight is something no parent should have to experience.

Good jaw and palate development (see the preceding section) may help protect against SIDS, because abnormal development can interfere with a baby's airway. In addition, breastfed babies are generally lighter sleepers than bottle-fed babies, and they experience a faster development of the central nervous system; both factors may help decrease sleep apnea associated with SIDS. Antibodies imparted through breast milk may also play a part in decreasing the rate of SIDS.

REMEMBER

SIDS is most common between the ages of 1 month and 6 months. Although research into the cause and prevention of SIDS is ongoing, breastfeeding during that time may significantly decrease your baby's risk of becoming a tragic statistic.

Protecting against asthma and allergies

Asthma is the leading chronic childhood disease, with 5 million children in the United States affected. If you've ever suffered from shortness of breath, you can appreciate the trauma this causes in babies too young to express what they're feeling.

Allergies and asthma are closely related; substances such as cigarette smoke, pollen, and certain proteins (including eggs, peanuts, and dairy) are often associated with asthma development.

The best way to avoid allergies in children is to breastfeed exclusively for the first six months, giving no supplements of any kind. This not only avoids exposure to trigger foods but also stimulates the baby's immune system to mature more rapidly.

Breastfeeding certainly isn't a cure-all: One large study showed that breastfed children and bottle-fed children were at equal risk of developing asthma. However, the same study showed that the onset of asthma symptoms was delayed in breastfed children.

Other studies have shown that breastfed children are less likely to develop allergies to pets, which could be a major consideration if Fido is an important part of your family.

Respiratory illnesses, such as chronic bronchitis, are twice as common in bottle-fed babies as in breastfed babies. Acute illnesses such as Respiratory Syncytical Virus (RSV) are also decreased in breastfed babies, although they can still occur.

A large Australian study involving more than 2,000 children, which was presented at the 1999 conference of the American Lung Association, theorizes that small amounts of breast milk enter the baby's lungs during breastfeeding and deliver antibodies to the respiratory tract, which may explain the decreased chance of respiratory irritation or infection.

Decreasing diarrhea and other stomach woes

Severe diarrhea can easily land a small infant in the hospital with dehydration; about 200,000 U.S. infants are hospitalized with dehydration each year. Babies who are breastfed have healthier guts in general, possibly due to the presence in breast milk of *lactobacillus* — a substance that reduces the growth of harmful bacteria. Also, breast milk is always clean, because it comes directly from the "container" to the baby, without the possibility of contamination from water or from the bottle. Studies have shown that feeding only breast milk for the first year can reduce the incidence of diarrhea by as much as one half.

Breastfed babies generally spit up less than bottle-fed babies as well, either because breast milk is more digestible or because bottle-fed babies swallow more air as they feed. (Breast milk stains are also easier to get off clothes than formula stains!)

Research indicates that breastfeeding may also decrease the chance your baby will develop *pyloric stenosis,* a condition that causes projectile vomiting and needs to be surgically corrected; pyloric stenosis occurs in 1 out of every 500 to 1,000 births.

For premature babies born after 30 weeks of gestation, the incidence of *Necrotizing Enterocolitis* (NEC), a very serious gut infection that can cause death or loss of a large part of intestine from gangrene, is over 20 times higher in babies fed formula than in breastfed babies. (See Chapter 9 for more on breastfeeding your premature baby.) NEC occurs in approximately 2 percent of the neonatal intensive care population.

Breastfeeding decreases the incidence of NEC not only because of the immunoglobulins it contains but also because it has a low pH, which slows bacterial growth in the intestines.

Considering other health benefits

No, breastfeeding won't bring about world peace, but new studies are constantly linking breastfeeding to additional health benefits. Consider the following:

- **Because breastfed babies have fewer allergies than bottle-fed infants, they have fewer rashes.** Your breastfed baby may even have less diaper rash, due to the lower pH of breastfed babies' bowel movements.
- **Breastfeeding may prevent "picky eater" syndrome later in life.** Because breast milk changes taste depending on what you eat, breastfed babies tend to be more adventurous in their eating habits and accept different tastes more readily.
- **Breastfeeding could have an impact on your child's weight later in life.** A very large German study showed that babies

fed only breast milk for 3 to 5 months were 35 percent less likely to be overweight at age 6. Of course, obesity is a complicated issue, and many factors contribute to children being overweight.

TIP

Another possible cause of obesity is the "clean your plate" syndrome, which may be more prevalent among bottle-fed babies. Parents sometimes push an infant to finish a bottle even if the baby seems disinterested in the last ounce or two.

- **Breast milk may help prevent childhood leukemia.** In a study of 2,200 children in 1999, babies who were breastfed for at least a month were 21 percent less likely than bottle-fed babies to develop childhood leukemia, one of the most common cancers in children. Breastfeeding was also found to reduce the risk of other childhood cancers, such as lymphoma.
- **Breastfeeding impacts a baby's IQ.** Many studies have shown a small increase in IQ for babies who are breastfed for six months or more compared to bottle-fed babies. Those extra five to ten points on the IQ scale may not guarantee acceptance into Harvard, but they certainly won't hurt! Breastfeeding promotes nervous system maturation and brain growth and development, so you'll be doing your best to develop your baby's potential.

Reviewing Mom's Health Benefits

Although many breastfeeding advocates focus on the positive effects for the baby, moms also reap physical benefits from breastfeeding. For starters, breastfeeding is the best way to get your body back into its pre-pregnancy state. (Be honest, you can't wait to fit back into your favorite pair of jeans, right?)

Benefits from breastfeeding come in many packages. You'll find short-term benefits (like uterine contractions so you don't bleed heavily immediately after delivery) and long-term benefits (like not developing osteoporosis when you're old and gray). Let's start in the delivery room.

The incredible shrinking uterus

Picture yourself after delivering your baby. You put her to your breast, your lower abdomen goes into a giant spasm, and blood starts flowing like Niagara Falls. You look down at the clot you just passed, wonder if you've given birth to a second baby, and remember vaguely reading about afterpains. (If you haven't read about them yet, pick up *Pregnancy For Dummies,* 2nd Edition.)

Afterpains are contractions of the uterus caused by the release of the hormone oxytocin. When you breastfeed, oxytocin is released into your body, which triggers these uterine contractions. Afterpains are necessary to shrink the uterus down to its previous size and to expel blood and clots, but they can be very uncomfortable; they also tend to be stronger after each delivery.

TIP

All women have afterpains, whether they breastfeed or not, but breastfeeding mothers usually experience stronger afterpains. I know what you're asking yourself: Why is stronger pain a good thing? Because the more acute the afterpains, the faster your uterus returns to normal.

Weight loss after delivery

Your first glance in the mirror after delivery may have you planning a carrot and prune juice diet to rid yourself of the excess weight. Breastfeeding can help you shed your excess weight while eating your regular diet. Producing milk uses 200 to 500 calories a day, on average. That may not sound like much, but it equals the calories burned running a couple miles a day or doing 30 laps in the pool.

However, be realistic: Don't expect to be back at pre-pregnancy weight within a week after delivery. When you're pregnant, you may brainwash yourself into thinking that this weight will come off as easily as it went on, as if your 7-pound baby is going to account for a 30-pound weight loss. For most women, this doesn't happen.

TIP

If you breastfeed and you maintain your pregnant caloric intake after delivery, you'll lose around a pound a week. But remember, just as pregnancy requires a certain amount of calories to create a healthy baby, you need a specific amount of calories to produce milk.

You need to consume a minimum of 1,800 calories per day in order to produce milk for your baby. Cutting your calories lower than that while nursing won't be good for you or your milk supply. Let your increased activity level and the milk-making calories help get the weight off. And don't worry about whether you'll have an "increased activity level" after delivery — when the baby comes, you won't remember what a sedentary day is.

REMEMBER

Don't cut down on your calories until the baby is at least 6 weeks old to make sure that you get your milk supply established and help your body heal after delivery.

Reduced cancer risks

TIP

Decreasing your risk of breast cancer is one of the most important benefits of breastfeeding. Studies show that breastfeeding decreases your chances of developing premenopausal breast cancer by nearly 25 percent. This benefit is strongly connected with the length of your breastfeeding experience. Two weeks is good, four months is better, and more than six months is best as far as protection against breast cancer goes.

Of course, nothing can completely eliminate this risk; family history is always an important factor in developing breast cancer.

Some studies have also shown a decrease in ovarian and uterine cancers in women who breastfed. One thought is that when a woman is nursing she is not getting her period as often, because nursing often delays the return of menses after delivery (see Chapter 16). Less menstrual cycles overall means less estrogen exposure, which may lead to reduced cancer risk.

Increased bone density

Chances are that you haven't yet thought about *osteoporosis,* the thinning of bones that often happens to women after menopause. But now *is* the time to think of it, because what you do during your younger years determines your bone density in the future.

While you're nursing, your bone density actually tends to decrease. However, this effect is temporary. Research has shown that after weaning, many women's bone density actually increases. This means that breastfeeding may help reduce your future risk of osteoporosis.

A reason to rest

Maybe you know this new mother: She's got a coffee cup in one hand and the phone in the other as she races from room to room. Her baby is propped up in an infant seat, a bottle wedged up to her mouth with a blanket. As mom runs past, she straightens up either the baby or the bottle, as both have a tendency to fall sideways.

REMEMBER

One of the best things about breastfeeding is that it can't be done long distance. You need to sit down and take a breather while you nurse, at least at first. Later on, perhaps you'll learn to breastfeed while carrying the baby in a sling through the grocery store, but that's your choice.

Breastfeeding enforces rest. And goodness knows, you'll need it.

Getting Emotional

You start nurturing months before your baby is born. From the day you found out your pregnancy test was positive, you've probably been talking to your child — even before he had ears!

You and your baby have an emotional bond, even before birth. Can this emotional high get any better? Yes! Nursing does more than supply nutrition; it helps increase the bond between you and your baby.

Bonding with your baby

Your new baby is totally dependent on you. This fact inspires a fierce protectiveness and desire to care for her. Hormones released during breastfeeding, coupled with the knowledge that you are directly responsible for your baby's growth and development, enhance your bond.

The release of the hormone oxytocin during breastfeeding (see Chapter 1) stimulates nurturing, loving feelings. *Prolactin,* the other hormone released to stimulate milk production, is known as the "mothering hormone" because of its calming effect. Anything that stimulates these feelings is good for both you and baby!

As early as four days after birth, a breastfed baby prefers the smell of his own mother's milk to others'. His bond to you has already begun. We're certainly not saying that women who don't breastfeed don't bond with their babies — of course they do. But we believe that a special connection occurs between a mother and baby when she breastfeeds.

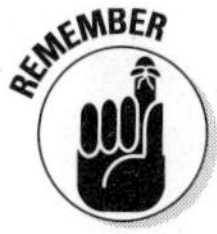

Breastfeeding won't turn your life into a fairy tale — you'll still have plenty of trials and tribulations of motherhood to overcome. But the difficulties fade in importance the first time your baby pulls back and smiles up at you, milk running out of both corners of his mouth — or when she stares into your eyes while she eats, one tiny hand cupped around your breast. These are the moments that bind you forever.

Helping Mother Earth

Breastfeeding is good not only for baby and mom, but also for the environment. One study showed that bottle feeding every baby in the United States would result in more than 86,000 tons of waste tossed into landfills in the form of cans and packaging. That doesn't include the tons of paper and other materials used to advertise different kinds of formulas and bottles!

Knowing you're giving the best

Pregnancy probably has you reading all kinds of books, taking classes, talking to friends, and watching The Baby Channel for hours at a time. You do these things so you can learn how to take the best possible care of your baby. And that feeling of wanting to give your baby the best doesn't change after delivery.

Breastfeeding has been the best method to feed a baby since the beginning of time, and all the brightly colored baby bottles and cute formula cans don't change that fact. Breastfeeding gives your baby food custom-designed just for her. We've seen a bumper sticker that says "Breast is Best!" It is.

Saving Money and Time

Breastfeeding certainly saves you money, assuming you resist buying every nursing shirt in the Motherhood store. You can expect to save enough to buy the baby every music-playing, light-flashing, sight-and-sound-stimulating toy on the market, which will certainly help with his physical and brain development as well!

Adding up formula and bottle costs

Formula costs vary depending on where you buy it and whether it comes ready to feed (the most expensive), in a concentrated form that requires adding water (less expensive), or in powder form (the cheapest, but the biggest pain to mix). You can count on spending between $1,000 and $3,000 a year on formula; the higher amount reflects the cost of specialty formulas for hyperallergic children.

You can buy bottles that can be cleaned and reused, or you may opt to use plastic liners that are discarded after each feeding. If you clean and reuse bottles, you may want to invest in a sterilizer (around $30), unless you use a dishwasher. If you choose plastic liners, they'll probably cost you several hundred dollars per year.

A starter set of bottles with colored nipples or cute designs painted on them costs around $30; plan on spending another $10 or so for extra nipples (because inevitably the dog will chew some of them, and some will melt in the dishwasher).

To be fair, if you breastfeed, you need to eat some extra calories; figure on spending a few hundred dollars per year for the additional food. And you'll want to invest in a few nursing bras and some disposable pads (see Chapter 5). Even so, breastfeeding saves you at least $1,000 per year, enough to buy the Cadillac of carriages and still have money left for the college fund.

Safety issues with formula

Because formula is a manufactured product, it can potentially be contaminated with bacteria at (or after) the time of processing. Formula recalls are not uncommon, for reasons such as the following:

- The formula may be contaminated with bacteria.
- The formula is not sterile.
- Post-processing contamination has occurred.
- Cans are mislabeled.
- Preparation instructions written in Spanish are incorrect.
- The formula has a lumpy, curdled appearance.

If you choose powdered formula, follow the instructions exactly so that the mixture isn't too thin or too thick. If it's too thin, the formula may not be nutritious enough; too thick, and it may have too high a concentration of certain ingredients and could make the baby ill.

If you mix concentrated or powdered formula with water, keep in mind that water can also be contaminated. Using bottled water should reduce this risk, although even bottled water isn't risk-free.

Always check the expiration date on the formula can to be sure what you're buying is fresh.

Comparing medical costs

Studies have shown that medical costs for breastfed babies run around $200 less per year than those of bottle-fed babies, because of the health benefits of breastfeeding detailed earlier in this chapter. This figure includes only office visits and prescriptions; it doesn't include time lost from work or the cost of hospitalization.

Preparing breast milk — a piece of cake!

Your mother or grandmother may have not-so-fond memories of sterilizing bottles using a rack that had to be put into a big pot full of boiling water. With luck, none of the nipples would melt, and no one would suffer second-degree burns from the whole experience.

These days, sterilizers plug into the wall, and dishwashers can eliminate the need for sterilizers altogether. Still, nothing is as easy to prepare as breast milk. Pull up your shirt, and there it is. No fuss, no muss, unless you have a really powerful let-down reflex (see Chapter 6) and squirt everything in sight before the baby latches on.

In addition to being easy, breast milk is always prepared perfectly: It comes out the right consistency and with the right balance of nutrients.

Traveling with a breastfed baby is also easier than packing a diaper bag with bottles. You don't need to beg the flight attendant to heat up your baby's bottle. You don't need to carry cans of formula through metal detectors or convert ounces to milliliters because you forgot to pack the bottles and have to buy more in Switzerland. (We talk more about traveling while breastfeeding in Chapter 14.)

Breastfeeding really is the easiest way to go!

Chapter 3

Is Breastfeeding Always Best?

In This Chapter

- Weighing the risks of chronic health conditions
- Using medications while breastfeeding
- Curbing bad habits
- Considering the impact of breast surgery
- Worrying about failure

Is breastfeeding *always* best? Of course not. Breastfeeding is best for the baby if it's the best choice for *you.*

You may find that for physical or other reasons bottle feeding fits your needs better than breastfeeding. For example, you may have a health condition that makes breastfeeding difficult, if not impossible. Perhaps you've had breast reduction surgery and have heard that it interferes with breastfeeding. Or you could find yourself surrounded by family members or coworkers who are less than supportive of your desire to breastfeed.

In these situations, the benefits of breastfeeding may possibly be outweighed by other factors. In this chapter, we help you sort through the facts and apply them to your particular situation so you can determine whether breastfeeding is your best choice.

Considering Your Health Issues

You may think your particular medical or personal circumstance means you won't be able to breastfeed, but the information in this section may surprise you. Here we give you the facts on how some common health problems really affect breastfeeding.

Women with chronic diseases are getting pregnant and delivering healthy babies today in larger numbers than ever before, thanks to improved prenatal care. And more moms with chronic conditions are able to breastfeed, as long as their own health is preserved. You must, of course, always ask your doctor if the general rules we discuss in the following sections apply to your situation.

Diabetes

Babies born to diabetic mothers can have more trouble than other babies stabilizing their blood sugars after delivery. If you are diabetic, your hospital may insist that your baby be monitored in the neonatal intensive care unit for several hours to a day after delivery. This separation may make initiating breastfeeding more difficult. If you intend to breastfeed, make that fact clear to the staff and explain that you don't want the baby given glucose or formula unless it's absolutely necessary.

If you breastfeed, your insulin requirements may fluctuate more than usual, so you need to keep a close eye on your blood sugars. Most breastfeeding moms need less insulin than they normally do. Your doctor or a nutritionist may need to help you revise your diet while you're breastfeeding to avoid becoming hypoglycemic.

REMEMBER

Your milk may be slower to come in if you're diabetic; it can take as long as five to six days. (Usually, a new mother's milk comes in within three to four days after delivery.) Don't let this potential delay discourage you.

Injected insulin isn't excreted in breast milk, so it won't affect the baby's blood sugar levels. If you're taking oral antidiabetics, Orinase is acceptable for breastfeeding. Glucophage, Avandia, and Actos have a higher potential for serious side effects to the baby (such as lowering blood sugar too much) and should be avoided until they've been studied further.

REMEMBER

On the plus side, nursing may lower your baby's chance of developing childhood diabetes. And if you have gestational diabetes, breastfeeding may decrease your chance of developing adult onset diabetes in the future.

Cancer

If you're a cancer survivor, you can breastfeed as long as you're not currently undergoing chemotherapy or radiation treatment. If you've had a biopsy or a lumpectomy (both of which involve cutting out a piece of breast tissue to check for cancer cells), you can generally breastfeed if less than 30 percent of the *areola* (the brownish area around the nipple) has been cut.

If you've had a *mastectomy* (the removal of one breast), you can nurse with your remaining breast. Breastfeeding does not increase the risk of cancer returning; in fact, breastfeeding may offer some protection against recurrence.

Hepatitis

If you have any type of chronic hepatitis, you need to discuss breastfeeding thoroughly with a doctor familiar with your particular circumstances.

Hepatitis B can be transmitted through breast milk, but many doctors believe that because the baby has already been exposed in utero to the virus, breastfeeding won't increase the risk to the baby. If the baby has had a shot of Hepatitis B immunoglobulin and also has received the first of three doses of the Hepatitis B vaccine, research shows that breastfeeding is safe for the baby. Both injections are normally given shortly after delivery.

Hepatitis C is also transmitted through body fluids, but the Centers for Disease Control believes that breastfeeding with Hepatitis C is safe for the baby. In several studies of breastfeeding moms with Hepatitis C, none of the babies became Hepatitis C positive. If you have Hepatitis C, have blood tests done while you're breastfeeding to make sure your disease hasn't become active, and check with your doctor and pediatrician to be sure they consider breastfeeding to be safe in your particular case.

Herpes

The herpes virus isn't transmitted through breast milk, but the baby can be infected if you have a herpes blister on your breast. It would be safe to breastfeed on the unaffected breast. *Acyclovir,* a drug commonly prescribed for herpes outbreaks, is considered safe to take while breastfeeding.

Polycystic ovary syndrome (PCOS)

PCOS has received a great deal of attention as a cause for infertility in the last few years, and recent studies have shown that women with PCOS may have difficulty breastfeeding as well. PCOS is a hormone imbalance; because breastfeeding is dependent on a delicate balance of hormones, some doctors theorize that PCOS may cause a decreased milk supply. The only way to find out if you'll have trouble breastfeeding with PCOS is to try it; many PCOS patients breastfeed without any problem at all.

Lupus

Systemic Lupus Erythematosus (SLE) is an autoimmune disease often found in young women of childbearing age. Lupus can damage connective tissue and cause problems in every part of the body. Most cases are mild and not life-threatening. Your baby can't catch lupus from you by breastfeeding, although about 5 percent of children born to moms with lupus eventually develop lupus themselves.

Some new moms experience a lupus *flare,* or a worsening of symptoms, after delivery. Some commonly used lupus medications, like corticosteroids, shouldn't be taken in high doses if you're breastfeeding because they pass through breast milk and could affect the baby's growth. Steroids can also decrease your milk supply. Discuss with your doctor whether the benefits outweigh the risks of steroids in your particular case.

While breastfeeding, also avoid frequent use of some nonsteroidal anti-inflammatories, such as naproxen (Aleve), which are often used for joint pain in lupus; they may affect the baby's cardiovascular system. The American Academy of Pediatrics approves the occasional use of naproxen while breastfeeding. Aspirin is another substance to avoid because it could cause bleeding. Ibuprofen is safer than naproxen because it has a shorter half-life (it leaves the baby's system faster). Cytoxin and Imuran, used if you're having a severe lupus flare, are also not safe for breastfeeding.

Thyroid disease

If you have an underactive thyroid (a condition called *hypothyroidism*), you can safely breastfeed while taking medication to regulate thyroid function. You should have blood tests done after delivery to make sure your level of medication is still appropriate. If your thyroid levels are abnormal, you may have trouble maintaining your milk supply.

If you have an overactive thyroid (*hyperthyroidism*), check with your doctor before trying to breastfeed. The American Academy of Pediatrics approves the medications Tapazole and PTU (propylthiouricil) for use by nursing moms.

One test often performed to determine thyroid function is a scan of the thyroid itself. Usually, the scan requires the patient to consume a small amount of radioactive iodine. If you're breastfeeding, you shouldn't have a thyroid scan done with radioactive iodine. If the test is absolutely necessary, ask your doctor about using *technetium* — another type of radioactive substance — for the scan, because your body completely excretes it within 30 hours. You may need to *pump and dump* (pump your breast milk and dispose of it) during that time period.

Multiple sclerosis

Multiple sclerosis, or MS, is most common in women between the ages of 20 and 40 — also, of course, the most common childbearing years.

MS, which affects muscles, can be severe at times and less severe at others. Pregnancy and delivery may exacerbate MS; you have a 20 to 40 percent chance of experiencing a flare-up after delivery. Many of the drugs used to treat MS, such as Avonex, Belseron, Rebif, and Copaxone, are considered to be moderately safe for breastfeeding. Consult your doctor for the best advice on whether breastfeeding will work for you.

HIV

Breastfeeding if you're HIV positive is a controversial issue. Some studies have shown that 20 percent of children born to HIV positive mothers contract the disease in utero, while 10 percent more are infected through breastfeeding.

The current recommendation of most doctors is that HIV-positive mothers should not breastfeed, because nearly all doctors believe that HIV can be transmitted through breast milk. Breastfeeding in this situation carries unnecessary risk to the child.

Epilepsy

Anti-epileptic drugs such as Dilantin and Tegretol do pass into breast milk, but most doctors believe that the benefits of breastfeeding outweigh the risks to the baby. Phenobarbital and Mysoline, also commonly prescribed anti-epileptics, are more likely to cause sedation in the breastfed baby and should be avoided if possible.

If you choose to breastfeed while on anti-epileptics, watch for signs of increased drowsiness in the baby; if this occurs, he may be getting too high a dose of the medication. Your doctor may advise you to frequently monitor the levels of the drug in the baby's blood.

Breastfeeding won't increase your baby's chance of having epilepsy, which is around 3 percent. Some babies whose mothers take anti-epileptic drugs have withdrawal symptoms when they are weaned off the breast; discuss what to watch for with your doctor before you wean the baby.

Active tuberculosis

If you have an active case of tuberculosis, discuss breastfeeding with your doctor. Tuberculosis isn't transmitted through breast milk, but the close contact with the baby could result in infection. If you've been on treatment for two weeks or more, breastfeeding is safe. Depending on your circumstances, your doctor may recommend immunization or prophylactic treatment for your baby.

Weighing the Impact of Medications

Many women take prescription drugs to control chronic health conditions. Many more of us rely on short-term prescriptions or over-the-counter medications to combat common illnesses. But what impact do these substances have on your baby if you breastfeed? The following sections provide general information, and you should always discuss your particular situation with your doctor before breastfeeding.

For the American Academy of Pediatrics' list of medications and their effects in breast milk, go to `www.aap.org`.

Taking prescription drugs

Always tell your doctor that you're breastfeeding before filling any prescription; she may have forgotten or may not think to ask. It doesn't hurt to also ask the pharmacist if the prescription is safe to take while breastfeeding. You may also want to check with your lactation consultant regarding possible effects on the baby or your milk supply.

Antibiotics

In general, any antibiotic that is safe to give to a baby directly is also safe if you're breastfeeding. If possible, avoid taking antibiotics in the category called *tetracyclines* because they can stain the baby's forming teeth. (The calcium in breast milk limits the drug's absorption, so damage to the teeth is unlikely. However, to avoid any possibility of staining, another drug can be substituted.) Also avoid newer drugs such as doxycycline (Vibramycin) or minocycline (Minocin) because they can cause tooth staining as well as decreased bone growth in the baby.

Also try to avoid the sulfa class of antibiotics, such as Bactrim, when the baby is less than 2 months old, because the baby's immature liver may not be able to break these substances down well. Taking them while breastfeeding could result in the baby becoming jaundiced.

Flagyl, an antibacterial used for certain vaginal and urinary tract infections, as well as other infections, is considered safe for breastfeeding but doesn't yet have AAP approval.

Antidepressants and other psychotropic drugs

Between 10 and 20 percent of all new moms suffer from postpartum depression, and many women are already on antidepressants during their pregnancy. If you need to take an antidepressant, doctors recommend Zoloft as the safest option. If Zoloft doesn't produce good results, most doctors then move up to Paxil, using Prozac as the last choice in this category. (Prozac has a longer half-life than the others, which means it stays in the baby's system longer. In some studies, Prozac has occasionally been associated with slow weight gain, colic, and irritability in infants.) See Chapter 7 for more information about coping with postpartum depression.

Older antidepressants called *tricyclics* are acceptable to use if you're breastfeeding. However, because tricyclics have more side effects than newer drugs such as Zoloft, most patients prefer the newer drugs.

Lithium, usually given for manic depression, shouldn't be taken while breastfeeding if at all possible. If you do take it, make sure your baby's blood levels are monitored frequently. Likewise, take Valium only when absolutely necessary while breastfeeding, if at all.

Asthma and allergy medications

Very little medication from inhaled steroids used to treat asthma and allergies passes into breast milk, so inhaled steroids such as Flovent are considered safe for breastfeeding. If you take oral steroids, your doctor may recommend prednisolone (Delta-Cortef) over prednisone (Deltasone) if you need large amounts of the drug.

Nasal sprays such as Flonase are safe for use while breastfeeding, as are eye drops.

Birth control pills

Birth control pills are generally considered safe to take while breastfeeding, although they may cause a decrease in milk production and the amount of protein found in your milk. Birth control pills may also occasionally cause breast enlargement in the baby. See Chapter 16 for much more information about birth control and breastfeeding.

Blood pressure medications

Because so many categories of blood pressure medications exist, you must check with your doctor about the safety of breastfeeding while taking your anti-hypertensive medication.

In general, low doses of diuretics such as Dyazide are considered safe, as are some beta blockers (Inderal, Lopressor, and Normodyne). Others, such as Tenormin, Corgard, and Betapace, are excreted in larger amounts in breast milk and could cause low blood pressure or a slow heart rate in the baby; these medications are not recommended for breastfeeding mothers. Procardia XL, Capoten, and Vasotec have all been deemed safe in breast milk by the American Academy of Pediatrics.

Pain medications and anesthetics

Demerol has a long half-life, which means it can make the baby sleepy in the first few days after delivery, but the American Academy of Pediatrics does consider it safe for use by breastfeeding mothers. Morphine, codeine, and hydrocodone are considered safe for short-term use if you need surgery, break your foot, or need pain medication for any other reason while you're nursing. If you take narcotics on a regular basis, discuss the pros and cons of breastfeeding with your doctor.

The use of morphine and fentanyl in epidural injections is also considered safe, as is the use of Marcaine or Xylocaine for epidurals.

Anesthetics such as Diprivan, Ethrane, and Pentothal are excreted rapidly and result in negligible exposure to the baby. Breastfeeding can resume as soon as you're awake and alert.

Using over-the-counter medications

Before you take any over-the-counter medication while breastfeeding, read the information inserts and the package. Also discuss their use with your doctor or lactation consultant. Many over-the-counter drugs can interfere with your milk supply or are not recommended while breastfeeding.

Antihistamines and decongestants

Antihistamines are considered safe to take while breastfeeding, although nonsedating drugs (such as Claritin and Allegra) are preferred. Any drug containing pseudoephedrine, such as Benadryl, may make your baby sleepy or irritable and also may decrease your milk supply by as much as 30 percent. Drink plenty of extra fluids if you're on an antihistamine.

Although decongestants are considered safe for nursing moms, many decongestants also contain pseudoephedrine. Taking medications such as Sudafed or Actifed on a regular basis may dry up your milk supply.

If you need to use any antihistamines or decongestants, choose shorter-acting medications rather than longer-acting ones to minimize effects on your milk supply. Take them only when really necessary, drink plenty of extra fluids, and nurse the baby as often as possible to help keep the milk supply going.

Pain relievers

Avoid taking aspirin while breastfeeding; acetaminophen (Tylenol) is preferred. Some nonsteroidal antiinflammatories (NSAIDS), such as ibuprofen (Motrin), are poorly absorbed into breast milk; ibuprofen is considered the best NSAID for breastfeeding moms. Clinoril and naproxen (Aleve) have a longer half-life and may accumulate in a breastfed infant whose mother takes them frequently. Feldene also has a longer half-life but is approved by the American Academy of Pediatrics for breastfeeding.

Examining Your Lifestyle

Many women quit smoking cold turkey, stop drinking altogether, and eliminate any recreational drug use the minute they find out they're pregnant. Yet, as soon as the baby's born, some nursing mothers start smoking again, drinking socially, and using recreational drugs occasionally. You may rationalize that the substances you use don't pass through breast milk, or that they pass through in such small amounts that they're inconsequential. This couldn't be further from the truth.

Drinking alcohol

For years, women have heard that drinking beer helps stimulate milk production. This idea got started because beer's active ingredient is brewer's yeast, which supposedly increases the level of *prolactin* (the hormone responsible for milk production) in men and non-lactating women. Unfortunately, if you're a nursing mom, you don't fit into either of these categories!

The alcohol in beer is a problem for your infant, and the yeast may not do you any good. The American Academy of Pediatrics advises that you avoid excessive or regular drinking (having more than one glass of wine, beer, or mixed drink on a regular basis) while you're breastfeeding. Alcohol crosses into the breast milk and stays there for at least two hours.

Over the long haul, moderate to excessive drinking can affect the development of your baby's brain and motor skills. It may also affect your milk supply. Oxytocin release (see Chapter 1) is inhibited when you drink, so your milk won't let down properly. Excessive alcohol may also affect your ability to take care of your baby.

Doctors agree that one glass of wine or one bottle of beer won't harm you and your baby. If you do decide to imbibe occasionally, remember these things:

- Minimize your baby's alcohol exposure for as least the first three months. Babies' livers are immature, so they can't detoxify the alcohol well.
- Drink *after* you breastfeed, not before. You shouldn't nurse for at least two to three hours after you've been drinking.
- Choose low-alcohol drinks — skip the Long Island iced teas!
- Make sure you're not taking any medication that could be made more potent by alcohol, such as sedatives or sleep agents.

Smoking cigarettes

You don't need to read this book to know that smoking is bad for both you and your baby. Warnings are everywhere, including on the packs of cigarettes. Obviously, if you're a reformed smoker, the best thing for you and your baby is to stay reformed and not start your habit again.

However, if you do smoke, recent studies have shown that your baby still benefits from breastfeeding. Breastfeeding helps prevent some of the worst effects of growing up in a smoking household.

Because of exposure to secondhand smoke, children of smokers have more illnesses in general than children of nonsmokers, especially respiratory illnesses. But children of smokers who are breastfed are healthier than children of smokers who are bottle-fed. A study performed in 1999 found that children who are breastfed for at least four months have a reduced risk of developing asthma until 6 years old. Cigarette smoke is a leading cause of asthma; breastfeeding may help protect your child if you or someone else in the family is going to continue to smoke.

Facing powerful reasons to quit

We want to try to persuade you to quit, even though we know nicotine is extremely addictive. Consider a few of the effects smoking has on both you and your baby:

- Babies of smoking mothers are more likely to suffer from colic, whether you breastfeed or not. This alone should be sufficient reason to give up smoking!
- If the fear of colic isn't enough to convince you, consider this: Babies of smoking parents have a seven times greater chance of dying from Sudden Infant Death Syndrome (SIDS) than children of nonsmokers. (We discuss SIDS in Chapter 2.)
- Nicotine is found in breast milk up to 1½ hours after you smoke a cigarette. Breast milk has the flavor of tobacco for 30 to 60 minutes after you smoke.
- Smoking mothers tend to give up breastfeeding earlier than nonsmoking moms. Some possible factors may include:
  - Smokers experience lower milk production.
  - The *let-down reflex,* which releases milk from the glands at the back of the breast and forces it to the nipple area where the baby can get it, is inhibited in smokers.
  - Smoking interferes with the production of the hormone prolactin. As we discuss in Chapter 1, prolactin stimulates the breast to make milk and also helps you relax.
- Babies exposed to cigarette smoke have a higher incidence of pneumonia, asthma, ear infections, bronchitis, sinus infections, eye irritation, and *croup* (an inflammation of the throat that makes the baby develop a harsh, barking cough).

- Children of smoking parents are more likely to become smokers themselves. Although this isn't necessarily linked to your breastfeeding experience, it brings the big picture into view. Most people who smoke may not want to, but they find themselves not able to give it up. They certainly don't want their children to follow in their footsteps.

REMEMBER

Babies can't just get up and walk away from cigarette smoke. Only you can make the decision not to expose your child to this toxic substance.

TIP

Studies have proven that nicotine patches are safe to use if you want to try to quit while breastfeeding. The patches expose you to less nicotine than smoking does, so both you and the baby benefit. Don't use patches and smoke cigarettes at the same time, though; the baby's exposure to nicotine would be extremely high. You may want to remove patches at bedtime to reduce your baby's exposure to nicotine and reduce side effects such as nightmares for yourself.

Breastfeeding as safely as possible

What can you do if you want to breastfeed and continue to smoke? Remember, studies show that breastfeeding is still best for your baby. We can't say often enough that the best thing for both of you is to stop smoking. But if you can't do that, here are some suggestions:

- Cut down your cigarette intake. If you can't stop smoking altogether, studies show that smoking less than 20 cigarettes a day significantly decreases the health risks from nicotine exposure.
- If you have to smoke, do so right after you've fed your baby or at least 1½ hours before a feeding. Following these guidelines helps limit nicotine exposure for your baby.
- TIP: Turn your house into a nonsmoking house. Smoke on the porch, in the backyard, or (shades of your teenage years) in the basement or garage. This goes a long way to lessen your baby's exposure to secondhand smoke, and if you make having a cigarette inconvenient, it may help you cut down as well.

REMEMBER

Even if you can't quit smoking, breastfeeding is still best for both of you because the benefits of breastfeeding help negate the effects of nicotine and provide long-term health benefits to you and the baby that bottle feeding can't duplicate.

Drinking caffeine

You may not think of the caffeine found in a cup of coffee, soda, or tea as a drug. But it is, and it's certainly one of the most widely abused.

Perhaps you've given up caffeine during pregnancy, or at least cut back from four Mountain Dews to one a day. Try to keep your caffeine intake low while you're breastfeeding. When you breastfeed, you have a built-in relaxation system with the release of the hormones prolactin and oxytocin (see Chapter 1). Caffeine works against this tranquilizing effect. Instead of you and your baby feeling calm and restful as a result of breastfeeding, caffeine can cause both of you to become irritable and jittery.

Limit your caffeine intake to three or fewer cups a day, depending on your drink of choice. Avoid "high-octane" coffees or sodas altogether, and try to consume decaffeinated drinks. Try to limit your caffeine intake to 400 milligrams per day. According to the American Academy of Pediatrics, this level of caffeine should not affect your baby.

Some of the highest caffeine-containing drinks may surprise you. For example, a cup of tea contains between 20 and 110 milligrams (mgm) of caffeine, depending on the type of leaf and brewing method. By contrast, a can of soda has 30 to 60 mgm. Chocolate contains 10 to 50 mgm in 2 ounces, so if you're a chocoholic, watch your caffeine as well as your calories! Coffee contains anywhere from 50 mgm to 300 mgm per cup, depending on the way it's brewed and the size of the cup.

Diet sodas contain a reduced amount of sugar, not caffeine. The caffeine count on diet sodas is just as high as regular sodas.

Some pain relievers, such as Excedrin, also contain caffeine; don't forget to count this if you're trying to keep your caffeine intake to less than 400 mgm per day.

Using illegal drugs

It should go without saying that using illegal drugs during pregnancy or while you breastfeed has dangerous consequences for your baby. But in case you aren't convinced, the following sections provide an overview of those dangers.

Smoking marijuana

Marijuana is the most widely used illegal drug in the United States. When you smoke marijuana, *THC* (the active ingredient in marijuana) is stored in your fat tissues, including your breasts. With chronic use, THC builds up and is secreted in small to moderate amounts in breast milk, to be absorbed by your baby. Smoking marijuana may also decrease your milk supply.

THC can make your baby lethargic and weak. He may not nurse well, and if that's the case, your milk supply will decrease, and the baby won't gain weight well. This creates a vicious circle that may result in your failing at breastfeeding.

The long-term effects of marijuana smoking on a nursing baby aren't well documented. But we do know that a tremendous amount of brain cell growth occurs in a baby's first year. Marijuana may modify the normal growth of an infant's brain cells.

Another important issue with a nursing mother using marijuana is the potential decrease in your ability to properly care for your baby. Smoking marijuana typically induces a high followed by a lethargic period. Your behavior during either period could put your baby at risk for injury.

Also remember that street drugs are rarely pure. The marijuana you buy on the street could be laced with other substances that are very harmful to your baby, and you won't have any idea what they are.

If you're smoking marijuana around your baby, you are doubling his exposure. Not only is he ingesting THC through your breast milk, but he's also inhaling your secondhand smoke. Obviously, the best situation for you and your baby is not to smoke marijuana while you're nursing.

Using cocaine

If you nurse your baby while using cocaine, you're probably going to give your baby the same cocaine habit that you have.

Babies under the influence of cocaine are irritable and sleepless, have diarrhea, don't gain weight, and may have long-term behavior problems. If you have a cocaine habit, you need to make two decisions immediately. First, you need to seek help: Cocaine addiction and baby care don't mix. Second, until you're clean, you need to bottle feed your baby.

Taking methadone

If you're in a methadone program, most doctors believe you can safely breastfeed, although small amounts of the drug may pass through the breast milk. The American Academy of Pediatrics lists methadone in the "usually compatible with breastfeeding" group. You are still providing your baby with all the benefits of breastfeeding, plus you're slightly decreasing the withdrawal symptoms he may have if you took methadone during your pregnancy.

Your baby may need to remain in the hospital for several weeks after birth to have his dependence on methadone gradually decreased. During this time he may be irritable and agitated, and he may experience sleeping difficulties, diarrhea, or vomiting. You can still breastfeed or pump milk during this time.

TIP

Limit your baby's exposure to methadone by taking your dose just prior to your baby's longest sleep time. As your baby grows and begins to eat solid foods, he will gradually wean himself from the small amount of methadone in your breast milk.

Getting piercings

Body piercings are nothing new; the Egyptians and Romans were into pierced navels and nipples. If you like the look, wonderful — but you may wonder if you can breastfeed with pierced nipples. Generally speaking, the answer is yes.

TIP

If you haven't been pierced yet and you think you may want to breastfeed in the future, have the nipple pierced horizontally; it seems to be easier to breastfeed with a horizontal pierce. Give yourself plenty of time to heal — at least six months for nipple piercings.

Remove nipple rings before nursing; your baby could choke or have a poor latch on your breast if you leave jewelry in your nipple during feedings.

Eating a vegetarian diet

If you breastfeed while following a vegetarian diet, you need to plan your food intake carefully to make sure you're getting enough protein and vitamin B_{12}.

Vegetarian diets have some benefits over meat-based diets; the breast milk of vegetarians often contains less pesticide contamination. Vegetarians may also have higher levels of calcium, because a high intake of animal protein can wash calcium out of your body in your urine.

There are many types of vegetarians. The least strict — those who follow a semi-vegetarian diet using dairy products, eggs, fish, and poultry — have few or no problems getting all the nutrients they need. The strictest vegetarians, *vegans,* consume only plant foods; they don't eat any animal products.

If you follow a strict vegetarian diet, make sure you're getting enough of the following nutrients:

- **Complete proteins:** Animal proteins are considered *complete* because they contain all the essential amino acids, the building blocks of proteins. Plants may contain one type of amino acid but not another, so you need to balance your intake to receive all the essential amino acids. Soy protein is a complete protein; milk, yogurt, cheese, and eggs are all excellent protein sources.
- **Iron:** Iron is necessary to transport oxygen to your tissues. Two types of iron exist: heme iron, found in meats, and non-heme, found in plants. Non-heme iron absorption is enhanced if you eat foods rich in vitamin C at the same time. Whole grains, legumes, green leafy vegetables, soy products, kelp, and fortified cereals all are good sources of iron. Dairy products and tea can both interfere with your absorption of iron and are better taken separately from your iron-rich meals.
- **Vitamin B_{12}:** B_{12} is necessary for cell growth and for your nervous system. Plants contain no B_{12}, but it's found in all animal products, including milk. If you follow a vegan diet, you need to take supplements to get enough B_{12}.
- **Calcium:** Calcium is easily available in most vegetarian diets. Good sources are milk, cheese, yogurt, fortified orange juice, and dark leafy vegetables. Legumes, broccoli, almonds, and calcium-fortified soy products are also good.
- **Vitamin D:** You need vitamin D for bone development. Being in sunshine for a portion of the day ensures vitamin D intake. Fortified milk is another good source. Vitamin D also aids in calcium absorption.
- **Zinc:** Zinc is needed for cellular growth. Fish and poultry supply plenty of zinc. Other sources include hard cheeses, legumes, soy products, wheat germ, yeast, nuts, and seeds.

Taking herbal supplements

Many people take herbal preparations without giving much thought to their safety. These preparations are sold in health food stores or mixed into a special formula by herbalists. They don't require a prescription, and in general they seem to be more healthy and natural alternatives to prescription medications.

WARNING! While that may be true in some cases, in some instances herbal preparations can be quite dangerous. You should avoid the following herbs while you're breastfeeding. Keep in mind that this is by no means a complete list.

- **Aloe:** Can cause diarrhea in the baby
- **Chaste Tree fruit:** High alcohol content may affect your milk production
- **Coltsfoot leaf:** Can cause liver toxicity in the baby
- **Cascara bark:** May cause diarrhea in the baby
- **Ephedrine:** May overstimulate the baby's nervous system
- **Fenugreek:** Traditionally used to increase milk supply, but large doses may cause colic
- **Kava kava:** May depress the baby's central nervous system
- **Licorice root:** Can increase blood pressure
- **Milk thistle:** May cause diarrhea and allergic reaction
- **Parsley and sage:** May dry up your milk supply
- **Valerian:** May cause drowsiness in the baby

You can drink herbal teas in moderation as long as the ingredients are known not to have potential side effects.

Breastfeeding after Reduction or Augmentation

If you've had surgery to change the size of your breasts, you may be wondering if breastfeeding is even a possibility for you. Consider the facts in the following sections, and discuss your specific situation with your doctor.

Knowing the risks of reduction

Breast reduction may affect your ability to breastfeed, depending on how your surgery was performed. Your individual success at breastfeeding will depend not only on how the surgery was performed but also on your ability to work through the initial rough times that occur when *anyone* breastfeeds (see Chapter 8).

Determining whether you can breastfeed involves some investigation, starting with contacting the surgeon who performed the operation. Ask him directly if the surgery will affect your ability to breastfeed. If he isn't available, request a copy of the operative report from his office or from the hospital where the surgery was done. Take the report to another doctor who does breast reduction surgery. She should be able to give you an idea if breastfeeding is realistic for you. You may also want to keep the copy of the surgical report and show it to a lactation consultant (see Chapter 4).

Knowing the following information about your operation will help:

- **Did your nipple need to be relocated?** If so, nerves were cut, which could affect your ability to breastfeed. If any nerve damage occurred around the nipple, breastfeeding may be difficult. This is because nipple stimulation signals the release of *oxytocin,* the hormone responsible for getting your milk from the ducts in your breast to the nipple.
- **Were milk ducts severed during the reconstruction of the breast?** Although in some cases milk ducts seem to *recanalize* (grow back together), don't expect this to occur. If a lot of milk ducts were damaged, the milk cannot travel from the milk-producing glands to the nipple openings because the pathway has been interrupted, and you may need to supplement with formula.
- **How much breast tissue was removed?** If a lot of tissue was removed, the number of milk ducts you have has been reduced, and you may not be able to breastfeed without supplementing. The only way to see if you can breastfeed is to try.

When you start breastfeeding, watch for signs that your hormones are kicking into gear, which indicates that you're feeling enough nipple stimulation. If enough hormones are being released, you should feel relaxed and even sleepy when you breastfeed. You may also feel thirsty. As we explain in Chapter 2, shortly after delivery you'll also experience cramping (called *afterpains*) while you breastfeed because of the release of oxytocin.

How else can you determine if you're breastfeeding successfully? Look at your baby while you nurse. Do you see and hear him swallowing? Does he seem satisfied after nursing, or does he act like he is still hungry? Look for signs like inadequate wet and stooled diapers, and monitor your baby's weight gain at your pediatrician visits. See Chapter 8 for more about nursing difficulties.

TIP

If your milk supply is low, you can still breastfeed, although you may need to supplement. One way to supplement is to use a Supplemental Nursing System, or SNS. This is a feeding tube that attaches to a supplemental milk bag on one end and to your nipple on the other (see Figure 3-1). When the baby nurses, he stimulates your nipple to help milk production but also gets the nutritional needs from the supplemental formula. Remember, even partial breastfeeding will reap benefits for you and your baby.

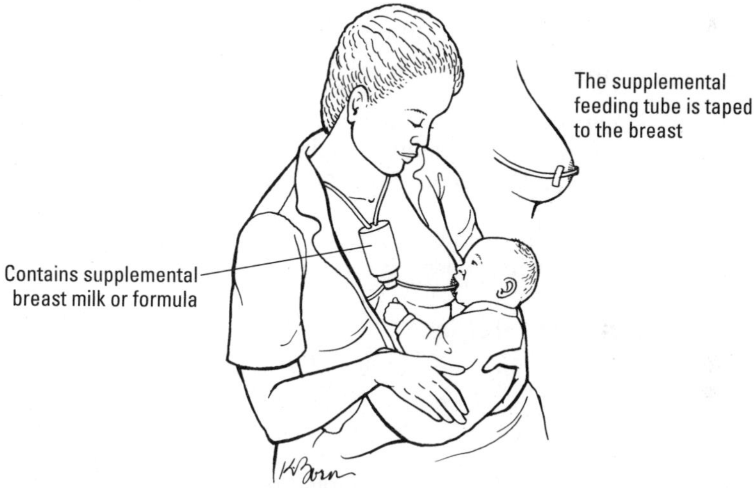
The supplemental feeding tube is taped to the breast
Contains supplemental breast milk or formula

Figure 3-1: Supplemental nursing systems help stimulate milk production while ensuring adequate nutrition for your baby.

Understanding the impact of implants

Breastfeeding after breast augmentation is a complicated issue. Can you successfully breastfeed with implants? The answer is a cautious yes, depending on your incision site, the size of your implants, and the reason you had them inserted to begin with. For example, you may not be able to exclusively breastfeed with implants if you have *hypoplastic tubular breasts,* which are underdeveloped and may contain fewer milk glands than normal breasts. See Chapter 4 for more details about this condition.

The silicone scare

A few years ago there was a great deal of concern over silicone implants and the possibility that silicone might find its way into breast milk. Newer studies have shown that silicone doesn't leak into breast milk even if the implant leaks. Here's why:

- Silicone molecules are too big to pass into the milk supply.
- Silicone isn't water soluble, so it can't dissolve into the milk.

Silicone is also found in larger amounts in formula than it could possibly be found in breast milk. The silicone controversy stems from a very small study (of 11 babies) done in 1994, which showed that 8 out of the 11 babies — all of whom had gastrointestinal problems and were born to moms with silicone implants — were breastfed. This was obviously a very small sampling and would need to be duplicated in a much larger study to prove that breastfeeding with silicone implants is harmful.

REMEMBER

Silicone is no longer routinely used in implants; saline, which would be harmless if it leaked into breast milk, is used instead.

Surgery specifics

Successful breastfeeding with implants depends on whether milk ducts or nerves were damaged during surgery. Surgery done through incisions around the nipple is more likely to affect breastfeeding. If your incision is under the breast or by your armpit, you probably will have no trouble breastfeeding.

If you have a nipple incision, you may have damage to the nerves in the nipple. During breastfeeding, those nerves signal the release of prolactin and oxytocin, the hormones that produce and deliver milk. If your nipples are numb or have decreased sensation, you may have difficulty breastfeeding.

Size can be an issue in breastfeeding as well. If your breasts are very large and your nipples very small, the baby may have trouble latching on properly (see Chapter 6).

WARNING!

If you have implants, when your milk supply comes in, you're more likely to run a fever and have more discomfort in general than women without implants. Some studies have shown that women with implants are three times more likely to have low milk supply than women without implants. You're also more likely to develop *mastitis,* a breast infection (see Chapter 8), or a *galactocele* (a milk-filled cyst in a blocked milk duct).

As with breast reduction surgery, if you've had breast implants, you need to watch carefully for signs that your baby isn't getting enough milk.

Tackling Common Fears

Pregnant women worry about everything, from getting through labor to whether the baby will have Uncle Theo's nose, and how to feed the baby is no exception. We hope that by sharing a little more information about breastfeeding, we can help you worry less about your chances of success.

Some of your concerns may stem from not knowing anyone who has successfully breastfed, so start asking your friends and neighbors if they nursed their babies. Find out if they enjoyed the experience, how long they breastfed, and what their general attitude toward breastfeeding is. Each breastfeeding mom is unique, of course, but for simplicity's sake we can group them into the following broad categories:

- **The fervent breastfeeder:** Often found at La Leche League meetings (see Chapter 4), the fervent breastfeeder is very serious about breastfeeding and may nurse her child well into toddlerhood.
- **The casual breastfeeder:** This mom breastfeeds because doing so means she doesn't need to buy formula or prepare bottles. She's generally pretty laid back about breastfeeding, does it because it's convenient and good for the baby, and doesn't get too sentimental about it.
- **The average breastfeeder:** Most women fall into this category. They breastfeed mostly because they want to do what's best for the baby, and they recognize the benefits to their health and the baby's. They usually breastfeed for 6 to 12 months, shed a few tears when they stop, and then go on with their normal lives (like putting up the potted plants so the baby stops eating the dirt out of them).

TIP

Make friends with someone who has successfully breastfed and whose general philosophy about breastfeeding is similar to yours. When you have a real idea about what breastfeeding involves and know someone who has succeeded at it, your anxiety will decrease.

Doubting your ability to breastfeed

You may have specific doubts about your ability to breastfeed; for example, you may have small breasts, flat nipples, or two or three extra nipples. (This isn't uncommon, by the way — many women have extra nipple tissue, usually in line with their "real" nipples.) Or you may be worried about your crazy work schedule, or how you'll watch your 3-year-old triplets and breastfeed your expected twins at the same time.

Everyone has specific issues that may seem to them more difficult than everyone else's. Again, the biggest source of help is to talk with other women who have been in the same boat and nursed successfully. The Internet is full of chat groups, and we list some of them in Chapter 18. La Leche League, an organization that promotes breastfeeding worldwide, holds meetings in almost every city, and many hospitals have lactation consultants on staff (see Chapter 4).

Your concerns about breastfeeding may be more general: Will you have enough milk? Will you have enough time? Will your mother discourage you? Remember that the decision to breastfeed isn't written in stone. You can always change your mind if you start and find you hate it, or discover that it doesn't fit your lifestyle. On the other hand, you can't easily decide to breastfeed when the baby's a month old.

Breastfeeding right after delivery isn't a life-long commitment; try it, and you may love it. If you never try, you'll never know what you may have missed.

Feeling modest

If you have a modesty issue, one of your authors — Sharon — can certainly relate. Your other author, Carol, on the other hand, didn't have a problem with breastfeeding in public. Everyone is different, and especially in this day of family restrooms in public places, you can find a way to be modest and successful at breastfeeding at the same time.

Breastfeeding in public doesn't mean that you must completely disrobe. With time and practice, you can learn to be discreet. As you get more comfortable with the technique of breastfeeding, it becomes easier to nurse publicly without anyone even realizing that you're feeding your baby. See Chapter 14 for tips on nursing in public.

Listening to other people's opinions

Whether you're a 19-year-old mom-to-be or pregnant for the first time at 46, you can be sure that your friends and relatives all have an opinion on breastfeeding that they'll be happy to share with you.

The fact that your best friend squirted breast milk all over the bride at her sister's wedding or that your mother got so weak from nursing you 24 hours a day that she passed out on the kitchen floor makes a great (and undoubtedly exaggerated) story, but it doesn't mean the same thing will happen to you. In fact, after reading this book, you'll be so well prepared for breastfeeding that chances are you'll be able to avoid your own horror story.

Should you tune everyone out? Not necessarily. If you have well-grounded acquaintances whose judgment you truly value, ask them about their experiences. As for dealing with your mother, sister, and best friend, you've got to listen to them, but you don't have to do what they say.

Most relatives and friends really do want what's best for you, even if they have a funny way of showing it sometimes. Keep in mind that they all have your best interests at heart.

Dealing with your partner's fears

You and your partner are supposed to be a parental unit, and if he expresses disapproval of your desire to breastfeed, you've got a big issue to deal with. The topic of breastfeeding will arise every few hours for months, so you need to work out your differences, as much as possible, before you walk in the hospital door.

Why would your partner not want you to breastfeed? Maybe he's afraid he'll be shut out of your relationship. Or he's afraid the baby will like you more than him. Or he's afraid your breasts will be ruined, or that he'll be jealous of the baby.

We're sure you get the idea here; the operative word is *afraid.* Your partner is worried about how breastfeeding will affect your relationship together. Your job is to convince him that breastfeeding won't come between you or prevent him from developing a good relationship with the baby. And if he reads the section in this book about physical changes after breastfeeding (see Chapter 7), he'll worry less about that, too.

Breastfeeding is a family experience, and with some up-front discussion and preparation, everyone in the family can have a positive experience.

Chapter 4

Preparing Physically and Mentally for Breastfeeding

In This Chapter

- Watching your breasts grow and change
- Planning ahead for your first weeks of breastfeeding
- Finding lactation consultants and support groups
- Picking doctors who support breastfeeding

We're going to assume that if you're reading this chapter, you've probably weighed the positives and negatives of breastfeeding and have decided to at least try it. We applaud that decision!

In this chapter, we describe the breast changes you can expect during pregnancy and the steps you can take to ready your breasts and nipples for nursing. We also help you look at your post-delivery schedule and how breastfeeding will fit into your life. We introduce you to lactation consultants and breastfeeding support groups, and we offer insight into the professionals who can make breastfeeding either much easier or much harder: your doctors.

Rolling with the Changes

Some pregnant women notice changes in their breasts even before they miss their period. The normal tenderness many women feel right before their periods is exaggerated in pregnancy; some women describe the feeling as tingling, and others say their breasts actually hurt — they can't stand the pressure of a bra on them.

Almost immediately after you become pregnant, your breast size increases; you may go up a cup size or two in the first two months. Some of the fat in your breasts is gradually replaced by glandular tissue, which grows and multiplies in preparation for nursing.

Glandular tissue is firmer than fat, which accounts for some of the size change. Increased blood volume and more water retention account for the rest. Progesterone and estrogen are the hormones responsible for your newly acquired cleavage.

Blood vessels in your breasts also increase in size; veins become more visible, especially if you're fair-skinned. The nipples become larger and more erect, the areolae (the dark areas surrounding the nipples) become darker and larger, and Montgomery's glands (see Chapter 1) are more noticeable.

Even before you deliver, you may leak *colostrum,* a yellowish liquid that contains a high level of antibodies and nourishment for your baby's first few days (see Chapter 1). You may also notice red stretch marks called *striae* on your breasts toward the end of pregnancy, if your breast size has increased dramatically. These stretch marks eventually fade to a silvery color.

Big, Small, Unusual: Does Breast Appearance Matter?

REMEMBER

In general, the size of your breasts has no impact on your ability to breastfeed. So if your Aunt Martha is clucking her tongue and saying that your breasts aren't big enough to feed a baby, feel free to ignore her naysaying.

Less than 10 percent of all women are unable to breastfeed at all; rarely is this inability related to the shape or size of the equipment. However, a few exceptions exist, which we discuss next.

Hypoplastic breasts

Hypoplastic tubular breasts are breasts that are underdeveloped; they appear long, thin, or cone-shaped and may be spaced widely apart. Sometimes one breast is considerably larger than the other. Hypoplastic breasts have fewer milk ducts than other breasts, which means you may not make enough milk for your baby. You may still be able to breastfeed, but you may need to supplement; the odds are about 50–50 that you'll make enough milk.

Hypoplastic breasts stay soft during pregnancy and don't become visibly engorged after delivery. The only way to see if you can successfully breastfeed with hypoplastic breasts is to give it a try. You need to watch your baby carefully to be sure she's getting enough milk.

Breast size

Very large breasts can be difficult for a baby to latch on to. If your breasts are very large and firm, breastfeeding may be a challenge. (See Chapter 6 for more about latching on.)

Your milk supply keeps up with your baby's needs whether your breasts are large or small. Women with small breasts may feel fullness in their breasts more frequently than women with large breasts, but milk production is continuous regardless of bra size.

Extra nipples

Some women have extra nipples, which usually aren't fully developed; they're more like dark, rough skin tags than the real thing. Extra nipples have no impact on your ability to breastfeed. (Unfortunately, you can't breastfeed triplets all at once if you have an extra nipple!)

Readying Your Nipples

Like breasts, nipples come in a multitude of shapes and sizes. A normally protruding nipple needs no help to get ready for nursing. The only time you need to bother your nipples before delivery is if they don't protrude but are flat or turned inward (*inverted*).

Giving your breasts a break

In years past, some doctors recommended toughening your nipples prior to breastfeeding by rubbing them with a rough cloth, pinching them, or pulling on them. An old wives' tale even suggested putting clothespins on your nipples to toughen them up! None of this torture is necessary.

The most common cause of sore nipples when you start nursing is improper latch-on. See Chapter 6 for more on nipple care and common nipple problems after delivery. And put the clothespins away!

Working with flat or inverted nipples

Flat or somewhat inverted nipples are very common; 10 to 30 percent of new moms have them. When your baby breastfeeds, the nipple needs to touch the baby's *palate* (the roof of his mouth) to stimulate a sucking response. If the nipple doesn't extend past the areola when the baby pulls the areola into her mouth, the nipple won't stimulate the palate. However, if the baby can pull the breast tissue into her mouth easily, her sucking often pulls the nipple out.

WARNING! When your milk first comes in, flat or inverted nipples can be difficult for the baby to latch on to, because the breast is so firm and taut that the baby can't easily pull the areola into her mouth. That's why some advance work may be necessary.

TIP You can check to see if your nipples are truly inverted by pinching firmly on both sides of the nipple, about an inch away from the center, at the same time. If the nipple pops out, it's not really inverted. If your nipples respond to cold by becoming erect, they're not truly inverted either.

If your nipples fail the pinch and cold tests, you may want to start working with them before you really need them, in the last few months of pregnancy.

Flat and inverted nipples (see Figure 4-1) are caused by *adhesions:* bands of tissues at the base of the nipple sticking to the tissue underneath them. Drawing out nipples requires gentle pressure to break or loosen the adhesions. From simplest to most complicated, the following methods help accomplish this:

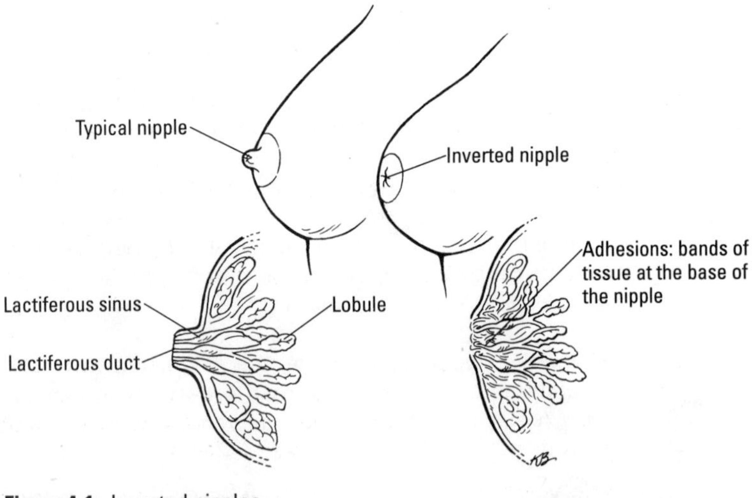

Figure 4-1: Inverted nipples.

TIP

- The simplest method of breaking down adhesions — called the *Hoffman technique* — requires only your own two thumbs. Place your thumbs at the base of the nipple on opposite sides of the nipple. Press in firmly while pushing your thumbs outward. This helps stretch the nipple and loosen the adhesions. Move your thumbs clockwise around the nipple and repeat this technique. You can do this several times a day.

- *Breast shells* are plastic cups that put gentle but constant pressure on the areola to break up adhesions. These fit inside your bra; to wear them, you may need to buy a bra one size larger than normal. Start by wearing them a few hours a day, and increase the time gradually. (We discuss breast shells more in Chapter 5.)
- La Leche League markets the Evert-it Nipple Enhancer, which puts uniform suction on the nipple, similar to a breast pump. Go to `www.lalecheleague.org` for more information.

Evaluating Your Postpartum Schedule — Realistically!

What do you imagine happening after you deliver your baby? If your life were a TV show, you might find yourself in a dreamy haze, sitting in a rocking chair with your baby sleeping peacefully in your arms. Perhaps you'd wear a long dress and have your hair pulled back in a soft, matronly style. Your baby would be dressed in a rose pink (or sky blue) handmade outfit. The hard work would be over, and you'd finally be able to relax.

Well, forget it. The end of pregnancy is the start of your new, sleep-deprived existence. Yes, new motherhood is an exciting, sweet time, but then there's all the rest. Many women go wrong by setting themselves on a post-delivery course that no woman could possibly maintain without a staff of four to help.

TIP

The time to consider postpartum time management techniques is long before you ever feel the first labor pain. Consider these examples:

- You may be feeding the baby every two to three hours when you first get home, so don't plan to host a major event — your parents' 40th anniversary party or a Cub Scout Jamboree — in your house for at least several weeks.
- If you have older children in school or daycare and belong to a carpool, try to beg off for a few weeks. Your coauthor Sharon will never forget how grateful I was when my friends took my 3-year-old to nursery school for a month after my fourth son came home. If your child's nursery school has after-school care, you may want to consider utilizing it a day

or two each week so you can catch up on sleep — or at least get the kitchen cleaned!

- Ask your partner to take time off work if his workplace offers paternity leave. If that's not possible, ask your mom, sister, or best friend to help out for a few days.
- If your church or another social group has a program that provides meals for the sick, take advantage of it; a casserole or two may last through the better part of the first week home.
- Hire a cleaning service once a week for the first few weeks. Looking at dust and clutter can push you over the edge when you're sleep deprived.
- Don't view your maternity leave as a wonderful time to get major household projects done, such as remodeling the bathroom. You may think you'll have lots of time for this sort of thing, but we guarantee you won't!
- Sleep whenever possible. We can't stress this enough.

We can't overemphasize the need to rest and not jump right back into your old routine the minute you get home. Too much running around decreases your milk supply, slows your healing, and makes you cranky!

Considering Your Return to Work

The last thing you may be thinking about as you prepare to deliver your baby is what life will be like when you have to go back to work. But continuing to breastfeed after you return to work is a challenge, so you'd be wise to consider your situation before you go on maternity leave.

Ask yourself these questions:

- Where is the best place to pump? An office with a door that locks is ideal, but if you don't have that luxury, you'll need to get creative.
- Are your supervisors and coworkers supportive of breastfeeding? If you don't know the answer to that question, now is the time to start having conversations about your plans.
- Can you arrange your schedule to go home at lunchtime and nurse?
- Has anyone in your office ever breastfed? If so, ask that person for advice.

We talk much more about working and breastfeeding in Chapter 13.

Seeking Support from a Lactation Consultant

If you have a lactation consultant in your area, you're fortunate. Certified lactation consultants are healthcare professionals who specialize in the management of breastfeeding; they offer current, research-based information on all aspects of breastfeeding.

Certified lactation consultants undergo rigorous training in every aspect of breastfeeding. Certification in the United States is done though the International Board of Lactation Consultant Examiners (IBCLE). Many consultants have a nursing background; some are dietitians or other healthcare practitioners. Some have no previous healthcare experience at all, just a passion for breastfeeding. Ask your obstetrician if your hospital has a lactation consultant on staff.

To qualify to take an exam to become a board-certified lactation consultant, a candidate must complete 900 to 4,000 hours of breastfeeding consulting and 45 hours of lactation education, as well as take classes in anatomy and physiology, sociology, and psychology or counseling. IBCLE members also take 75 hours of additional lactation education every 5 years to renew their certification, and they take a recertification exam every 10 years.

Some lactation consultants have private practices, while others are on staff at local hospitals. Many maintain a 24-hour-a-day "hotline" to help with those questions that plague you in the middle of the night.

If a lactation consultant is available to you, make sure you meet with her before you leave the hospital; in some hospitals, this is required. Even if your first attempts at breastfeeding go extremely well, you want to have personal contact with someone you may need desperately at 3 a.m. two weeks down the road!

Try to arrange a meeting with a lactation consultant before the baby's even born. She can assess your breasts, answer your questions, and (most of all) give you the initial enthusiasm you may need to start breastfeeding in the first place. She can answer all the questions you feel too dumb to ask anyone else, besides answering some you haven't even thought of yet!

Some women who are very interested in breastfeeding but haven't taken the IBCLE certification advertise themselves as lactation consultants. If a certified lactation consultant isn't available in your area, a noncertified consultant can still be very helpful. It helps you to know what that person's credentials are, so be certain to ask.

For a list of IBCLE-certified lactation consultants, go online to `www.breastfeeding.com` or `www.ILCA.org`. You can also check your local phone book, call 1-800-LALECHE, or contact the Breastfeeding National Network at 1-800-TELLYOU.

Meeting with a Support Group

Support groups are wonderful for new mothers. Call it a playgroup if it makes you feel less conspicuous, but think about organizing a breastfeeding support group before you deliver, even if the group consists of just you and two friends. Only other nursing mothers are going to understand and have suggestions when you feel like hanging a sign around your neck that says "Eat at Mom's."

The right support group can keep you strong when facing a whole aisle of formula cans covered with pictures of smiling, thriving babies, while yours has been up screaming for the last three nights straight, and your mother is accusing you of starving your baby.

La Leche League

The best-known breastfeeding support group is La Leche League. La Leche League is the foremost authority on breastfeeding worldwide and has been supporting breastfeeding mothers and babies for many years. You can find out more information about La Leche League online at `www.lalecheleague.org`, or call 1-800-LALECHE to find a support group in your area.

La Leche League's support groups offer mother-to-mother advice on breastfeeding, parenting, and nutrition. La Leche League leaders are trained in *non-medical* breastfeeding advice and can be extremely helpful in guiding you through a difficult time.

You may think that La Leche League is only for fervent breastfeeders, but this isn't the case. Each La Leche group has its own personality, so if the first one you attend is too fervent for you — or not fervent enough! — try another. Like many organizations that have a passionate message, La Leche is best approached from a "Take what you like and leave the rest" approach. La Leche leaders know their stuff, and if you don't have a lactation consultant nearby, they may be the only people around who can help you through really difficult breastfeeding problems.

You may find yourself becoming pretty zealous about breastfeeding yourself, or you may not. If your group is full of zealous breastfeeders and you don't feel comfortable expressing your views to them, don't. Get the help you need, ferret out a few people who seem fairly laid back, and get your own support group going on the side. (See Chapter 18 for more suggestions on organizing a support group.)

Additional options

The Nursing Mothers Advisory Council (`www.nursingmoms.net`), another breastfeeding support organization similar to La Leche League, has chapters throughout the United States and other countries. Counselors, who have no clinical training, offer mother-to-mother breastfeeding advice and telephone support. Your local hospital may also have a breastfeeding support group.

TIP

If you can't find a support group or any new moms to share experiences and woes with, get on the Internet. Type in *breastfeeding* and join a colony of nursing moms all sitting in front of their computers chatting about Johnny's strange rash. Check out the message board at `www.breastfeeding.com`, which has more than 6,000 messages, or just go to Google or another search engine and type in *breastfeeding bulletin board.* Sites exist to suit everyone's needs, including one site titled "Breastfeeding Militants"!

Dissecting Your Diet

If your daily breakfast includes Twinkies and your idea of a food group is peanut butter and chocolate, you may think your diet won't be good enough to make good milk for your baby. Rest assured that poor nutrition, while not optimal for *you,* probably won't interfere with breastfeeding.

REMEMBER

We're certainly not advocating a diet of junk food for any mom-to-be or nursing mother — we discuss your nutrition needs in much more detail in Chapter 7. But you probably already realize what you should be eating: proteins, green leafy vegetables, fruits, and whole grains. We all know that Snickers bars, although they do contain peanuts, do not constitute a good dinner. But we also know that many women have poor eating habits, and we don't want you to assume you can't breastfeed unless you drastically change them.

Many studies have shown that even malnourished moms make healthy breast milk. The person who suffers the most if your diet is inadequate is *you.*

We want both you and your baby to be healthy, so we suggest trying to stick to a varied diet, including foods from all the food groups — with an occasional Mars bar thrown in, of course. Your nursing baby will take what he needs from you, just like he does while you're pregnant. If you don't have enough nutrients left over to keep yourself healthy, that could spell trouble. You don't want to start losing your teeth at the age of 30, do you?

Picking a Positive Obstetrician

If you want to breastfeed, having a supportive obstetrician is a big help while you're in the hospital. A good OB can run interference with unhelpful hospital staff and may be able to bend rules for you if, for example, your hospital is back in the Stone Age regarding having the baby room with you. (See Chapter 6 for more information on rooming in.)

A good OB also knows where to find help if you're having difficulties; she'll set you up with a lactation consultant, if the hospital has one, or a representative from a breastfeeding support group.

Asking about her breastfeeding stance

If you already have a gynecologist who also does obstetrics (not all do!), make sure you ask questions about where she delivers and how supportive she is of breastfeeding before you even get pregnant. Doing so will avoid a situation where you feel forced to find another doctor when you're four months pregnant and discover your gynecologist isn't as supportive as you'd like. For more on picking an OB, check out *Pregnancy For Dummies,* 2nd Edition.

You may not realize how susceptible to suggestion you are when you're pregnant, especially if the suggestion comes from an authority figure like your doctor. It's not hard to pick up the unenthusiastic attitude of a doc who thinks breastfeeding is for cows. "Well, sure you can *try* breastfeeding," she may say, shaking her head a little at the same time. Or, "Aren't you going back to work? Why struggle with breastfeeding for only six weeks?"

This type of OB isn't going to be too helpful in the delivery room and beyond. And because breastfeeding should start in the delivery room (see Chapter 6), you need an ally to support your first attempts.

Choosing between doctor and hospital

Unfortunately, when you find Dr. Right, you may realize that he works at Backward General Hospital, where the babies are brought out of the nursery at four-hour intervals no matter what anyone says. This can put you in a real quandary. Do you keep a doctor you love even if he practices at a hospital you hate?

Some doctors deliver at more than one hospital, although for convenience they may prefer to keep most of their deliveries in one place. Sometimes your doctor's location on the night you deliver depends on who goes into labor first. If you're the first delivery of the night, he goes where you want to go. If another lady in labor beats you to it, she may prefer a different hospital, which means your doctor follows her. Some offices call in a second OB if you want to go someplace else; others insist that you come to the hospital where your doctor is stationed that night. Obviously, this is something you need to discuss with your doctor long before you go into labor.

If you really don't want to change doctors because he's been your gynecologist since your first embarrassing exam and knows you inside and out (literally!), talk to him in advance to see if he can bend the rules for you. Some hospitals are ruled by Nurse Ratched's cousins, and many doctors won't rock the boat for fear of reprisals down the road. (Nurses can make life tough for doctors if they want to — ask any doctor!)

If you're going to be stuck in a rotten place and really don't want to change doctors, ask if your doctor will at least let you go home early, assuming your delivery goes smoothly.

Choosing a Supportive Pediatrician

Next to a supportive OB, a helpful pediatrician can be your biggest ally both in and out of the hospital. If you want to know who's supportive and who's not, ask a few maternity nurses. Or ask the local breastfeeding support group; they can probably give you a rundown on every pediatrician in town.

You can still breastfeed with an unenthusiastic pediatrician if you're strong enough to stand up to the suggestion that everything that happens to your child, from diarrhea to a staple in the roof of his mouth (honestly, it happened to one of our sons!), is a result of your breastfeeding. If you're still nursing at three months, an unsupportive pediatrician will suggest that you wean. If your baby has jaundice or loses weight after delivery — both of which are common (see Chapter 6) — an unsupportive pediatrician will have the formula truck backing up to your hospital door.

This is Sharon speaking: When I had my second son, I went to the only OB in town who was willing to let me do natural childbirth, instead of knocking me out the minute I walked in the door. Like every other doctor in town, his attitude toward breastfeeding was somewhat behind the times. I had no choice but to work with the pediatrician who was on staff at the place of delivery, so I got my doctor's best friend.

My son lost a little weight after delivery and was jaundiced. I'll never forget the two doctors and the nurse circling my bed one day informing me that if my son didn't gain weight at the *next feeding*, they were going to give him a bottle.

I was still young and didn't know my rights in this world, so I meekly agreed and told the kid he'd better hop to it. And he did! We avoided the bottle police in the nick of time with a gain of 2 ounces.

After that, I found my own pediatricians and paid for them out of my own pocket. And they were worth their weight in gold. Finding a supportive pediatrician these days is probably a much easier task; ask good questions ahead of time, and you'll find one worth his weight in gold as well.

Chapter 5

Setting Up and Stocking Your Breastfeeding Space

In This Chapter

- Designing your breastfeeding spaces
- Buying bras, shirts, and gowns
- Picking the best breast pump
- Choosing breast pads, nipple shields, and breast shells
- Deciding whether to buy bottles and pacifiers

It's time to go shopping! You need to buy some essential equipment for breastfeeding, and you may want to consider getting some nice-to-have but not essential things.

In this chapter, we help you set up a functional nursery and discuss the pros and cons of nursing in the "public areas" of your home — the living room or family room. We also help you find the most comfortable nursing chairs, the best nursing bras, the most efficient breast pumps, and all the accessories you need to make breastfeeding a pleasure.

Arranging Your Space

At your coauthor Carol's house, the standing joke is that things run under the *form over function* rule: Appearance is more important to me than performance. When I decorated the nursery, I kept in mind that this wasn't just a baby's room. I knew that the two of us would spend lots of time together there, and I wanted it to be pleasing to both of us. Night feedings can be exhausting; why not do them in a place that's both comfortable and pleasant?

When you start arranging your nursing space, you'll probably set up two areas. First, of course, is the baby's room. You'll probably do most of your night feedings here, and visitors usually want to see this space first so they can oooh and ahhh over the cute wallpaper. During the day, you may spend most of your time in your family room or living room. Depending on whether you decide to co-sleep with your baby (an issue we discuss in Chapter 6), you may need to set up a nursing space in your own bedroom as well.

Nesting in the nursery

Curtains that match the crib bumper pads are very nice and will satisfy your *form over function* needs, but other items are more essential for a comfortable breastfeeding experience:

- Topping the list is a comfortable place to sit, whether you prefer an upholstered chair, a wooden rocker, or a glider. See the section "Rocking Through Nursing" later in this chapter.
- A footstool or ottoman elevates your feet and knees, bringing the baby closer to your breasts. This position can reduce neck, shoulder, and back strain. Some ottomans are too high for comfort, so you may want to look for a special nursing stool. You can find handmade stools at `www.thisbabyofmine.com` or `www.nursinggear.com`. Medela also makes a nursing stool, available at `www.medela.com`. Alternately, you can get creative and make your own from a kitchen step stool.
- A table by your chair is a must, because you need burping cloths, baby wipes, a clock, and receiving blankets within arm's reach. And having a drink next to you at each feeding is a great reminder to keep your fluid intake up while you're breastfeeding. If you're tight on space, get creative: Your coauthor Sharon used a wicker plant stand!

Setting up space in the family room

Hide and seek is fun when you're 10, but not when you're a new mom and you have to disappear into the nursery to breastfeed every time company arrives. Arranging your nursing space in the family room is the start of public breastfeeding (which we discuss in detail in Chapter 14). Setting up a comfortable spot allows you to feed the baby discreetly and still be part of the action in the house.

REMEMBER

Having a nursing spot set up in the middle of the action is good only if you're comfortable with it. When you first come home from the hospital, you may feel comfortable nursing only in front of your partner — and maybe not even him! Be direct about your needs for privacy, even if that means kicking everyone out of the family room for a while. Ask your partner for help telling your family and friends to give you space; he may enjoy having an active role to play as "keeper of the gate." (But don't go overboard, unless you never want to see your Aunt Susie again!)

If you have other children, you need to decide if you're comfortable nursing in front of them. Of course, depending on their ages, you may not have a choice.

If you have toddlers, arrange your nursing area so they can sit next to you. That way, they won't climb on top of the kitchen cupboards every time you nurse. Have favorite books or puzzles handy, prepare a snack for them before you begin nursing, and encourage them to watch the baby make funny faces. (We discuss handling siblings and breastfeeding in Chapter 14.)

If you plan to nurse in front of your children or other people, you may want to arrange the furniture in your family room so your nursing chair isn't center stage. Perhaps set your table and chair behind the couch, or in a corner. Unless you want all eyes on you, definitely don't put your chair right next to the TV! Keep in mind, also, that as the baby grows, he'll be distracted by what's going on around him. He may nurse better if you're away from the action.

Your furniture and equipment needs for the family room are similar to those in the nursery:

- A comfortable chair is still a must, although you may choose to use the corner of the couch. Your impulse might be to go for a great overstuffed chair, but be warned: Many overstuffed chairs are too deep to sit in comfortably, unless you're tall. If you're short (like your coauthor Sharon is), your feet will stick straight out in front of you — not comfortable for the long haul!
- A table within easy reach will hold not only the breastfeeding essentials but also the remote control, a magazine, the TV guide, and a snack or two!
- A simple basket, like a wicker laundry basket, comes in handy for holding all the baby care equipment you need each day — diapers, wipes, spare outfits, and small toys, for example. Fill it in the morning so you don't have to run back and forth to your baby's room for these things all day long. Visiting even the prettiest nursery gets old after your tenth trip up the stairs for something as simple as a washcloth!
- Lots of extra pillows are helpful, especially when you're just learning how to nurse (see the section "Pumps, Pillows, and Paraphernalia" later in the chapter).

Breastfeeding in your bedroom

We discuss the pros and cons of co-sleeping in Chapter 6. If you do chose to share your room with your baby, at least for the first few months, keep the following in mind:

- An overstuffed reading pillow provides back and arm support for feedings. You'll also need pillows under your arms to help lift the baby up to the breast.
- A bedside *bassinet* (small crib) helps you scoop up the baby easily, if you don't plan to have the baby in your bed. Many bedside cribs are designed to line up at the same level as your bed so you can reach the baby without any barriers. Look at `www.armsreach.com` for ideas.

  A cradle or a regular bassinet in your room also allows easy access to your baby for night feedings.
- Keep spare diapers, clothing, washcloths, and wipes in your room, or carry your basket full of goodies from the family room into the bedroom each night or during naptime.

Rocking Through Nursing

"Rock Around the Clock" should be the theme song for the nursing mom. You can nurse your baby in bed or in a regular chair, but most moms prefer the comfort of a rocking chair or glider. Babies love to be rocked, whether the person holding them is sitting in a chair or standing up swaying. (The next time you're in a grocery checkout line, look around and see if you spot a woman swaying back and forth — chances are she's a mom whose body can't break the habit, even if the baby has long since grown up!)

Choosing the right rocker can be difficult, because so many types are available. Rockers can cost upwards of $500, so this is no small purchase. Before you buy, ask about the company's return policy in case the chair isn't right for you. And definitely keep your receipt!

Glider-type rockers with matching gliding ottomans can feel like heaven to a nursing mom, but they can also cost up to $1,000 depending on the manufacturer, the chair's design, and the fabric you choose. These chairs often have padded arms, which may be removable for washing. Dutailier (`www.dutailier.com`) and Shermag (`www.shermag.com`) are popular manufacturers of glider and ottoman combinations. Many department and furniture stores carry these brands.

Carol's rock-a-bye babies

For the first few months of their lives, we kept each of our boys in our bedroom in a cradle that my dad made. Each time I made the transition of putting them to sleep in their own rooms, the change was traumatic — for me, not for them! However, I grew to enjoy spending time with each child in his own room. I would nurse him on one side and then change his diaper to prepare for the return to the crib. But after I sat back down in the rocking chair to nurse him on the other side, inevitably I would not want to put him back in the crib. I would just rock and rock.

That was 28 years ago. I still have my rocker and so many memories of our nights together!

Whichever type of rocker you choose, it should be wide and comfortable enough to hold your baby with some extra pillows under your arms for support, as well as behind your upper and lower back. (We discuss where to place pillows later in this chapter.)

TIP

Look for a rocker that has a solid back and arms. It should give you adequate back support, and your feet should touch the floor when you sit back. (You don't want to have to constantly lean forward in the chair, because that changes the configuration of your breasts and makes it difficult for the baby to latch on properly.)

A plain wooden rocker, whether antique or brand new, is the classic baby soother. Your coauthor Sharon still has the rocking chair her mother used, and it was second-hand when she got it! It has very high arms (good for holding a baby) and a nice rounded back.

TIP

Some experts suggest not nursing in a rocking chair when you first start breastfeeding, because it may be more difficult to nurse if you're a moving target. After you have breastfeeding down to a science, the rocking chair will be fine. Keep in mind that some rockers make using a nursing pillow difficult, because the chair arms are too high to rest your arms on comfortably. Test the chair before you buy!

REMEMBER

Even if you decide not to nurse your baby in the rocker, you can still use it for comfort. Studies show that babies like rocking at a pace of about 60 beats a minute; they're used to hearing a ticking heartbeat of the same rate, so the rhythm is familiar. Rocking the baby to sleep leaves only one trick that you need to master: getting him into his bed without waking him up!

Breastfeeding with a Baby Carrier

Think about walking into a room with conversations going on all around you, but you're not part of any of them. No one even acknowledges your presence. This is how babies must feel when they're down in a stroller and the rest of the world is so far above. To bring the baby up to eye level, think about "wearing" your baby by using a sling-type carrier. It brings him closer to you so he is able to listen to your heart, your voice, and your breathing, like he did before he was born. Most babies find this very soothing.

A study published in the journal *Pediatrics* in 1986 documented that wearing your baby reduces crying and fussiness by 43 percent. This may seem extremely important to you someday when you're trying to make (and eat!) dinner while keeping your baby occupied.

Don't get us wrong: A sling isn't your ticket to baby bliss 24 hours a day. But it offers you more flexibility when it comes to caring for your baby and getting a job or two completed at the same time.

Many types of carriers are available. The best type for nursing is a sling that you wear across the front of your chest (see Figure 5-1). A sling is a simple piece of fabric with a couple of sliding rings to hold it together. It can be worn with the baby on your back, in front, or to the side. Obviously, for breastfeeding, you want the baby in front (unless you have very large, flexible breasts!). By simply pulling up your shirt, your baby can nurse discreetly.

Slings cost $25 to $50 if purchased new and can often be found for much less in consignment shops. They are usually washable — a big plus with breastfed babies who can have loose stools.

You can also find slings online if your local baby store doesn't carry them; just type in "sling breastfeeding" on your favorite search engine. Some brands to look for include Huggababy, Maya, New Native, and Over the Shoulder Baby Holder.

Carriers that are more rigid than simple slings, such as Baby Bjorn carriers, can be used for nursing as well, but they're a little more complicated to use because you need to let down one side of the carrier.

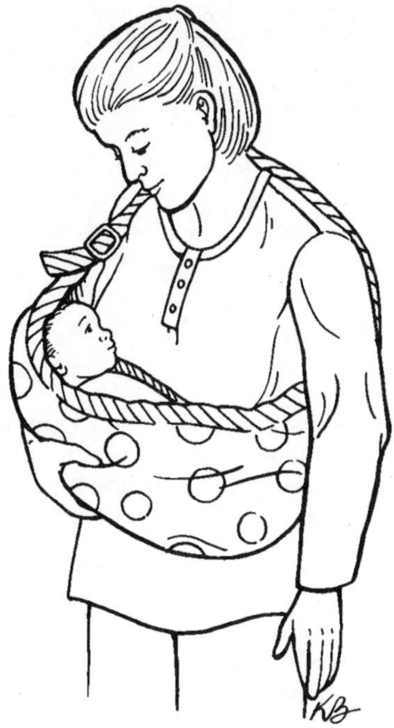

Figure 5-1: Sling-type carriers let you carry the baby and nurse while freeing your hands.

Stocking Your Wardrobe

No one ever said nursing shirts and nursing bras were glamorous, but they've made great stridesover the last 20 years. Whether you're a stay-at-home mom or chairman of the board, you need to get dressed in the morning in clothes that are comfortable and conducive to nursing.

Trying on nursing bras

If you're well along in your pregnancy, you're probably not hanging out at Victoria's Secret too much these days. Lacy, flowery little wisps of material have probably disappeared from your lingerie drawer, replaced by massive white tents stitched together in the middle. You may shudder to think what comes after this, with the start of breastfeeding.

Wearing the proper nursing bra provides breast support and makes you more comfortable. You should buy two or three *all cotton* nursing bras in the final weeks of your pregnancy. At this time, your cup size will be its closest to your post-delivery size.

Most maternity shops, department stores, and undergarment specialty stores carry nursing bras. Wherever you go, make sure that the person helping you knows how to measure and fit you. Proper fit is the key to comfort with any type of bra.

If a salesperson isn't able to help you, find your bra size by following these steps:

1. **Measure around yourself just under your armpits with a measuring tape.** Keep the tape snug, but not tight. If the measurement is an uneven number, round it up to the next even number. This is your *band size.*
2. **While wearing your best-fitting unpadded bra, measure around the fullest part of your bust.** The difference in the band and bust size in inches is your *cup size.* Up to 1 inch, the cup size is A; 2 inches, size B; 3 inches, size C; 4 inches, size D. Nursing bras go up to J!

For example, say your band size measurement is 39 inches. Add an inch to round up to an even number: 40. Your bust size is 43 inches. Subtract the difference (3 inches). Your bra size is 40 C. Simple!

When you try on a nursing bra, bend over and gently "shake" your breasts into the cups. A well-fitted bra should cover the entire breast; no part of the breast should spill out. The bottom band should be snug, but the bra shouldn't put pressure on your breasts. If the bra is too tight, it could cause a milk duct to become plugged or *mastitis* (infection) to develop. The bra shouldn't ride up in the back, and the straps should keep your breasts elevated without cutting into your shoulders.

When considering cup size, keep in mind that you may need room for a breast pad or breast shell (both of which are discussed later in this chapter). For band size, buy a bra that you can fasten on the inside row, so you have more hooks to expand to after your milk comes in.

Make sure your bra flaps (see Figure 5-2) are easy to open and close. You don't want a bra that requires neighborhood assistance to open! Opening the flap should be a one-hand operation; you want to be able to hold your baby in one arm and slip up your top and undo the flap with the other. (This is probably the only time in Carol's life that *form over function* went out the window!) Some bras have clips and some have snaps to hold the flap up; you may want to try them both to see which is more maneuverable for you.

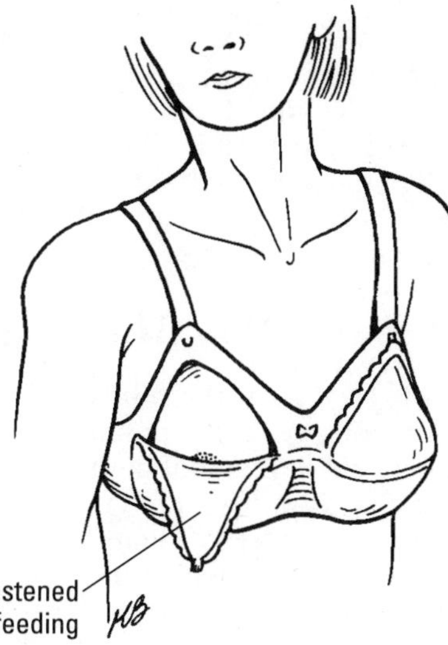
Flaps can be unfastened for breastfeeding

Figure 5-2: Nursing bras with flaps are a wardrobe essential.

Nursing bras can be expensive but are worth the investment. Don't be surprised if you need to buy bras in different sizes as time goes by. You may even find yourself back in your regular bra months down the road. At this point you can use the *lift and load* routine — just *lift* your bra up off the breast and *load* the baby on.

If you want to try on bras at home, check out some of the following Web sites where name-brand nursing bras can be purchased:

- `www.motherwear.com`
- `www.bravadodesigns.com`
- `www.bosombuddies.com`
- `www.medela.com`
- `www.birthandbaby.com`
- `www.mybreastpump.com`

TIP

Most of these sites have return policies that allow refunds, although some may charge a small restocking fee. When you try on a bra, wear a breast pad in case you leak breast milk. Some online stores allow returns even if the bra has been worn, if you're unhappy with its comfort or performance. Make sure you read the return policy before you purchase!

Some well-known names of nursing bra manufacturers are Olga, Fancee Free, Bravado, Leading Lady, Goddess, Decent Exposure, and Melinda Gros.

REMEMBER

You don't have to wear a bra. Some women like that *born free* (or *hang free,* at least) feeling. But wait until you're an advanced breastfeeder before ditching your bra. Your breasts need support in the beginning — at least for the first month. We found ourselves even wearing bras to bed in the beginning, because it was more comfortable.

Looking chic in nursing shirts

Nursing shirts (and gowns) can be helpful, especially at first. When you wear a nursing shirt, you don't have to bare all to feed the baby. There's a slit in the front of the shirt (see Figure 5-3); you just slide the slit over your breast to give the baby access. The time may come when you feel so comfortable with nursing that you wouldn't care if the President of the United States was in the same room with you. But until then, these "peek-a-boob" aids are helpful.

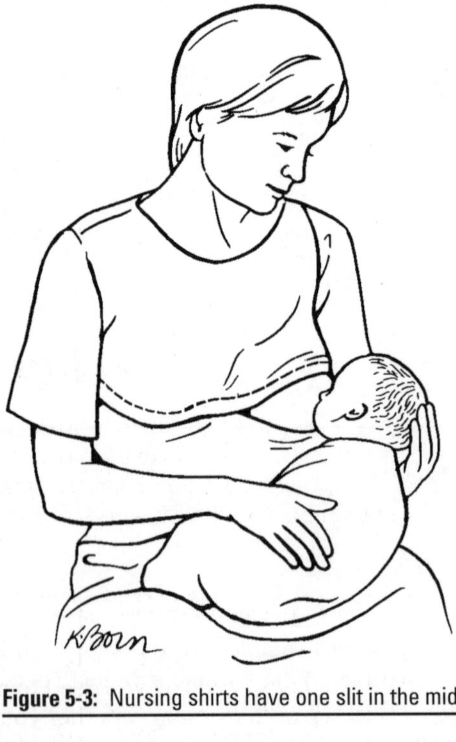

Figure 5-3: Nursing shirts have one slit in the middle.

Mothers of twins may not find nursing shirts helpful because most have only one slit in the front, making it impossibly to nurse two babies at one time. If you want some two-slit shirts, get creative. Simply buy two large T-shirts and cut two slits at breast level in the first one. Wear the second, unaltered shirt over the one with slits. When you nurse, lift up the top shirt while placing the baby on the breast. You can nurse comfortably without exposing your entire chest or belly.

Of course, you don't need special shirts to nurse. If you're comfortable, just place a receiving blanket over your baby, and he'll cover the rest. If you're really embarrassed about nursing in public, you can throw another blanket over your own head! (That won't make you too conspicuous, will it?) You can also sew two blankets together and make a poncho.

Your coauthor Carol *loved* flannel nursing gowns, especially in the winter. On those chilly nights, you'll find that a nursing gown keeps you a little better covered than a shirt you have to pull up.

You can buy nursing shirts and gowns at maternity stores or in most department stores. Web sites for purchasing nursing outfits include `www.AllegroMedical.com`, `www.flannelnightie.com`, `www.lactationconnection.com`, `www.maternitystop.com`, `www.momstobefactoryoutlet.com`, `www.momshop.com`, and `www.motherwear.com`.

One alternative to wearing nursing shirts is using a "peek-a-boo," a piece of Velcro that holds your shirt out of the way while you're nursing or pumping. Check out the Web site `www.mommysthinkin.com` to see this item. The cost is around $6 for one; they come in several different colors.

Pumps, Pillows, and Paraphernalia

You still need a few more things to stock your breastfeeding nursery. Some, like nipple shields and breast shells, may not be necessary for you. Breast pads, on the other hand, are an essential for nearly every nursing mom, at least in the first few weeks.

Buying or renting a breast pump

One of the most complicated items you need is a breast pump; you may be surprised at the number of choices you need to make before purchasing one. Every nursing mom, whether you're staying at home or going back to work, should have one. How exotic the pump is up to you. You can buy a manual or electric breast pump, or you can rent an electric one.

If possible, don't start pumping until your milk supply is well established — at least four weeks after delivery.

What you buy or rent depends on your needs. Are you going to pump only occasionally, like when you go out to dinner with your husband and want someone to give the baby a bottle of breast milk? Or are you going to pump on a regular basis because you have to return to work?

If possible, discuss pumps with a lactation consultant before purchasing one; she'll probably recommend that you get your feet wet with breastfeeding before investing in a pump. Pumps can be expensive, and you can't return them after they've been used, so you want to make as informed a decision as possible.

If time is money for you, get a fully automatic electric double pump; you can pump both breasts completely in 10 to 20 minutes. Using a semiautomatic pump takes 15 to 30 minutes; a battery-operated pump takes 20 to 30 minutes; and a manual pump (or hand expressing milk) takes at least 20 to 30 minutes. The following sections explain what each type of pump is.

If you're establishing your milk supply for a preemie or an adopted baby (see Chapter 9), you almost certainly need a fully automatic electric pump. Other pumps probably won't give your breasts the stimulation they need to establish your milk supply.

Manual pumps

Manual pumps (see Figure 5-4) may work for occasional pumpers. They're easy to find and easy to assemble, but they're not always easy to use.

Several types of manual pumps exist; the most common are a piston-type pump and a pump that consists of two cylinders. With the cylinder type, one cylinder slides back and forth, creating suction, and the other stores the expressed milk. This type holds only a small amount of milk, so you need to stop and empty frequently. You may find the cylinder type of manual pump hard on your nipples.

Some manual pumps, like the Avent Isis, Medela Harmony, and Ameda One Hand, have soft silicone breast shields that are easier on your nipples. They operate by squeezing a handle, so they require only one hand to use. You can nurse on one breast and pump on the other at the same time.

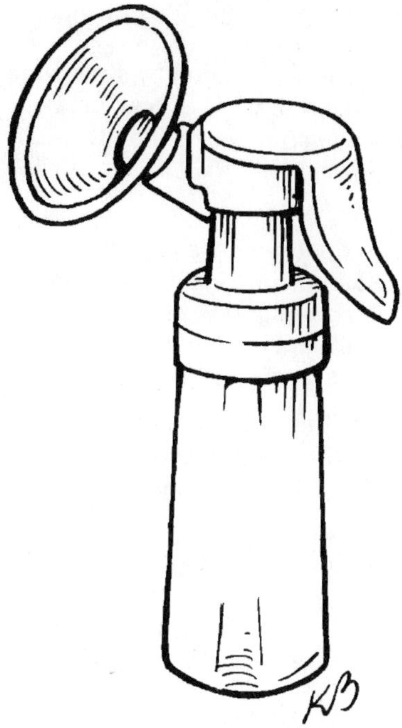

Figure 5-4: A manual breast pump.

Breast pumps are very personal items. What may work for one mom may not for another. The big plus of manual pumps is they are inexpensive, so if you have to try a few different ones, it won't be too traumatic to your pocketbook.

The other advantages of manual breast pumps are that they're compact, portable, and quiet. They don't have moving parts that could break, and they don't require electricity or batteries to operate. They're also easy to find; most pharmacies have them in stock.

Some manual pumps are very easy to use and effective; others are less so. Many women are able to get only a scant amount of milk using a manual pump, and some pumps can bruise or scrape your nipples. You also have to be a juggler to pump and hold the equipment at the same time, and you may find your arms getting tired because you hold the pump in one hand and manipulate the bulb, cylinder, or piston to form the suction with the other hand.

If you have carpal tunnel syndrome or are prone to repetitive stress injury in your hands and are planning to pump frequently, don't buy a manual pump! These pumps are very hard on your hands if you use them on a regular basis. Look for a semiautomatic or fully automatic electric pump instead.

Readily available manual pumps include the following:

- **Ameda One Hand:** Suction is created by squeezing a hand grip; cycling speed and amount of suction can be controlled by how hard and fast you squeeze the handle. Cost runs approximately $50 to $60. Visit www.ameda.com for more information.
- **Avent Isis:** This pump operates by squeezing a handle. Its claim to fame is the soft silicone insert that compresses the breast and causes less trauma to the breast and nipple. Cost is approximately $40. To find a supplier for Avent products, call 1-800-542-8368 or visit www.aventamerica.com.
- **Evenflo Manual Breast Pump:** Widely available, it creates suction by the use of a plunger pulled up and down. Visit www.evenflo.com. Cost is approximately $18.
- **Medela ManualEase:** This pump uses the cylinder mechanism to start the flow, but a spring in the plunger makes the release automatic. Milk flows into an attached bottle. This pump can be adapted to an electric pump. Cost is approximately $50. Call 1-800-435-8316 to find a supplier for Medela products, or visit www.medela.com.
- **Medela PedalPump:** This pump may be less tiring to use because the suction comes from a foot pedal, not your arms. You can pump two breasts at once. Cost is approximately $50. See the previous bullet for contact information.

Battery-operated pumps

Battery-operated pumps tend to have more disadvantages than advantages. Their energy is supplied by AA batteries, so you may need to buy stock in a battery company. It takes eight to ten seconds to build up suction, so a battery-operated pump takes longer to use than a regular manual pump. Most are *semiautomatic,* which means you need to use one hand to create suction. They're also slower than electric pumps because they have less power; they cycle around 12 sucks per minute.

The advantage of a battery-operated pump is it's easier to maneuver than a manual pump and just as portable. If you don't think that you'll need to pump on a regular basis, a battery-operated pump may work for you.

Some battery-operated pumps include the following:

- **Evenflo Comfort Select Auto-Cycling Breast Pump:** This pump has a soft breast cup and an adjustable vacuum dial to set a vacuum level that's comfortable and functional. This product contains everything you need for pumping away from home included in a carrying case. The price is approximately $45. For more information, see www.evenflo.com.

- **Gentle Expressions (Lumiscope):** This pump is semiautomatic and costs around $35 — a good value for the money. You can purchase a separate AC adapter to save on batteries. This pump does not come with a carrying case. Visit www.lumiscope.net/gentle_expressions.html for details.
- **Medela MiniElectric:** The only battery-operated pump that sucks and releases automatically, this pump is faster than most other battery pumps. You can pump both breasts at the same time. Many lactation consultants recommend this pump for their clients. The cost is around $75. Call 1-800-435-8316 to find a supplier for Medela products, or visit www.medela.com.
- **Whisper Wear:** This is an interesting concept; you insert the pumps into your bra and attach them to a collapsible collecting bag. The cups must be placed correctly, or the suction doesn't work well, but you can wear this pump without taking off your clothes. (Some users we know recommended wearing a tight bra.) The cost is around $200 for a double pump, $99 for a single. For details, visit www.whisperwear.com.

Electric pumps

If you pump frequently, an electric pump (see Figure 5-5) is the only way to fly! It has limitations (like you need to be near electricity), but it far outperforms a manual pump. Some pumps have AC adapters, making them more portable. However, the cost may make you think twice; don't be surprised to see prices as high as $200 to $300. Some smaller, mini electric pumps are a little less expensive.

TIP

Check with your health insurance carrier if you're pumping because your baby is premature or ill. The cost of a breast pump rental may be covered under your policy. Hospitals and lactation consultants often rent electric pumps. If your hospital does rent them, you may find a good price there due to its high volume of business.

You can rent a pump for $1 to $2 per day. Monthly rates decrease if you keep the pump longer; costs range from $48 per month for up to three months down to $40 if you're using it for a longer period. We found some pumps for as little as $31.50 a month. It pays to go shopping if you decide to rent, but make sure that you know exactly what you're renting. A cheaper price may add up to a less powerful pump with additional equipment that you have to purchase.

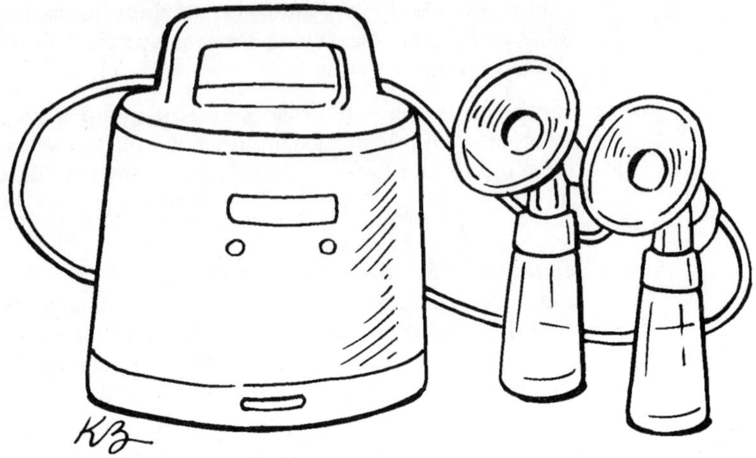

Figure 5-5: An electric breast pump.

A fully automatic electric pump offers several advantages:

- It requires only one hand to use. This may not seem like an advantage until you're trying to pump your milk and eat lunch at the same time because the baby is *finally* sleeping.
- Most women find electric pumps more effective than other pumps in getting milk out of their breasts.
- Many women find electric pumps gentler on their breast tissue than other pumps. However, this is not true for everyone; again, your breast pump preference is a highly personal one.
- This type of pump imitates your baby's sucking action, even down to number of sucks per minute (48 to 60).
- Many fully automated electric pumps allow you to pump both breasts at one time, which means you can finish pumping in half the time.
- You can usually regulate the speed and vacuum pressure.

Disadvantages of a fully automatic electric pump include the following:

- These pumps tend to be on the larger side, making them less portable and more conspicuous.
- This type of pump is more expensive to buy than others.
- *Quiet* is not in the vocabulary of most of these pumps, no matter what the manufacturers say. These pumps are work

horses, and they often sound like it! If you're interested in a quiet electric pump, consider a smaller, handheld battery/electric pump.

If you want a quiet electric option, consider the Medela Symphony, which sounds like a clock ticking. However, there's a heavy price to pay for silence; this pump runs about $1,250.

- Some pumps can be hard to take apart and put back together again when you wash them.

Some electric pumps are *semiautomatic;* they require you to create suction by holding down a button. The big plus for these pumps is that they're cheaper than fully automatic pumps. However, they aren't as efficient.

Electric breast pumps you can purchase include:

- **Medela DoubleEase:** This affordable, fully automated pump is a little slower than most fully automated pumps. It comes with a carrying case that has an insulated area for your pumped milk. This pump can run off of C batteries as well as electricity; the cost is about $200. Call 1-800-435-8316 for suppliers, or visit www.medela.com.
- **Hollister/Ameda Purely Yours:** With this automatic/semiautomatic double or single pump, you control the frequency and vacuum by placing your thumb on top of the bottle. The cost is about $110; adding an AC adaptor and backpack case raises the price to approximately $220. Check carefully when purchasing this pump, because three versions exist that offer different options. Call 1-800-413-3216 for more information.
- **Medela Pump In Style:** This fully automated double pump is described as "near hospital grade," and it does a quick and efficient job. The cost is around $250 with the carrying case, storage, and cooling system. Call 1-800-435-8316 for information, or visit www.medela.com.
- **Nurture III (Bailey Medical):** The cost for this fully automated double pump, with adjustable suction and cycling speeds, is around $160 with carrying case, cooler, and storage system. Visit www.baileymed.com.
- **Whittlestone Breast Pump Expresser:** This pump massages the breast with soft liners for more natural stimulation. It contains all the accessories to pump away from home. The cost is approximately $300. Visit www.whittlestone.com for more information.

Electric breast pumps you can rent include the following:

- **Ameda SMB and Lact-e pumps:** These heavy-duty hospital pumps rent for $1 to $2 a day. Call 1-800-323-4060 to find a rental station near you.
- **Ameda Elite:** This pump is electric but has a built-in battery pack. Call 1-800-323-4060 to rent.
- **Medela Classic:** This heavy-duty pump weighs about 20 pounds. Call 1-800-TELLYOU to find a rental station.
- **Medela Lactina Plus and Lactina Select:** You can vary the speed on these electric pumps, which can be used on both breasts at one time. They're great for the working mom because they weigh only 4 pounds. Call 1-800-TELLYOU to rent.

TIP

If you need to pump exclusively for a preemie baby or an infant in intensive care, the Medela Classic and Ameda SMB/Lact-e pumps are good choices because of their great suction. However, many rental stations do not have them available because they are much heavier and less portable than other pumps.

The Medela Symphony is now available for rent as well. As we mention earlier in this section, it is very quiet and effective. Originally marketed to moms with babies in intensive care, this pump is now being marketed more broadly because moms love it. Check the Medela Web site, `www.medela.com`, for more information.

How to choose?

TIP

It may make you tired even thinking about the choice between manual versus battery-operated versus fully automated versus semiautomatic breast pump. With so many choices, your best bet is to contact a lactation consultant or childbirth educator to help you make this decision. Explain how you'll use the pump, and she can suggest the best one for you. If possible, rent the one she suggests; if it turns out to be the wrong choice, you can trade it in for a better one.

Some online sites for checking out and buying breast pumps are `www.affordablebreastpumps.com`, `www.mybreastpump.com`, and `www.nursingbaby.com`. An excellent Web site for comparing ratings and prices of many breast pumps on the market is `www.nextag.com`. (Click on "Baby" from the home page.)

TIP

You can find users' opinions of various pumps on `www.epinions.com` and `www.amazon.com`. The most popular pumps have lots of reviews, which contain valuable information on the pros and cons of each.

Used breast pumps

If you're a bargain shopper, you may wonder about buying a used breast pump in order to save money. A word of caution: Most pumps are made to be used by one person only, because breast milk can get into the pump motor or contaminate the internal parts of the pump. Bacterial and viral infections can be transmitted through a breast pump that isn't manufactured for use by more than one person.

The following breast pumps are FDA-approved for *single use* only: Avent Isis, Evenflo Manual Breast Pump, Gentle Expressions, Gerber Precious Care, Hollister/Ameda Purely Yours, MagMag Mini Electric, Medela MiniElectric, Medela Pump In Style products (Original, Advanced, and Traveler), Medela DoubleEase, and The First Years' Simplicity pump.

These breast pumps are FDA-approved for *multiple use,* meaning they can be adequately cleaned to prevent cross contamination: Ameda Elite, Ameda Lact-e, Ameda SMB, Medela Classic, Medela Lactina, Medela Symphony, and Bailey Nurture III.

If you use a pump at the hospital or decide to rent one, the pump you use should obviously be approved for multiple use and sterilized between users.

Hands-free pumping

If you'd like to be able to talk on the phone, read a book, or use the computer while you pump, a rather strange-looking but effective undergarment called *Made by Moms Pumping Band* may work for you. It looks like a giant Velcro bra, with slits that the horns that attach to your nipples fit through. Everything is held in place, leaving your hands free to do something else. This product sells for around $35 and can be found at `www.babycenter.com`.

Resting on nursing pillows

To be comfortable while nursing, you'll probably want to tuck pillows behind you for back support and under your arms to help support the baby. A pillow on your lap brings your baby closer to the breast.

You can use plain bed pillows for this purpose, or you can splurge with special nursing pillows — good items to put on your registry (see Figure 5-6). Whether you use bed pillows or a $40 specialty model is up to you; either can help you get the baby in the correct position to nurse and make you more comfortable.

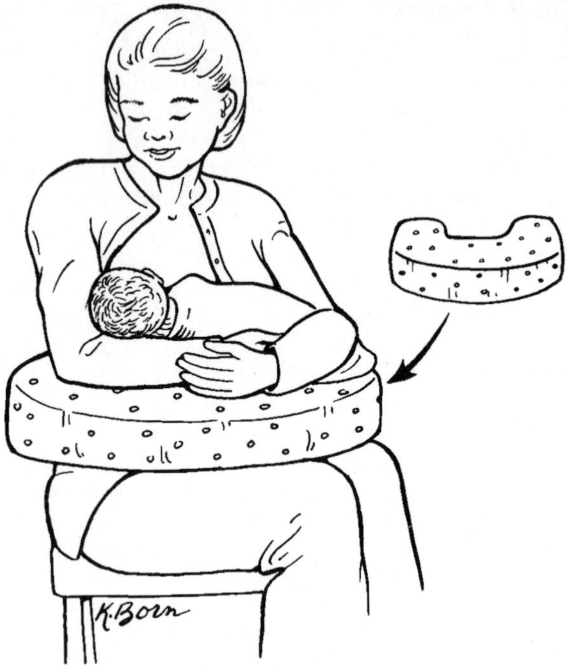

Figure 5-6: A nursing pillow can make it easier for you to support and position the baby.

Most official nursing pillows are U- or C-shaped and fit around your waist. Some completely encircle you and fasten with Velcro; others go only partway around you. The ones that go all the way around and fasten are easier to walk around with and also provide some support to your back.

TIP

Make sure the pillow you use is firm; if it's too soft, the baby will sink into it and not get any higher on your lap. A plastic cover over the pillow is essential. (No matter how much disposable diapers improve, they still can leak!) Most nursing pillow covers are washable, and some pillows are as well.

The following nursing pillows are readily available:

- **Boppy:** The Boppy pillow, made by The Boppy Company (`www.boppy.com`), is a semicircle that fits around your waist. People either love it or hate it. Designed originally as an aid to prop up babies and give them tummy time, the Boppy has become the most popular nursing pillow in the United States. The baby rests on the semicircle, turned toward you in position for nursing. The Boppy should put the baby's mouth at nipple level. Some moms find the baby stays in place easily, leaving their hands free. Others find that the baby slides down too easily, ending up between you and the Boppy. Some plus-size women say this pillow is too snug; some thin women say it's not snug enough.

The Boppy is reasonably priced; you can find it for less than $25. The pillow is not machine-washable, although you can buy removable washable covers, which come in a variety of patterns. Having an extra cover or two is a good idea.

TIP: If this pillow doesn't work for you for nursing, you may still find it worthwhile as an aid to prop the baby. You may also find it helpful to sit on after delivery, if your stitches are uncomfortable.

- **Nurse Prop R Pillow:** This pillow is made by Leachco, a company that makes several nursing pillows. It has a bend in it so you hold the baby at a 45-degree angle or higher. Leachco's Natural Boost pillow also can be angled. Leachco's pillows cost between $20 and $35 and can be seen online at `www.leachco.com`.
- **My Brest Friend Pillow:** Sharon's daughter-in-law used one of these pillows and swears by it! Made by Zenoff, it's fairly large, but very firm and supportive. It has Velcro attachments so that it completely encircles your waist; you can move around and have a free hand because you don't have to hold the pillow in place. Pockets on the side can hold a water bottle, a paperback book, a washcloth, or some wipes. The cost is around $39.

  TIP: The same company makes an inflatable version called "My Best Friend," which can be carried anywhere and inflated when you need it. Zenoff pillows can be found online at `www.zenoffproducts.com`.
- **Boston Billow:** This pillow is a little different because it's stuffed with small polybeads that mold to you and the baby — unlike foam, which is hard to adjust. Because the pillow molds to the baby, the baby stays in one place with less adjusting. Both the inner and the outer pillow are washable. The pillow weighs only a pound and costs around $32. Boston Billow products can be found at `www.bostonbillows.com`.

TIP: If you want a pillow and cover-up in one, the Mother Cover Nursing Pillow, made by Leachco (`www.leachco.com`), may be for you. The pillow is used for support, and the cover can be put over your shoulders to cover the baby. A space at the top allows you to see the baby. The pillow can also be used without the cover-up portion.

Some pillows are made especially for nursing twins, such as EZ-2-Nurse and the Twin Nursing pillow. They cost around $50, and they let you feed both babies at the same time and keep your hands free. You can find twin pillows at many Web sites, including `www.twinstuff.com` or `www.doubleblessings.com`.

Filling your bra with pads, shields, and shells

Breast pads, nipple shields, and breast shells all fit into your bra, but they have very different functions. We start with the simplest, and the one almost everyone needs: breast pads.

Stopping leaks with breast pads

Breast pads are absorbent cotton pads that collect milk that leaks out of the nipple until your let-down reflex (see Chapter 6) is better controlled. In the first few weeks of nursing, you may experience a considerable amount of leakage! Breast pads (also called *nursing pads*) bear a strong resemblance to sanitary napkins, which can actually be cut down to size and used for this same purpose.

TIP: You can purchase boxes of disposable breast pads, or you can choose washable cotton pads, which are more cost-effective if you don't mind adding to your laundry pile. A box of 50 or so disposable pads costs around $5; you can buy a pack of four washables for around the same price.

Should you choose washable or disposable? Disposables are more convenient, because you use them once and throw them away. They're also more expensive, for the same reason. Some other disadvantages to disposables are that they bunch up more easily and tend to be more visible in your bra. They also may shred more easily, leaving little pieces of cotton stuck to your nipples. Some have a thin plastic outer coating, which holds moisture in rather than letting it evaporate; this may keep your nipples wetter longer. Wet nipples are more prone to developing a yeast infection (see Chapter 8).

If you choose washables, you need to buy several pairs — at least two, and preferably four. They should be washed every time they get wet, not just dried and reused.

Some pads are contoured, and some are more like flat circles. If you buy contoured, keep in mind that the contour of the pad may not fit your particular contour! On the other hand, flat pads slide around more easily and are more noticeable through your shirt. Some brands come with sticky strips to hold them in place in your bra.

If you're looking for flesh-colored pads, Medela makes a beige, lace-covered washable pad. The lace covering on the outside is nice, but with frequent washings, you may find the lace unraveling.

The best-known breast pad manufacturers include the following:

- **Avent:** Avent's disposable Ultra Comfort pad has a nipple indent. The company's washable pads come in a package of six with a laundry bag — essential if you want to keep track of the pads in the washer!
- **Evenflo:** This company's disposables are flat; its washables are contoured and have a lace covering. The disposables don't have anything on the back to hold them in place.
- **Gerber:** Gerber's new disposables are contoured and have an adhesive area to hold them in place. They come in three types: slow, medium, and heavy flow. They also have absorbent gel inside to decrease wetness.
- **Johnson & Johnson:** This company makes two types of disposable pads. The Healthflow Ultra pad is contoured and somewhat small in diameter, has a nipple indent, and has no tape or plastic backing. The Super Absorbent pad is flat and textured on the back but not covered with plastic.
- **Lansinoh:** Both its disposable and washable pads are contoured. The disposables come with a tape that helps keep them in place. Lansinoh products are very highly rated by nursing moms.
- **Medela:** Medela's washables are lace-covered, contoured, and available in white or beige. The disposables are a closed U shape so they can be contoured to your shape.

Many other brands of nursing pads are available, including Leading Lady, Nursing Mother, and Sweet Cheeks. Experiment until you find a brand you really like.

Covering your nipples with a shield

Nipple shields are sometimes recommended to help draw out flat or inverted nipples (see Chapter 4) or protect sore nipples. The shields are made of soft plastic or silicone and fit over the entire areola (see Figure 5-7). You need to moisten the back of the shield to help it adhere to your skin. You wear the shields while breastfeeding. Nipple shields should be used only as a last resort and only under the supervision of your lactation consultant or physician.

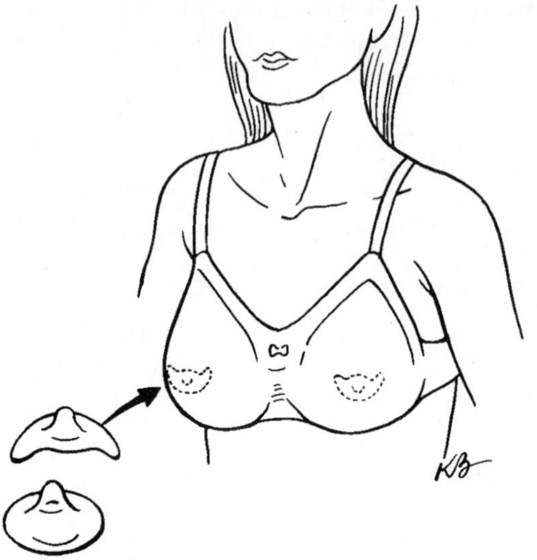

Figure 5-7: Nipple shields should be used only as a temporary solution.

Most lactation consultants agree that sore and cracked nipples are caused by poor positioning and/or improper latch-on (see Chapter 6). Nipple shields are only a temporary measure to help your nipples heal or help your baby latch on when all else fails. Using shields for long periods may decrease your milk supply, so use them only with the supervision of a lactation consultant.

Several well-known makers of baby goods make nipple shields. Avent and Medela are both known for their high-quality products. Newer shields made by La Leche League and Medela are made of thin silicone and allow more skin-to-skin contact than other shields.

Wearing breast shells

Breast shells are quite different than nipple shields. Shells are never worn while nursing; they're used between feedings or before the baby arrives to help draw out flat or inverted nipples or to collect leaking milk.

Shells come in several pieces, as shown in Figure 5-8. The piece that fits next to the breast puts gentle compression to help draw out flat or inverted nipples (which we discuss in Chapter 4). The outer piece fits over the top and usually has air holes to allow circulating air to keep the nipple drier. Leaking milk collects in the shell; some brands have a little spout you can use to pour the milk into a bag or bottle if you're storing breast milk.

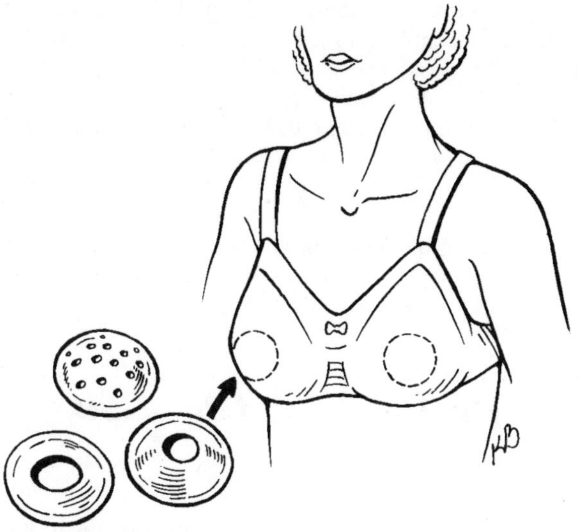

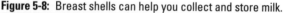

Figure 5-8: Breast shells can help you collect and store milk.

WARNING!

Unless you're able to dump the milk immediately after it leaks, don't save it. Milk that sits in the shell may grow bacteria.

TIP

Make sure the spout points upward when you put the shell on, or milk will pour all over you when you remove it! Also make sure the air vents are at the top; if they're on the bottom, milk comes right back out through the little holes.

During nursing, you can wear a breast shell on the breast you're not using, to prevent you from getting soaked during let-down and also to help collect milk.

Avent and Medela make several types of breast shells, which cost around $10 a pair.

Coating your nipples with creams

Sometimes all you need to heal sore nipples is a little air drying; other times, you may need lotions or creams. Most creams are food grade and lanolin-based. *Food grade* means the cream doesn't need to be removed before you feed the baby. Lansinoh and Medela make excellent lanolin creams.

One disadvantage to creams is that they're often yellow and somewhat greasy, meaning they can stain your clothes. Wear a breast pad, unless you're not concerned with staining your nursing bras, and try to keep the baby's clothes away from the cream. You need to use only a tiny dab of cream; it spreads a little easier if you warm it by rolling it between your fingertips before applying.

Some types of creams absolutely should not be used on your breasts when nursing. Among them are alcohol-based products, which make nipples more prone to crack; petroleum-based products, which don't allow the skin to "breathe"; and vitamin E–based products, which may be toxic to the baby. Look for ultra-purified lanolin ointment, which is pharmaceutical grade and safe for breastfeeding.

One of the best things you can use to help heal your nipples is free — your own breast milk! Dab a little of your milk on sore nipples and let it dry thoroughly.

Buying a Few "Just in Case" Bottles

You may feel conflicted about buying a few bottles to have on hand in case you need them. If having them in the house is going to tempt you to use them the first time you have a problem nursing, then by all means don't buy any!

A three-pack set of bottles costs between $2 and $5, depending on which brand you choose. Don't be surprised to get a few sets as shower gifts, even if you've made it perfectly clear that you're going to breastfeed.

Many years ago, buying bottles was easy. The bottles were clear glass, and the nipples were rubber. The bottles broke if you dropped them, and the nipples got soft and/or melted in the sterilizer. Today, bottles come in many styles. You can use angled bottles, meant to be easier to hold and prevent the baby from swallowing air. You can use disposable bottles, where a plastic sheath fits over the lip of a plastic reusable holder. You can buy bottles with clowns on them, bottles in designer colors, nipples made of rubber, nipples made of silicone. . . . How do you choose?

Going with the slow flow

Most lactation consultants highly recommend silicone slow flow nipples. These were first made by Avent and Medela, but now nearly every baby company offers some type of slow flow silicone nipple. These nipples are designed to prevent nipple confusion (which we discuss in the nearby sidebar "Avoiding nipple confusion") by imitating the suck needed to breastfeed. The baby needs to work

Avoiding nipple confusion

Nipple confusion may arise when a breastfed baby is fed with a bottle or given a pacifier. Breastfeeding requires a strong coordinated suck. The tongue is placed below the nipple, and the jaw muscles are used to massage the milk ducts to keep milk flowing. When the baby stops sucking, the milk flow stops. If you watch your baby when he nurses, you can see the muscles in his face moving.

If you give your baby a bottle, the milk flows quickly and constantly. The baby grasps only the nipple to suck and uses his tongue to compress the nipple to stop the milk flow.

Because milk from a bottle flows much faster, the baby may learn to prefer the bottle and refuse to nurse, or he may not nurse as strongly. This is why you should avoid using bottles or pacifiers for at least the first four to six weeks, if possible.

harder to obtain milk from these nipples, like he does when breastfeeding. The silicone nipples are also less prone to collapse during feeding. (When the nipple collapses during bottle feeding, the baby may suck air into his belly, which can cause gas.)

Realizing that size really matters!

Some bottles have short, stubby nipples on a very wide base; Playtex nursers were the first type of nipple with this design. Although the design looks somewhat like a breast, it's actually one of the worst nipples for breastfeeding moms to use because the nipple is so short.

TIP

Look for longer nipples — the longer, the better. You want the baby to stimulate his palate with the nipple, just like he does when breastfeeding. A longer nipple also deposits milk further back in the baby's mouth, more like breastfeeding does.

Making the Pacifier Decision

Pacifiers are a source of heated debate when you're breastfeeding because most pacifiers are shaped to encourage a totally different sucking mechanism than the suck used in breastfeeding. Many studies have shown that moms who use pacifiers may breastfeed for a shorter period of time overall, have more problems breastfeeding, and have less confidence in their ability to breastfeed than moms who avoid pacifier use. As with bottles, you should try to avoid pacifiers for the first four to six weeks of breastfeeding.

Yet, like everything in life, exceptions exist. If you have a baby with a constant need to suck, you may end up using a pacifier on occasion because you do have to carpool, make dinner, and use the bathroom from time to time. You can't nurse every minute of the day; a pacifier may be the answer if you have this type of baby.

Part II

Putting Breastfeeding into Action

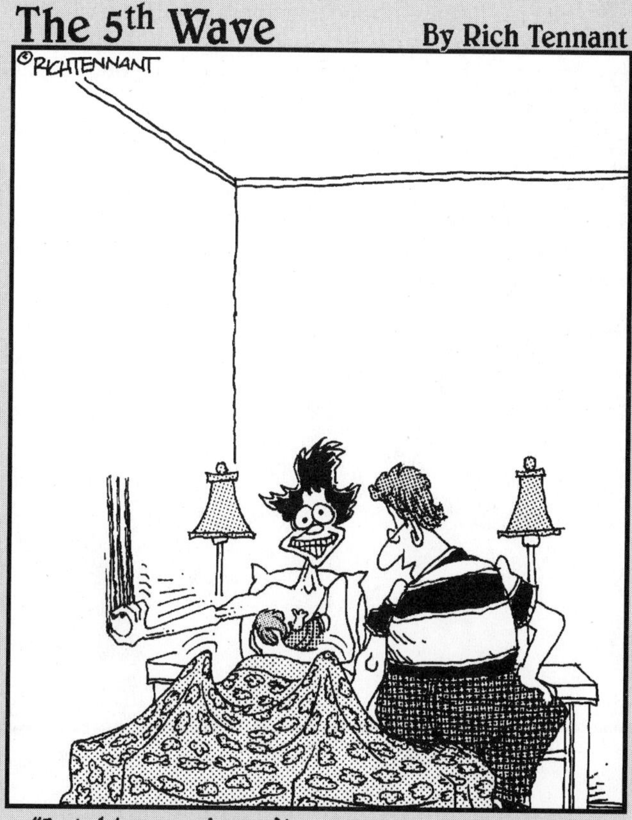

"Latching on doesn't seem to be a problem."

In this part . . .

Welcome to parenthood! Sleepless nights, new fears, frustrations, and worries are all part of the territory. Sometimes breastfeeding goes well while you're in the hospital, but everything falls apart when you get home. Sometimes nursing is a challenge from the beginning, because your baby is ill or has special needs. Only the rare parent breezes through breastfeeding without needing a little help or reassurance along the way. This part helps you find solutions to breastfeeding problems you're likely to encounter.

Chapter 6

At the Hospital: Beginning to Breastfeed

In This Chapter

- Making your first attempt at breastfeeding
- Nursing after a cesarean section
- Coaxing your milk in and handling engorgement
- Breastfeeding after your baby's circumcision
- Coping with jaundice
- Dealing with hospital rules and staff

By the time the information in this chapter is important to you, you'll be a mom — congratulations! Whether this is your first baby or your tenth, the hormonal changes that come with the cutting of the cord will have you on an emotional high one minute, and turn you into an emotional wreck the next. This is normal, so ride with the changes, both emotional and physical.

You deal with many new tasks in the first hours after delivery, from episiotomy care to nursing the baby for the first time. Don't expect to be perfect at everything right away. The hospital staff should help you learn your new role, and we give you lots of suggestions here.

In this chapter, we explain what happens to your body right after delivery, help you through the first breastfeeding, and suggest ways to make your hospital stay a good one. For additional information about what to expect during and after delivery, see *Pregnancy For Dummies,* 2nd Edition. Welcome to parenthood!

Producing Milk after Delivery

Not long after you deliver your baby, you also deliver the *placenta* — the organ that nourishes the baby during pregnancy. The minute the placenta is delivered, your body undergoes huge hormonal readjustments that may have you feeling like you're caught in a giant earthquake of emotions. Your levels of the hormones estrogen and progesterone drop, while the level of prolactin remains high. This combination of events triggers your body to start producing milk.

REMEMBER

Your milk supply doesn't come in full force until the third or fourth day after delivery. The first day or two after delivery, the baby receives *colostrum,* a yellowish fluid that is high in protein and antibodies. With today's short hospital stays, you may already be home before your milk comes in.

When your milk comes in, you'll definitely know it: Your breasts become hard and tender, and you may even experience shooting pains in them. You may also feel feverish. The veins on your breasts may appear even more prominent than they did when you were pregnant, and you may actually be able to feel the outline of milk ducts as they enlarge and fill.

This stage of *engorgement,* as it's commonly called, may last a day or two. Engorgement is caused not only by the increase in milk in your breasts but also by the increased amount of blood and fluid from lymph nodes in your breasts. (See the section "Dealing with Engorgement" later in this chapter.)

WARNING!

If you experience a fever after delivery that lasts more than 12 hours, report it to your doctor; the mild feverishness you feel with engorgement should subside within 12 to 24 hours.

As your milk comes in, it changes appearance. The thick, creamy, yellowish colostrum changes to a thinner, pale white or bluish milk. Although this milk may not look as nourishing to you, it is!

Nursing for the First Time

In some hospitals (or if you deliver at home), your baby is placed on your naked abdomen immediately after delivery. With your doctor, nurse, partner, and mom all staring expectantly at you, you try to position the baby to nurse. Watch out — he's slippery! What on earth is your doctor doing down there? Is that the placenta? This tender moment may be a little awkward, with everything else that's going on distracting your efforts.

Starting off on the right foot

TIP

Try to ignore everything else going on around you and concentrate on the baby. Eye-to-eye and skin-to-skin contact are the best ways for you and the baby to get acquainted. If at all possible, don't be rushed. Sometimes nurses want to give you a one-minute token bonding session, and then grab the baby away to be weighed, measured, eye-dropped, cleaned, and brought back after the doctor has put you back together. We blush to admit we were guilty of this in our own nursing careers. Sometimes space is tight in labor and delivery, and two or three more couples are waiting for your room.

Obviously, if your baby isn't breathing well or needs to be evaluated immediately, you won't be able to hold him right away. But if at all possible, hold him for a little bit. He may or may not be ready to nurse right after delivery; watch for clues, such as *rooting* (turning his head looking for the nipple) or sucking his hands, which show he's ready to start nursing. Doing so may save you from some frustrating first attempts to nurse before he's ready.

If your baby is taken to the warmer to be cleaned up first because that's the way things are done at Rules-Oriented Hospital, don't get upset. When the nurses finish, they'll bring the baby back to you.

TIP

If you're too distracted by the doctor pulling and tugging as he sews up your episiotomy or any tears, wait to start breastfeeding until he's finished. Try to concentrate on one major event at a time. Some women are uncomfortable and afraid to hold the baby while the doctor is stitching; if that's the case, ask your partner to hold the baby close to you so you don't have to worry about dropping her.

Sooner or later your doctor will finish putting you back together, and you can concentrate on the baby. After a minute or two of gazing into each other's eyes, you're ready for the big moment: your first breastfeeding.

Positioning the baby for comfort

Right after delivery, a healthy baby who is left alone will crawl up to his mother's breast, find his own position, latch on, and begin suckling. If you're giving birth in a hospital, your baby probably won't be given that opportunity.

Most likely, a nurse will hand you your baby after the initial weighing and measuring rituals are out of the way. Unless you've had a cesarean section (which we discuss later in this chapter), you'll probably be sitting up or semi-reclining, and you'll naturally cradle the baby in the crook of your arm to get ready to breastfeed.

You can position the baby for breastfeeding in many different ways, and changing positions helps the baby empty different duct areas in the breast. The positions described here are most commonly used, but as you become more experienced, you can certainly try others.

The cradle hold position

The cradle hold (or *Madonna position*) is the traditional baby holding position. With the cradle hold, the baby's head rests on the crook of your arm, and you support his legs and back with your forearm (see Figure 6-1). If you're using the left breast, his head is in your left arm. Turn the baby toward you, chest to chest. (Skin to skin is wonderful if you can manage it.) You may want to put a pillow under the baby to support his weight and bring him up to breast level. Fold a pillow in half and place it under your arm, with the fold up along your side. This keeps your arms at breast level and supports them comfortably during the feeding. Use your free hand to position and support your breast.

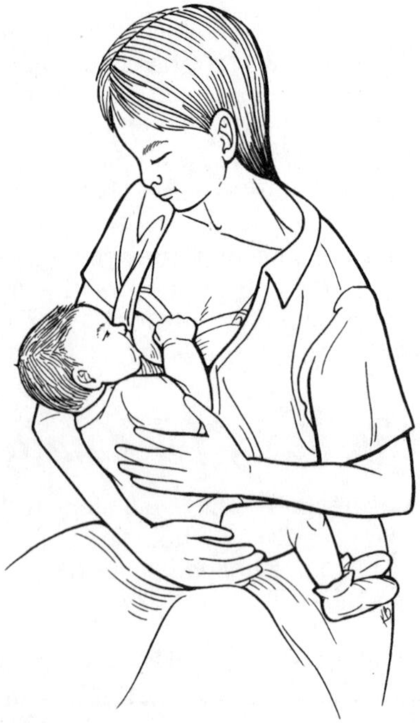

Figure 6-1: The cradle hold, or Madonna position.

The cross cradle hold

With the cross cradle (or *reverse cradle*) hold, the baby's head is supported with the left hand if you use the right breast. The baby's body is supported by the rest of your arm (see Figure 6-2). If you're feeding off the right breast, your right hand supports the breast. Turn the baby toward you, chest to chest. This position works well for a baby who has trouble latching on, because you have control of her head and can see her mouth better. This is also a good position if your baby arrives early; a preterm baby's head is big in relation to the rest of her body, and her neck muscles are weaker.

Latching on properly — the key to breastfeeding success!

Getting the baby to latch on to your breast properly is crucial. Latching on properly helps prevent sore nipples and ensures that your baby gets enough milk.

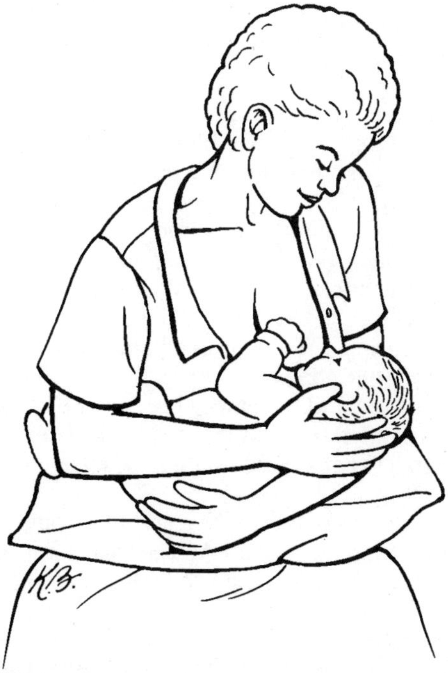

Figure 6-2: The cross cradle position gives you better control of the baby's head.

Make sure you're comfortable in the bed. If you're lying at a funny angle or don't have a good grip on the baby, adjust yourself. Hold the baby on his side, so he doesn't need to turn his head to reach the nipple. You and the baby should be chest to chest. Bring the baby close to your breast, with his nose lined up with your nipple.

You may need to use your fingers to support your breast and make it easier for the baby to grasp the nipple. Place your thumb on the top of your breast and, forming a *C,* place your other four fingers below the breast to lift up. Make sure your fingers and thumb are resting on the breast tissue, not on the areola. If your breasts are very large, place a rolled-up towel in the fold underneath to give support.

TIP

Don't touch both the baby's cheeks at the same time in an effort to turn his head in the right direction. He'll turn toward anything touching his cheek, and if you touch both you confuse him. Tickle his lips with the nipple; don't try to force it into his mouth.

Some babies bobble their heads back and forth wildly, looking for the nipple; others find the nipple easily but don't seem all that interested in sucking. Try to calm the bobbler down by teasing his lower lip with the breast, so he'll turn toward it. If you have a bobbler, try using the cross cradle hold, which gives you better control to guide his head where it needs to go. If he finds the nipple but doesn't seem all that interested, give him a little time. Some babies want to lick the nipple for a few minutes before they nurse.

When your baby opens his mouth wide, move his mouth toward the nipple. Move the baby, not the breast. If you have a perfect baby who's read all the books, he'll turn slowly toward the nipple, open his mouth wide, pull the areola and the nipple into his mouth, and begin sucking. We've seen one or two babies like this in our lives. More likely, he'll find the nipple, open his mouth halfway like a guppy, and get frustrated and turn away because he can't get it into his mouth. Or he'll root wildly, passing the nipple a dozen times but never grabbing onto it. Keep trying — it'll happen eventually!

TIP

If you have trouble seeing the baby's face and positioning his mouth properly, the football hold, described later in this chapter, may help you line him up with your nipple so he can latch on more easily.

When the baby is latched on well, an inch or so of the areola is in his mouth. His lips are rolled out, his tongue is under the breast, and his chin is touching your breast. His nose should be resting on top of your breast, not buried in it. Figure 6-3 shows what a proper latch-on looks like.

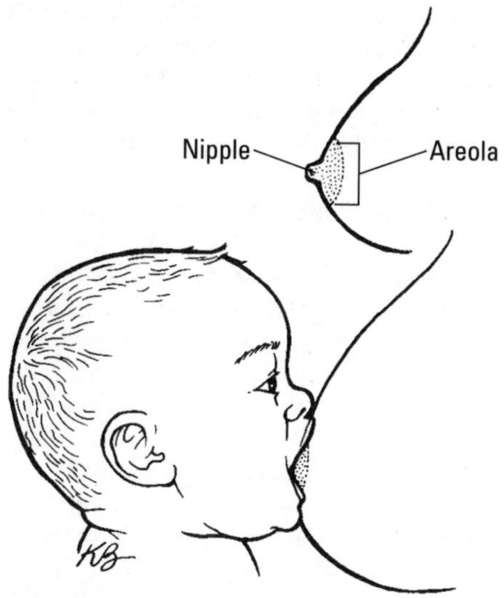

Figure 6-3: Latching on properly is the key to successful breastfeeding.

Several things need to take place in a perfect latch-on:

- The baby needs to open his mouth wide.
- He needs to close his mouth onto the areola, not just the nipple.
- He needs to begin sucking so that the nipple and areola are pulled into his mouth to form a teat. The nipple makes contact with a spot where the baby's hard and soft palate meet; touching this spot stimulates more sucking.
- The baby needs to coordinate his ability to suck and swallow.

Dealing with flat or inverted nipples

Most women with flat or inverted nipples (see Chapter 4) are able to nurse well immediately. A baby with a strong suck draws out the nipple easily, as long as he can latch on to the areola. If your breasts are fairly soft and not overly large, you can compress a good portion of the areola between your fingers so the baby can grasp it. His sucking will then draw the nipple out so that it stimulates the roof of his mouth properly.

If your breasts are large or very firm, the baby may have a harder time grasping the tissue. Engorgement makes this even more difficult. Avoiding engorgement helps tremendously if you have inverted nipples, and the way to avoid engorgement is to nurse frequently. This is a catch-22 if the baby isn't latching on well.

REMEMBER

The baby needs something to latch on to, and if your breast resembles a taut beach ball, there's nothing for him to grab. Before each feeding, roll your nipples between your fingers, if they protrude even a little. If they're really inverted, put one finger above the nipple and one below, on the areola, and gently compress the tissue; this may help the nipple pop up a bit. Hold a cold washcloth to the nipple for a minute to stimulate it to keep protruding.

If it sounds like you need three hands to get the baby latched on while working your nipples, you're right. You may need your partner's or a nurse's help at first. Some women use a breast pump for a few minutes to pull the nipple out before feeding; ask if your hospital has a commercial-grade pump you can use. Nipple shells and shields (see Chapter 5) may also help you draw the nipple out.

If you have flat or inverted nipples after delivery, don't despair. Almost all moms with inverted nipples are able to breastfeed; it may just take a little extra work to get things going. You'll make just as much milk as moms with protruding nipples.

REMEMBER

Nipples are often unequal, with one being less inverted than the other. If one nipple turns out to be impossible to work with, you can nurse using just one breast. However, this is very rarely the case.

Removing the baby from the breast

TIP

If you need to remove the baby from your breast, break the suction by inserting your finger between your breast and the baby's mouth. Press gently on the areola, and remove the nipple from the baby's mouth (see Figure 6-4). If you pull the baby off without breaking the suction first, you could injure your nipple.

Feeling frustrated? It's normal

If your baby hasn't read any of the books and doesn't seem to understand the concept of nursing at all, don't worry. If your baby is the wild man type, throwing his head back and forth like the MGM lion but never getting near the nipple, don't worry. If she just brushes past the nipple without even opening her mouth, don't worry. Immediate success is nice, but it's not essential.

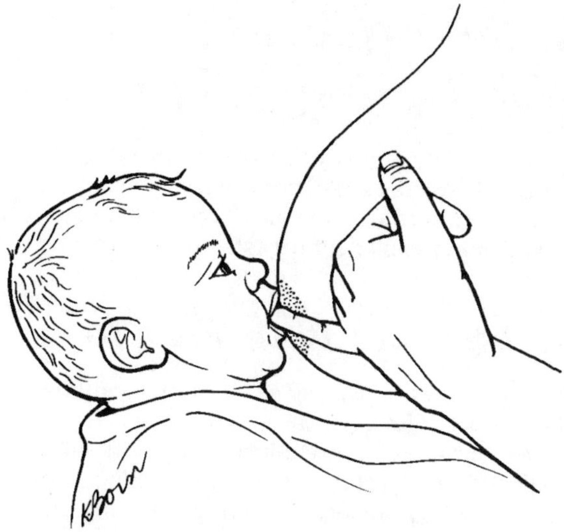

Figure 6-4: Always break suction before removing baby from the breast.

Try not to get upset at yourself or the baby. You're both brand new at this, and breastfeeding is a coordinated, learned activity. Remember how long it took you to learn to ride a bike? Think of nursing the same way.

Relaxing during the first feeding

The point of the first nursing is for you and your baby to get to know each other. You're not going anywhere, and neither is the baby. You don't absolutely need to complete the first feeding in the first hour after delivery, although the baby may be very alert in the first hour or two and then sleep deeply for several hours.

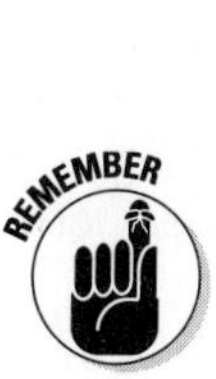

If you feel as though you're accomplishing nothing in your first feeding, rest assured that's not the case. You're establishing contact; the baby begins to know your smell. You're starting the bonding process. If your baby nurses well, he gets some high-calorie colostrum to carry him through the next few hours and begins to learn the mechanics of breastfeeding. Even if the baby just licks the nipple, you're starting to stimulate milk production, and you're stimulating your uterus to contract (see Chapter 2).

All that, on top of labor and delivery! You've had a busy day, so have something to eat and drink and take a nap. Your next nursing attempt will go better if you're taking care of yourself.

Knowing the Effects of Medication During Labor

Sometimes the medications you have during labor affect your first nursing attempt. Some medications make the baby sleepy; some make you sleepy. Here's how some of the most common medications given in labor can affect breastfeeding.

Inducing labor with Pitocin

Many women today are *induced* — given medications that jump-start labor — either for their own convenience, the doctor's convenience, or because of a possible problem with mom or the baby. A drug called Pitocin is commonly used to induce labor. Pitocin induction has been associated with breastfeeding problems.

Pitocin has an *anti-diuretic effect* (it decreases your production of urine), which may cause you to retain fluid, creating severe engorgement or a delay in milk production. It can also contribute to newborn jaundice (which we discuss later in the chapter in the section "Breastfeeding through Jaundice"). If you're induced, you're also more likely to receive epidural anesthesia, and epidurals may also interfere with breastfeeding (see the next section).

You probably don't want to be pregnant for one more minute than necessary. However, try to let the baby decide the timetable for delivery rather than the doctor's golf conference in Scotland or your nursery school carpool schedule. Every breastfeeding obstacle that you avoid may make the difference between success and failure.

Of course, many inductions are done for medical reasons; if your doctor feels you need to be induced, don't throw in the towel on breastfeeding. Most likely you and your baby will have no long-term negative effect from an induced labor. Remember, your doctor knows your case best!

Nursing after an epidural

No one ever said labor was painless. If anyone actually does say this to you, they're either suffering from memory loss or trying to ensure that you're not scared of labor.

If you deliver in the hospital, you have a 50 percent chance of receiving an epidural anesthesia. Epidurals are given through catheters placed in the epidural space near the spinal cord; the medication injected usually consists of a numbing anesthetic and a pain killer, such as fentanyl. An epidural gives very good pain relief from your abdomen down to your legs by numbing the nerves that reach those areas.

For years, childbirth educators and lactation consultants, including La Leche League instructors, have believed that the use of epidurals affects breastfeeding. Recent studies show that this may be true.

If you have an epidural, some of the medication enters your blood stream, where it passes across the placenta to the baby. Because the baby's immature liver can't break it down quickly, the effects of the medication — such as having difficulty coordinating sucking behaviors — may linger in the baby longer than they do in you. The effects generally wear off in 24 to 48 hours. Some studies also show that epidurals interfere with the release of *oxytocin,* the hormone responsible for your let-down reflex.

Epidural anesthesia may lengthen labor and may increase the chance that you or your baby will run a fever after delivery. If either of you runs a fever, you're more likely to be separated from each other for longer times. (The baby may be sent to the neonatal intensive care for IV antibiotics if he runs a fever.) Several studies have also shown that epidurals as more likely to result in jaundiced babies (see the section "Breastfeeding through Jaundice" in this chapter).

Keep in mind that the side effects from epidurals are generally temporary, and epidurals provide very helpful pain relief to many women. The bottom line: Talk with your doctor about possible risks and benefits of epidurals well before your due date! For more info about epidurals, see *Pregnancy For Dummies,* 2nd Edition.

Using narcotics during labor

Narcotics in labor are often given intravenously, which means their effects wear off within a few hours. But if you deliver your baby shortly after receiving an IV narcotic, the baby may be very sleepy. Every labor and delivery nurse has seen babies in this situation who are sleepy enough to require resuscitation.

Some studies have shown that Demerol is more likely to depress the baby than morphine. Both these drugs are given during labor and after delivery, especially if you've had a cesarean section. If your doctor is willing to give you a choice of medication during and after labor, morphine may be a better choice.

Nursing after a Cesarean Birth

In developed countries, the rate of delivery by cesarean section (*C-section*) has soared over the last three decades. If you deliver your baby in a hospital in the United States, you have approximately a one in four chance of a surgical delivery.

You can nurse after a cesarean, but you may have a rougher road getting breastfeeding established. After you get over the initial hurdles, your breastfeeding experience will be no different than if you deliver vaginally.

Planning for a C-section

Perhaps you know in advance that you're having a cesarean delivery. Most planned cesareans are done because the baby's in a *breech* position (her feet are in a down position, rather than her head), or a *transverse* (sideways) position. If you've had a previous cesarean, you may be having another by choice or because your obstetrician recommends it.

Knowing ahead of time that you're delivering surgically allows you to sit down with your obstetrician and discuss some important issues related to breastfeeding. Talk to her about the following:

- **What type of anesthesia is available?** If at all possible, you want to avoid general anesthesia. You and the baby will both be sleepier longer if you've had general anesthesia, and you won't see the baby immediately after delivery. A spinal or epidural anesthesia allows you to see the baby right away and possibly begin breastfeeding soon after delivery.
- **Can I breastfeed on the operating room table?** In theory, this should be possible, but the hospital routine may come before your wish to breastfeed the baby. The staff's first priority is to make sure that you and your baby are okay. After the baby is examined, she'll be brought to you. Be prepared for the reality that most operating rooms are not set up for breastfeeding. You'll be lying flat on your back on a table not much bigger than a two-by-four; your hands may be restrained, and you may feel some tugging and pulling. Your doctor will be concerned about contaminating the sterile operating field and will warn you not to touch anything. Under these circumstances, breastfeeding may be difficult.

- **Can my partner be with me in the recovery room?** You may assume that this is a given, but not all hospitals allow support people in the operating room, even in this enlightened day and age! If your partner is in the room, he may be able to help you position the baby to breastfeed in the recovery room.
- **Will the baby have to go to the newborn nursery?** At some hospitals, babies born by cesarean routinely go to the nursery for evaluation. Ask if you can keep the baby with you, as long as she's doing well.

Coping with an unplanned C-section

If you have an unplanned cesarean, you have to roll with the punches. For example, if the baby is having distress, you may receive general anesthesia because it can be administered quickly. If you already have an epidural in place, you may be awake when the baby's born.

If the baby's heart rate drops or another problem occurs, the hospital staff will probably take the baby to the nursery immediately after delivery to be evaluated. If the surgery occurs because your labor hasn't progressed, but the baby's doing fine, you have a better chance of keeping the baby with you after delivery.

Recovering after surgery

When the cesarean is finished, you'll be moved to a recovery room. Hopefully the baby will be with you; if she's been taken to the nursery, ask if she can be brought back after you're settled.

REMEMBER

If you've been given spinal or epidural anesthesia, you may be unable to move yourself up in bed without assistance because you're still numb. You may also have uncontrollable shaking; this is a side effect of the anesthesia. These two things can make it hard for you to find a comfortable position to nurse, so you'll need the help of your partner or support person to get set up to breastfeed. Pry the cell phone from his hands and have him help you — he can call his bowling team to tell them about the delivery in a few minutes.

If you've had general anesthesia, you may be very groggy for the first hour or so after delivery. If you're holding the baby, someone needs to be with you at all times.

Despite all the obstacles, this is a good time to try to get the baby on the breast. Your baby's sucking urge is the strongest and the baby is most alert in the two hours after delivery. After this period, newborns fall into a very deep sleep. You may find it nearly impossible to interest your baby in nursing after this happens.

TIP

If you start nursing right after delivery, you also take advantage of the pain-free time zone, which usually lasts an hour or so before your anesthesia wears off.

After a cesarean, you'll probably remain in the hospital for three or four days. You've had major surgery, so you're going to be tired, and you're going to have pain. Both are obstacles to breastfeeding, so you need to minimize both as much as possible.

Don't be afraid to take pain medication. It will help you to relax, and you'll be more comfortable holding the baby. (We discuss different types of medications later in this section.) Try to take a pain reliever a half hour or so before you nurse, so the medication has time to work. Pain medication also can help you sleep, and you need all the sleep you can get to recover from the surgery.

Make sure that your partner or support person can stay with you while you're in the hospital, because you'll have a hard time jumping out of bed when the baby cries. If possible, arrange for a private room so you aren't kept awake by a roommate.

Keeping weight off your incision

After a cesarean section, you won't want to place any pressure on your incision area. Most cesarean incisions are low on your abdomen and horizontal, just above your pubic hair, but some incisions are vertical, extending up toward your navel. Having the baby press on your incision, as he will if you use the cradle position, is a sure way to end your breastfeeding experience way too soon! You can hold the baby in other ways to avoid this problem.

Pretending the baby's a football

The football, or *clutch,* hold is exactly what it sounds like. If you can't visualize this, ask a football nut to demonstrate! Think of how a football player looks as he runs down the field, clutching the football so he doesn't drop it. That's the position you and your baby will be in, although we don't expect you to go running anywhere.

In this position, you sit upright with pillows behind you for back support. Another pillow is placed at your side to support your arm and your baby. Place the baby at your side, chest level, on top of the pillow. His head should be facing your breast. Wrap your arm around him, using your hand to support your baby's upper back and neck. Support your breast with your other hand, using the C-hold we describe earlier in the chapter. In this position you can see your nipple and guide it into his mouth. Because the baby's whole body is to your side, he won't press on your incision (see Figure 6-5).

TIP

Bring your own nursing pillow or regular pillows to the hospital; hospitals are chronically short of pillows! And be sure to put your name on them.

Lying down on the job

This position is comfortable whether you've had a cesarean or are still just a little numb or exhausted from your delivery. Lie on your side, and get someone to place several pillows behind your back and a pillow between your legs for support. You also want a couple pillows under your head to make your neck more comfortable. Place the baby on his side, facing your breast. You may need to prop pillows behind the baby to keep him in place. Hold the baby with one arm; the other arm can be tucked under your head or around the baby's back (see Figure 6-6).

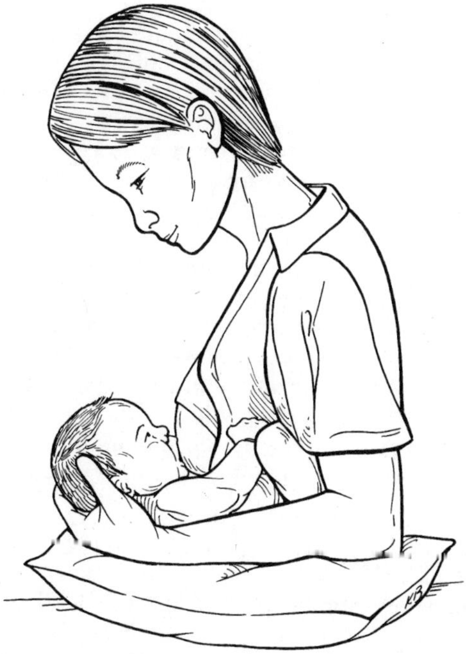

Figure 6-5: Using the football hold keeps the baby away from your incision.

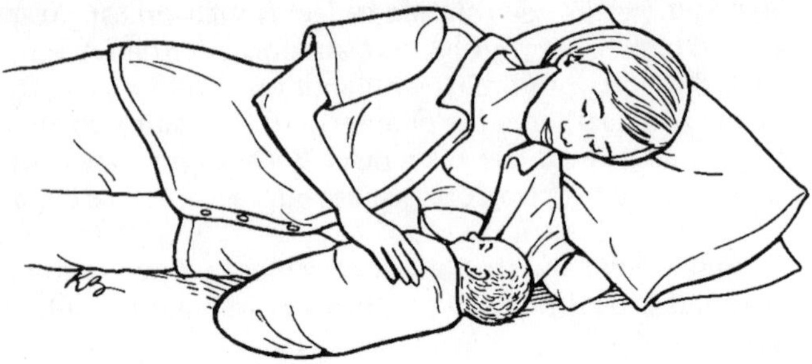

Figure 6-6: Position the baby away from your incision by lying down.

To prevent a major backache after you nurse, make sure that your back and hips are in a straight line. Bring the baby close to the breast; direct the nipple into his mouth. You can nurse from your other breast in this same position by elevating him on a few pillows.

TIP

Protect your abdomen with a towel or small pillow in case your baby decides to use your incision area for kickboxing practice.

Alleviating pain after delivery

The minute you deliver your baby, you undergo an attitude change. As soon as the cord is cut, your labor feelings of "it's all about me" turn into "it's all about my baby." You may be worried that the pain medication you need to make you comfortable will have a bad effect on your baby. We're here to reassure you that, although the most common pain medications may have some small effect on the baby, the benefits to you outweigh the risks.

REMEMBER

Milk production is triggered by hormones being released when your breasts are stimulated by sucking. This stimulation needs to occur as soon as possible after delivery to prime the pumps. If you're in a lot of pain, you won't feel like breastfeeding, which can delay the start of your milk production. You want to take the medication that has the least effect on you and the baby, of course. But the breast is a very good filter, and the amount of medication that passes to the baby is usually minimal and rarely causes side effects in the baby.

Epidural or spinal pain relief

If you had a cesarean with an epidural catheter in place or were given a spinal anesthetic, the anesthesiologist may give you medication for long lasting pain relief through the catheter. This medication, called Duramorph or Astramorph, is a single injection of a morphine-like medication.

Duramorph and Astramorph are given through the epidural catheter before the catheter is removed (if you had an epidural) or are given with the spinal anesthetic. Medication given *intrathecally,* as epidural or spinal injection is called, is absorbed less by your breast milk than medication given through your IV or by injection.

This medication usually provides very good pain relief for approximately 12 to 24 hours. The plus of this medication is the continuous pain relief that it provides, unlike the ups and downs that occur when you get injections of pain medications. One disadvantage to Duramorph is that you may have itching, and the antihistamines usually given to counteract itching, such as Benadryl, may make you drowsy. Some women also complain of nausea and vomiting with Duramorph. If you're nauseated, you won't feel like drinking, and you need fluids to build up your milk supply. Ask your doctor to prescribe something for nausea in this case.

IV or injections

If you had your cesarean under general anesthesia, you can't have Duramorph. Instead, you'll receive intravenous and intramuscular injections of narcotics like Demerol when you request them.

Don't hesitate to ask the nurse for pain medication the first few days after delivery. You'll be leaving the hospital soon enough, so take full advantage of this stronger pain medication while you can.

Unfortunately, nausea and vomiting can be side effects of injectable narcotics. Narcotic injections may also make you sleepy.

Some hospitals use a PCA (*Patient Controlled Analgesia*) pump after surgery. Narcotics such as morphine are given through a pump that's connected to your IV tubing. When you start feeling uncomfortable, you press a button and get a boost of pain medication. This machine gives you some control over how much medication you get. You can't overdose yourself, because limits are set on the machine by the nurses.

The On-Q system

The newest option for pain management after surgery is pretty clever, but it's not offered everywhere yet. The system is called On-Q. At the end of your surgery, the doctor places a tiny catheter with a balloon-like device attached to it into the incision. The balloon contains a numbing medication somewhat like Novocain. The catheter slowly drips the numbing medication into the incision until the balloon empties. This can last up to five days depending on the rate of flow that's set. Studies show that patients who use this device need much less oral or injected pain medication.

Meeting a lactation consultant

In Chapter 4, we discuss the role a lactation consultant can play during your pregnancy and after delivery. Many hospitals have lactation consultants on staff. Usually a consultant comes to see you before you go home.

If you have any questions or problems, write them down so you won't forget to ask the lactation consultant. If possible, have your partner there for the visit as well, because he may have questions and concerns that surprise you!

Your lactation consultant may try to see you during a feeding so she can assess how the baby latches on. This is especially helpful if your milk has come in, because the baby who latches on easily at delivery may have a harder time when your breasts turn into beach balls.

If your lactation consultant has regular hours for accepting phone calls, or if she does home visits, be sure to get her card. Sometimes problems don't arise until you've been home for a few days, and having that card (even if you never use it) may mean the difference between hysteria and calm problem solving the first time the baby spits up, refuses a feeding, or acts like he has colic.

Oral medications

When you go home, an oral narcotic such as Percocet or Vicodan can help you through the rough first days. Oral narcotics can make both you and the baby drowsy. Here's the catch-22 with narcotics: If you take them *after* you nurse, your baby gets the least amount of exposure to the medication. However, if you're uncomfortable when trying to nurse, you may not have a good let-down of milk. Take just what you need before a feeding to be comfortable, then take more after the feeding if necessary.

TIP

As soon as possible, stop taking narcotics and use acetaminophen or ibuprofen for pain control. Both of these medications are safe while you're breastfeeding.

WARNING!

Constipation is very common after any surgery, and narcotics can make it worse. Ask your doctor to prescribe something for you if over-the-counter agents aren't working. The best ways to counter constipation are to get up and move around as soon as possible after delivery and to drink lots of fluid.

Letting It All Out: The Let-Down Reflex

Anything called a *reflex* must come naturally, right? Unlike the immediate reflex reaction you get when you, say, hit your knee with a little mallet, the let-down (or *milk ejection*) reflex can be interrupted by pain or tension.

The let-down of your milk is essential to breastfeeding. Without it, your baby won't get enough to eat. This is how let-down occurs:

1. **Your baby starts to suckle, stimulating nerve endings in your nipple.**
2. **The hormone prolactin is released, stimulating milk production in the alveoli.**
3. **The hormone oxytocin is released, which squeezes the milk through the ducts to your nipple.**

Many women feel a pins-and-needles, or tingling, sensation when let-down occurs; you may also be able to tell when your milk is let down because the baby's suck–swallow pattern changes. She'll swallow more as more milk comes out. Remember that you may feel cramping when the baby nurses, or you may notice a gush of blood that's caused by your uterus clamping down (see Chapter 2).

If you're having trouble with let-down, make your feeding as stress-free as possible. If you're still having discomfort from the delivery, take pain medication an hour or two before the feeding.

How do you know if your let-down reflex is working? If your baby is gaining weight and having adequate urine and stool output (which we discuss later in the chapter), he's getting enough milk.

It may be helpful to establish a let-down conditioned reflex. Conditioned reflexes are taught; think of Pavlov's dogs, which developed conditioned reflexes and performed in certain ways in response to certain stimuli. You can help teach your breasts to let down milk by signaling that nursing is about to begin. The key is to follow the same routine each time you're about to nurse.

For example, try having something to drink while sitting in your nursing chair. Use visualization techniques to "see" your milk flowing through your breast. Or place warm washcloths over your breasts or take a warm shower just before feeding.

After nursing is established, you may face another problem: an overactive or hyperactive reflex, where too much milk is released too quickly. We discuss overactive let-down in the next section of this chapter and in Chapter 8.

Dealing with Engorgement

When your coauthor Carol taught childbirth classes, people would always ask, "How will I know that I am really in labor?" I'd always give the same answer: "Believe me, you'll *know.*" The same can be said about breast engorgement.

If you haven't delivered yet, your breasts probably seem humongous, and you may think they can't possibly get any bigger. The day or two after delivery, your breasts will feel fuller. As your milk comes in, this fullness can quickly turn into engorgement.

The "before" of engorgement

Almost every new mom experiences some degree of engorgement. Engorgement begins from two to five days after you deliver and lasts 24 to 48 hours if you treat it by nursing your baby frequently. Engorgement signals that *colostrum,* your baby's first food, is turning into a more mature milk.

Before your milk comes in, you produce about 1 to 2 ounces of colostrum a day. As your regular breast milk comes in, this increases to about 20 ounces a day. In addition, your breasts have an increased blood flow and enlarged milk ducts.

You may feel like you're producing milk up to the top of your chest and into your armpits. Your breasts may be hot, hard, and shiny. This is all normal, and feeding your baby frequently resolves it.

The "during" of engorgement

Engorgement occurs whether you breastfeed or not; in fact engorgement is usually worse in moms who don't nurse. According to lactation consultant Christopher Wade, M.D., engorgement is extremely high in western cultures because we tend to nurse less frequently in the first few days after birth. He states that in cultures where the baby is fed 8 to 12 times a day from the time of delivery, engorgement symptoms are minimal.

To help minimize engorgement,

- Begin breastfeeding as soon as you possibly can, preferably in the delivery room.
- Breastfeed 8 to 12 times in a 24-hour period to prevent milk from accumulating in the breasts. Nurse at least 10 to 15 minutes on one breast (and as much as 30 minutes) before switching sides. The baby may need to nurse for longer time periods in the first few days because your milk volume is low.
- Initially, breastfeed from both breasts at each feeding; alternate the side you start with.
- Make sure your baby empties your breasts. If he doesn't, use a breast pump to complete the job. Contrary to previous beliefs, experts now say that pumping after nursing if you're engorged does not stimulate more milk production and may help keep your milk production from decreasing due to increased swelling in the ducts.
- Before you leave the hospital, have a lactation consultant or another nursing expert confirm that your baby is latching on correctly.
- Avoid supplemental feedings in the beginning. Your payback in engorgement may not be worth the night's sleep that you get. If you miss a feeding, pump both breasts so they aren't twice as full for the next feeding.

Treatments for aching breasts

Although the steps in the previous section can minimize symptoms of engorgement, they probably won't eliminate them. Following are suggestions to make you more comfortable when you're engorged:

- Apply a hot towel to your breasts for five minutes or so, or take a warm shower. This softens the breast tissue and makes latch-on easier. A hot towel also helps get your milk flowing and catches dripping milk; the resulting increase in comfort will help with your let-down reflex.
- Give yourself a gentle breast massage or hand-express some milk in order to improve your milk flow (see the next section). Try these techniques before you start nursing; sometimes a

  few drops of milk on your nipple remind the baby what he's supposed to be doing. Continue the massage while you nurse your baby, massaging the breast the baby is nursing from. Massage the breast during the pause he takes between sucks.

  Milk production is directly related to milk emptying. If you don't take it out, Mother Nature won't put it back.

- Wear a good supportive bra, but make sure it's not too restrictive. A too-tight bra could decrease your milk flow and cause a blocked milk duct or mastitis (see Chapter 8).
- Use deep-breathing techniques to relax and increase let-down. Maybe you thought you were done with breathing techniques after delivery, but they may work better for you here than they did in labor. Sometimes, when the baby first latches on, you'll feel a pain akin to his twisting your nose off your face. This can last until your milk starts flowing.
- Cabbage leaves aren't just for Mr. McGregor's garden anymore! Place cold cabbage leaves on your breasts to reduce swelling in the breast tissue. You can put them directly on your breasts for 10 to 15 minutes before you nurse. Leaving them on longer may reduce your milk supply. Don't use cabbage leaves if you're allergic to cabbage or sulfa drugs, or if you develop a rash.
- Take ibuprofen to relieve discomfort and decrease inflammation in the breast tissue. But don't take it on an empty stomach.
- Use cold compresses after you nurse to reduce breast swelling. Keep them on for no more than 20 minutes. You can use an ice pack, but something as simple as a bag of frozen peas often works better because it molds to the shape of your breast.

Left untreated, engorgement can lead to *mastitis,* an inflammation or infection of the milk ducts or gland tissue that develops from incomplete emptying of the breast (see Chapter 8).

Expressing milk by hand

With time and patience, engorgement eventually subsides. In the meantime, you nurse as often as you can, but your breasts still look like watermelons and leak like an old faucet. And your baby is struggling to latch on to these beach balls. How can you make it easier for him and more comfortable for you? Hand expressing a little milk before starting to nurse decreases the tension in your breasts and gives the baby a softer target.

To manually express milk, follow these steps:

1. **Position your thumb above the nipple and your first two fingers below.** Position them about 1 to 1½ inches behind the base of the nipple (making a letter C with your hand). Your fingers should be placed over the ducts that lead to the nipple. Exact placement isn't critical; as long as your fingers are near the edge of the areola, you're close to the ducts.
2. **Press your thumb and fingers straight back toward your chest without squeezing your fingers together.** This stabilizes the breast while you express milk. To get milk out of the breast, you have to move it from behind the milk sinuses to the nipple area.
3. **Gently roll your thumb and fingers together toward the nipple.** This rolling motion compresses and empties the milk reservoirs. Repeat this movement until milk starts dripping from the nipple.
4. **Rotate your thumb and finger positions around your nipple.** You want to massage all the ducts so the entire breast is softened.

You can use a breast pump (see Chapter 5) to get the same results. Pump just enough milk to get the nipple and areola soft so your baby can latch on. Don't empty the breast — just soften it.

Don't squeeze, pull, or slide your hands over the breast tissue or nipple. You can damage the sensitive tissues by being too rough.

Slowing a too-fast flow

When you finally get your nipple and areola soft enough for your baby to latch on and start nursing, you feel like you're home free. Unfortunately, when you're engorged and your let-down reflex isn't well established yet, you may have another problem: too much milk coming out too fast at the beginning of a feeding. You'll know this is happening when the baby starts gulping, gasping, spitting up, or pulling away from the breast at the beginning of the feeding.

Before placing your baby on the breast, hand-express milk until you feel your let-down reflex occur. (Keep a towel handy to mop up Niagara Falls!) Start nursing when your milk slows from a stream to a trickle. Another trick is to place the baby on the breast, but when you feel your milk let down, take him off until the flow starts to slow. You can put him back on the breast as soon as this occurs.

Sometimes hyperactive let-down persists past the first few days of nursing. We discuss hyperactive let-down more in Chapter 8.

Nursing a Circumcised Baby

Circumcision — removal of the foreskin of the penis — is one of the most common elective surgeries in the United States; more than 1 million circumcisions are performed each year. Parents choose to have their sons circumcised shortly after delivery for two key reasons. One is that infant circumcision is far less traumatic than circumcision performed later in life, should it become necessary. The second (and probably most common) reason is that most men in this country are circumcised and want their sons to look like them.

Most babies are "circed" before leaving the hospital, which means you barely have time to establish breastfeeding before the surgery takes place. The shock and trauma of circumcision can disrupt breastfeeding at a time when it most needs to be reinforced.

Studies have shown that babies fall into a state of deep sleep after being circumcised and may not want to nurse for a time. When your milk supply is just being established, this may be detrimental to nursing, and, of course, the baby also needs to eat to gain weight. Try nursing him right after the surgery, before he falls into the deep sleep that often follows circumcision.

If you want your son circumcised, consider having the surgery done when the baby is a week or so old and breastfeeding has been fairly well established. The baby will be more likely to realize your breast is a comfort source and may nurse more quickly after the surgery. You need to discuss this option ahead of time with your obstetrician or pediatrician to see if you can bring the baby back to the hospital to have this done; also check with your insurance company to make sure it's willing to pay for it!

Breastfeeding through Jaundice

When the nurse brings your baby to you and she resembles a pumpkin, she has jaundice. Neonatal jaundice is very common; between 50 and 80 percent of babies are jaundiced to some degree. A jaundiced baby may appear quite yellow, or she may just have a little yellowish coloration to the whites of her eyes.

Understanding the causes

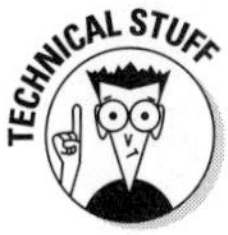

Before your baby is born, she has more red blood cells than adults do, because she gets her oxygen from your blood cells. Oxygen is carried in the hemoglobin portion of red blood cells. After delivery, when the baby begins to breathe oxygen on her own, she doesn't need as much hemoglobin, so some of it begins to break down into bilirubin. Bilirubin is broken down in the liver and excreted in bowel movements. Sometimes babies' livers aren't terribly efficient after birth, especially if the baby is premature or stressed in any way. If the liver isn't working efficiently, the bilirubin won't be broken down very quickly, and some will be stored in the skin.

Bilirubin gives the skin and whites of the eyes the yellowish coloration associated with jaundice. This type of jaundice, called *physiologic jaundice,* develops during the first few days of life; it may be slightly more common in breastfed than bottle-fed babies, because breastfed babies consume less fluid in the first few days of life (before moms' milk comes in) and don't have as many stools.

Babies who have a lot of bruising from the delivery, such as those delivered by forceps or vacuum extraction, may also have higher levels of bilirubin, because they have additional red blood cells breaking down from the bruising.

Jaundice is treated only if the levels of bilirubin become unusually high — over 15 mg/dl. When the skin becomes saturated with bilirubin, the bilirubin accumulates in other areas of the body. If it accumulates in the brain cells, they can be damaged, causing a condition called *kernicterus.* This doesn't occur until bilirubin levels are very high, over 25 mg/dl.

Treatment of jaundice involves *phototherapy* — putting the baby under intense light for a day or two. This light exposure makes the bilirubin water-soluble so it can be flushed out in the baby's urine as well as the stool.

Physiologic jaundice is rarely serious. If your baby experiences this condition, you should nurse as frequently as possible to get him through jaundice, which can last 10 to 14 days.

Following are two less-common types of jaundice:

- *Pathologic jaundice* is a different and much more severe condition, which is usually caused by a blood incompatibility between mother and baby. If you have Rh-negative blood and the baby's blood is Rh positive, you will be treated with *Rhogam,* an injection that prevents the development of Rh disease during your pregnancy. Doctors routinely test your blood type to prevent this type of jaundice. Otherwise, your blood cells may cross the placenta during pregnancy and destroy the baby's red blood cells.

This type of jaundice is caused by an immature liver being unable to eliminate the large number of broken-down red blood cells. The baby may become severely anemic and could need a blood transfusion. A usually less severe form of pathologic jaundice is caused by an ABO incompatibility, where mom has type O blood and the baby has A, B, or AB blood. ABO incompatibility rarely requires transfusion.

- *Breast milk jaundice* sounds quite frightening but isn't serious and definitely is not a reason to stop breastfeeding. Breast milk jaundice develops between seven and ten days after delivery. It occurs because some mothers' breast milk contains substances that seem to cause jaundice. This type of mild jaundice can last for months, is not harmful to the baby, and doesn't require treatment. Your doctor may want to make sure no other problems are causing the jaundice by taking the baby off breast milk for a day or two and retesting the levels. If they drop, the cause of the jaundice is breast milk. You do not need to stop breastfeeding if this is the case.

Nursing during treatment

Different pediatricians use different criteria for using *phototherapy* — exposure to ultraviolet light — to treat jaundice. Most babies who are put under *bili lights* (lights that help make the bilirubin in the baby's system water-soluble) aren't ill and should continue to breastfeed.

Obviously, having your baby under the bili lights can be a big obstacle to breastfeeding. The baby needs to eat so she'll urinate and stool out the bilirubin, but you may not nurse her as often as you would if she were in your room. This is because hospital staff watching her for hunger cues may not be able to pay as close attention as you can. Also, jaundice makes babies sleepy, so she may not demonstrate a strong appetite.

A baby under the bili lights has an increased need for fluid because the heat can cause dehydration. Frequent nursing is crucial. Your baby may need supplemental fluid if he's too sleepy to nurse well.

TIP

Be proactive by asking the nursing staff to bring the baby to you whenever she appears hungry — not just at four-hour intervals. Also, visit the nursery yourself so you can watch for signs of hunger, especially two or three hours after the previous feeding.

If for some reason your baby can't be removed from the warmer more often, pump your breasts at least every two to three hours to encourage your milk to come in. The more your breasts are stimulated, the faster your milk comes in. The more fluid the baby gets, the more he stools and urinates, the faster the bilirubin is washed out of his system, and the faster the jaundice disappears.

Anticipating Emotional and Physical Changes

Your body changes drastically right after delivery. Some changes, like the shrinking of your uterus (see Chapter 2), are outwardly visible. Others, like the hormone shifts that occur, can't be seen but are certainly felt. Each change has a potential impact on nursing; knowing what to expect can help you cope more effectively.

Crying with the baby blues

Almost all new moms suffer through a day or two of emotional highs and lows commonly called the *baby blues.* Baby blues are short-lived and completely normal.

You anticipate and plan for the birth of your baby for months. Suddenly, the anticipation is over and reality hits. Your long-awaited infant has a squashed nose and blotchy skin. You thought she'd be a redhead, and she has no hair at all. Maybe you expected a girl and got a boy. Even if you got exactly what you expected, the reality is you're not *expecting* any more. You've got him — or her. Many people experience the same letdown after the holidays, and they don't even have the excuse of rampaging hormones!

Be aware that you're going to have some sad, teary moments. If you don't fall madly in love with your baby the first time you see her, don't feel like you're a terrible mother. The majority of women probably have the same experience!

Keep in mind that *postpartum depression* is a very different animal from the baby blues — it lasts longer and may require intervention. If you find yourself dwelling on thoughts that you may harm the baby, having severe nightmares, or feeling overwhelming anxiety, tell your doctor, nurse, partner — anyone — immediately. We discuss postpartum depression in Chapter 7.

Bleeding and cramping

Your body releases the hormone oxytocin when you nurse, which causes muscles in your breast to contract (in order to move milk to the baby) and also causes your uterus to contract. As we explain in Chapter 2, this is a good thing — it helps your body get back to prepregnancy shape faster than if you don't breastfeed.

It's normal to bleed after delivery. The blood, called *lochia,* is bright red at first and contains the sloughed-off lining of the uterus. When you breastfeed, you may feel cramping and small gushes of blood; what you're experiencing is uterine contractions.

Put on a clean sanitary pad just before breastfeeding. You may also want to sit on a blue "chux" pad, which has a plastic backing to keep blood from leaking through to the sheets. Don't sit on your bathrobe or the back of your gown; fan them out to the side so only your bottom is resting on the chux.

Uterine contractions, often called *afterpains,* can be painful, so you may want to take a pain reliever before nursing. Otherwise, if you're worried about having pain while nursing, you may find it hard to let down your milk.

Between feedings, your nurse may press on your stomach at regular intervals. She's feeling to see if your uterus is firm, like it should be, or if it's boggy. If it's boggy, that means the uterus is not contracting well, so she'll firmly massage the uterus until she can feel it turning into a hard, roundish ball. You can do this yourself as well to speed the process along.

Getting an Uncooperative Baby to Nurse

The first days after delivery are exciting, as you and your baby start the process of getting to know each other. Intuitively, you'll start reading his movements, his facial expressions, and his verbal communications.

From day one, different babies have different ways of doing things. Your baby may wake up on schedule, eat, sleep, and generally be a pleasure. Or, he may be hard to wake up, hard to calm down, or hard to get interested in nursing. And you'll wonder how on earth to deal with a baby who doesn't seem to have any concept of eating.

REMEMBER

Your baby needs to nurse frequently in order for you to develop a good milk supply. In the first couple days of life, most babies are sleepy and nurse only six to eight times a day. By day three, they're waking up and eating more frequently. Try to nurse every two to three hours after the first few days (count the time from the start of one feeding to the start of the next), or 10 to 12 times in a 24-hour period. This is your full-time job right now, and the job description is simple: Get to know your baby and build up your milk supply.

But what if your baby hasn't read the job description and is too sleepy, too disinterested, or too frantic at feeding time? Don't get discouraged. Trust that perseverance will win out.

Looking for hunger signs

Newborns haven't quite mastered the art of letting you know when it's time to eat. Your baby's hunger signs may be subtle, such as:

- Sucking his lips, his tongue, his fingers, or his fists
- Starting to fidget (which indicates he's not in a deep sleep anymore)
- Turning toward your breast (especially if his mouth is open)

REMEMBER

Crying is a late sign of hunger. Try to read these earlier hints so your baby doesn't get too hungry. If he starts crying, you may have a harder time calming him down and getting him to nurse.

Nursing the sleepy baby

Contrary to popular belief, when your newborn sleeps, it doesn't necessarily mean that he's happy and satisfied. Most newborns sleep a lot after delivery; they're usually exhausted from the trip. But by the third day after birth, if your baby continues to be sleepy, you should examine what's going on. Following are some possibilities:

- A long, medicated labor and delivery can cause your baby to be sleepy. Your baby's liver is immature, which means he can't get medication out of his system as quickly as you can.

- He may be jaundiced.
- Circumcision can be an exhausting ordeal for your son. Be patient with him on the day of this surgery, but encourage him to find comfort in nursing.
- An over-stimulated baby may retreat to sleep. Keep noise and light levels low in your room; you may have to kick your nearest and dearest 12 visitors out for a while.
- Your baby may be getting too much or too little milk. When your milk comes out too fast, your baby can be overwhelmed and turn away from the breast. This can have the same effect as having too little milk: Either way, if your baby isn't getting enough calories, he may be weak and sleepy.

After considering why your baby may be sleepy, you need to know how to wake him up. Believe us, these tips come in handy even later in life — such as when your "baby" is 15 years old and you want him to cut the grass!

- **Pull the covers off him.** Loosen or even take off his clothes. If he doesn't have anything on but his diaper, he's more likely to stay awake. Holding him skin-to-skin is stimulating and will also help keep him awake. Remember, though, that newborns lose heat quickly. Make sure the room is warm enough and that he's not directly under an air conditioning vent or in a draft.
- **Dim the lights in the room.** If the lights are too bright, he'll close his eyes. Remember, he's used to being in the dark!
- **Talk to him and try to make eye contact.** Your baby responds to your voice even before he's born. He's going to be listening to you for the rest of his life; he might as well start now.
- **Watch for signs of a light sleep cycle.** Like adults, babies have sleep cycles, some of which are deeper than others. When your baby is in a light sleep cycle you'll see rapid eye movements under his eyelids, facial movements, movements of his arms and legs, and even sucking. You should have an easier time waking him from a light sleep cycle than from a deeper one.
- **Gently change him from a lying to a sitting position.** Like your old dolls, babies sometimes open their eyes when you sit them up from a lying position.
- **Stimulate him.** Rub your hand gently up and down his back, or rub his hands and feet. Move his legs in a bicycle motion. Tickle his spine lightly.
- **Wipe his face with a cool, damp cloth.**
- **Hold him in a football hold.** A cradle-type position encourages cuddling and sleeping.

Feeding the disinterested baby

If they're not medicated, most babies are interested in breastfeeding shortly after delivery. However, if you need pain medication during labor or require a cesarean delivery, your baby may not be as alert or interested in feeding immediately after delivery. It may take a while before your milk comes in and she's interested in actively breastfeeding. During this period (which can be as long as 10 days), your baby may seem disinterested and distant. Although this is very frustrating, remember that many babies react this way.

REMEMBER

Some moms feel rejected by this lack of interest. Keep in mind that your baby isn't consciously deciding she isn't interested in breastfeeding, and she isn't rejecting you or your milk.

Some babies won't nurse right after delivery if they've been suctioned vigorously and have an aversion to anything placed in their mouths. If your baby had some fluid in his nose and mouth that needed to be suctioned out right after delivery, he may not appreciate a nipple in his mouth, but this disinterest will be short-lived. Keep in mind that pacifiers will draw the same response. If someone jabs a pacifier into the baby's mouth too hard or too early when he's not ready to suck, he may feel startled and upset, setting up a negative reaction to mouth stimulation.

Remember also that, like you, the baby's been put through a complicated physical experience. Maybe her neck was at a funny angle during delivery, and the position you're holding her in is uncomfortable. Try changing positions before you throw in the towel on breastfeeding.

One thing you can do is to set the mood for nursing. No, the baby doesn't need wine and candlelight (although it might benefit you!), but you can do some things to encourage her to relax and breastfeed:

- **Talk to her.** Make eye contact.
- **Unwrap her so she's not quite as warm and cozy.**
- **Keep the lights dimmed.** She's very much like the sleepy baby who is retreating from activity.
- **Lay on your side to nurse.** This encourages you both to relax.
- **Take some time to stroke your baby.** Different from the stronger physical contact to wake your sleepy baby up, you want to gently rub her body. Skin-to-skin contact is a great way to entice and interest your baby.

- **Let her suck on your finger initially, stimulating her upper palate.** When she seems ready to nurse, try to put her on the breast.
- **Tease her with some drops of expressed milk on her lips.** Remind her what you're both doing here.
- **Encourage your let-down reflex.** Some babies get frustrated quickly — if the milk isn't pouring into their mouths, they're going to go somewhere else, like to sleep! Place a warm washcloth on your breasts to get your let-down engine running. Use breast massage while you nurse. Some babies start nursing eagerly but lose interest when the flow decreases; gently massaging the ducts helps keep a steady flow coming.
- **Try short, frequent nursing sessions.** Nurse whenever you can. If she seems even the slightest bit awake and alert, try to get her on the breast. Remember, this frequent nursing is necessary only until she gets with the program.

TIP

As with the sleepy baby, read her cues. Sometimes she's experiencing too much stimulation and retreating into her own little world. You may notice her yawning, hiccupping, even stretching her palms outward as if to say "no, leave me alone." Don't struggle with her if you see this happening; she'll probably win! Leave her alone, and try again in a half hour or so.

If she stays disinterested for more than 24 hours, you'll have to pump to get your milk to come in, and you may have to feed her the expressed milk through a cup, bottle, or lactation aid. If you persist in trying every few hours or so, she should get with the program.

If none of these suggestions helps, get the assistance of a lactation consultant or La Leche League leader.

Calming the frantic nurser

Some babies seem quite anxious to nurse but can't seem to grasp the mechanics. They brush past the nipple, mouth open, over and over until they become frustrated and start crying. This turns into a vicious cycle: The baby cries because he can't grasp the breast, and he can't grasp the breast because he's crying. What can you do to stop this merry-go-round without joining him in the frustration?

First, don't feed the fire. Take a deep breath and try to keep calm. Babies are very sensitive to their surroundings. (This is a good thing to remember throughout your motherhood career.) If you get upset about his behavior, he'll become tenser.

Don't throw in the towel at this point. Many women, including us, have experienced early nursing problems and managed to get through them. Have confidence that you can do it, too.

If he works himself into a real frenzy, help him calm down and start again. Try the following suggestions:

- **Walk around the room with him.** Babies love movement. He's used to it — he walked with you for nine months.
- **Cuddle him in the cradle position, or bundle him snugly with a lightweight blanket so his arms and legs are close to his body.** Some babies miss the tightly held feeling they had in the womb, so try to recreate it.

Many times a baby becomes frantic because he missed his early hungry stage while he was sleeping. When he wakes up, he's overly hungry. What can you do to prevent this?

- **Watch your baby, not the clock.** Feed him when you see early hunger signs; don't wait for him to cry.
- **Nurse your baby more frequently.** This prevents your baby from getting to the frantic stage if it's caused by hunger.
- **Hand-express or pump for a minute or so to get your milk flowing.** Express some drops of milk onto your breasts while your baby is attempting to latch on. This may help him find what he's looking for and settle down.
- **If he's becoming frantic before your let-down, squirt a little previously expressed milk into the corner of his mouth.** Remind him that there's more where that came from!
- **Take advantage of an open mouth.** Babies don't keep their mouths open wide for long. When the opportunity comes, get as much of your breast in his mouth as possible. If he won't open his mouth wide, try tickling his lips with your nipple.

If you're certain that your baby isn't overly hungry, but he's still frantic, explore other possibilities. Try changing his position; he may have a sensitive neck or a sore throat after delivery, or he may just prefer another position. Support his neck so his head doesn't wobble. It sounds simple, but sometimes simple things work.

As you attempt to soothe your baby, make sure you're not stroking both cheeks. Babies have a rooting reflex that causes them to turn their heads toward the source of the stroking. If you're touching both cheeks, you'll confuse and frustrate him.

Focusing on Baby's Weight

You've just gone through nine months of panic every time you got on the scale. Now, here you are doing the same thing, only this time you're worried about the baby's weight.

Don't obsess about your baby's weight loss after delivery. Weight loss in a newborn is normal within certain limits. If you breastfeed frequently, and if your baby latches on properly and nurses long enough to get the *hind milk* (the creamier milk that comes later in a nursing session), he'll regain weight very quickly.

Expecting weight loss

Weight loss in newborns is normal for several reasons:

- Your baby is born with extra fluid and fat stores in preparation for labor and the first days after delivery. These extra fat stores provide nutrition in the first days when mature milk hasn't come in yet, and he's not getting a large amount of calories.
- Some weight loss is due to your baby's shedding of fluid and through the passage of his *meconium* stool (the baby's first bowel movement).
- If you have an induced labor, epidural anesthesia, or a cesarean section, you receive a large amount of intravenous fluids. This causes both you and your baby to retain fluid. When your baby is born, his weight is inflated by the extra water. When he urinates or stools this fluid out of his body, his weight drops.

Weight gain is calculated from the baby's lowest known weight. For bottle-fed babies, a weight loss of 5 percent in the first week of life is considered normal. A weight loss of 7 to 10 percent is considered normal for a breastfed baby. (The difference is that a bottle-fed baby gets a calculated amount of calories every time he drinks.)

Helping baby gain

The first milk a breastfed baby consumes is colostrum. Quality, not quantity, is key here. You produce only 1 to 3 ounces of colostrum in a 24-hour period, and your baby's stomach at birth can hold less than an ounce. But as we discuss in Chapter 1, colostrum provides essential nutrition to get your baby off to a healthy start.

By the third or fourth day after birth, your mature milk comes in. Your baby's digestive tract is ready for this fluid and nutrition increase. Your baby should be nursing frequently and gaining her lost weight back by the time she's 2 weeks old.

REMEMBER

Some babies are a little slower to regain weight than others. If your baby is gaining weight slowly, ask a professional to assess her nursing skills. Together you can make sure your baby is

- Nursing often and long enough (at least every 2 hours, lasting at least 15 to 20 minutes on each breast).
- Sucking vigorously enough to cause a let-down reflex in your breasts. You should hear and see swallowing.
- Latching on properly to stimulate milk production.
- Emptying the breasts with each feeding and appearing satisfied after nursing.
- Looking healthy, bright-eyed, active, and alert.

A weight gain of 4 to 7 ounces per week or an ounce a day is considered normal for the breastfed newborn. However, this is an average: Babies don't gain weight back in a textbook perfect format.

REMEMBER

Babies who are larger at birth tend to regain weight at a slower pace. They should, however, regain and surpass their birth weight by 14 days. Baby boys gain weight a little faster than baby girls.

Keeping Tabs on Diapers

While you're in the hospital, the nurses will ask you how many wet and dirty diapers you've changed. They're not just keeping a supply list for reordering diapers! What goes in has to come out. If your baby is providing you with sufficient wet and dirty diapers, he's getting the nutrition he needs.

TIP

It's easy to remember what your baby should be doing in the wet diaper department:

- Day 1: Your baby should have at least one wet diaper.
- Day 2: Your baby should have at least two wet diapers.
- Day 3: Your baby should have at least three wet diapers.

This pattern continues through the sixth day. After the first week, your baby should have six to eight wet diapers a day.

Meconium is the first stool your baby passes; some babies pass meconium even before they're born. Don't be alarmed by the contents of a meconium diaper. Meconium is sticky, almost tar-like, and green or black in color. Meconium has been in the baby's intestines for months. Its contents are an awful-sounding combination of digested amniotic fluid, fetal skin, hair cells, enzymes, blood, and mucus. As disgusting as it sounds, meconium is considered sterile, unlike normal stool, which is filled with bacteria.

If your baby passes meconium a long time before birth, you may think you've given birth to a Martian, because her skin, nails, and cord may be stained green! Fortunately, the meconium supply is limited. Your baby's stool will progress to a slightly more pleasant color and texture.

After meconium comes the *transitional stool.* Transitional stool appears when your milk starts to come in and is greenish or yellow/brown. It's grainy, seedy, and more liquid than formed.

When meconium has cleared her intestines, your baby may have up to four stools a day. This increase in stools occurs because her milk intake is increasing. If your baby still has meconium stools after five days, she may not be getting enough milk.

Your baby should continue to have around four dirty diapers a day, with the stools remaining a liquid consistency. Breastfeeding stools tend to spread to fit the diaper, meaning they're usually somewhat of a mess to clean up! They can be yellow to bright green, loose (even runny), curdy, or creamy — resembling cottage cheese with mustard in it. A breastfed baby can have up to 12 "little squirt" stools per day.

Dealing with Hospital Routines

If you have a vaginal delivery, you probably won't be in the hospital more than two days. If you have a cesarean section, are having a tubal ligation, or have any complications like excessive bleeding or infection, you could be there for four or five days. While most hospitals these days are very supportive of breastfeeding, four or five days is plenty of time for the hospital routine to sabotage breastfeeding if you happen to deliver at Rigid General.

The ideal time to find out what your hospital considers a typical schedule for moms and newborns is *before* you ever set foot in the door. Tour the hospital, ask questions, and determine whether this facility is where you want to deliver your baby.

However, we know that geography, insurance, or other factors may dictate that you're stuck with Rigid General. Regardless, you can still make breastfeeding work for you and your baby.

Avoiding the four-hour schedule

A few hospitals are stuck in a time warp; you'll know you're at one if the nurse says that she'll bring your baby to you every four hours to be fed. You need to be clever to get around this mindset.

First, appeal to your pediatrician's or obstetrician's higher instincts: Ask her to write in your chart that you can have the baby brought to you on demand or can keep the baby in your room. If the doctor writes it as an order, the nurses have to do it.

If you still have problems getting the baby for more frequent feedings, get out of Dodge. Assuming you have an uncomplicated delivery, you can beg your doctor to let you go home immediately. Make sure to follow up with your pediatrician a few days after you get home so she can check the baby out; some health issues don't show up until a few days after delivery.

Keeping the baby in your room

Most U.S. hospitals have gone to a "rooming in" system, where the baby stays in the room with you all the time. In some circumstances, rooming in isn't the best option; if you have a complicated delivery, you may not feel well enough to take care of the baby around the clock. Be honest with the nurse if this is the case.

If your hospital allows support people to stay overnight, your partner may be able to take over some baby care. However, not all hospitals are set up for overnight visitors. (And if you have older children, your partner may not have the option of staying with you.)

REMEMBER

Be aware that your idea of rooming in and the hospital's may differ. The staff may keep babies in the nursery for several hours each morning and evening so the pediatricians can see all the babies in one place. Shortly after delivery, the babies may be required back in the nursery for a few hours of observation and care. If you have a boy, he may be taken for circumcision and then need to stay in the nursery for more observation. By the time the day is finished, the baby may have spent more time out of your room than in it!

Asking others to run interference

Whenever possible, let other people play the heavy while you're in the hospital. Whether it's going head-to-head with a difficult nurse or dealing with relatives who don't understand that a five-hour visit is too long, you shouldn't expend the energy to deal with them.

If your mother-in-law or best friend is openly disapproving of breastfeeding, you need to get them out of your room while you're feeding the baby. But you may not have the physical or emotional energy to deal with them when you're a melting puddle of hormones. So let other people handle it.

Consider asking your doctor to write an order restricting visitors. Enlist the lactation consultant to reason with your doctor about not giving supplemental water in the nursery. Save your energy so you can feed the baby.

Handling disapproving staff

Believe it or not, some doctors and nurses are not terribly supportive of breastfeeding mothers. Perhaps they didn't breastfeed their own children, so they can't see what the big deal is about breastfeeding. Or they think that your baby is losing too much weight or is too jaundiced and assume that breastfeeding is the culprit.

REMEMBER

Being medical professionals ourselves, we're not suggesting you throw what the staff says out the window. They may have legitimate concerns, so listen hard to what they're saying. This is where your partner can come in handy: He's not suffering from fluctuating hormones, so when the doctor says she thinks the baby needs more fluids, he won't jump to the conclusion that he's a terrible parent. You, on the other hand, may.

If you have a lactation consultant in the hospital, bring her in on conversations with your doctor or nurses so she can help you decide if you really should supplement, give the baby water, stop nursing, or whatever the staff suggests. If you deliver at Podunk General and have no access to a lactation consultant, call your nearest La Leche League leader and ask her to listen in on the conversation.

Chapter 7

At Home: Establishing the Breastfeeding Habit

In This Chapter

- Surviving your first days at home with your new baby
- Deciding where the baby should sleep
- Scheduling feedings — or not
- Checking out your postpartum body
- Eating to maintain your milk supply
- Supplementing with bottles

You're home! You've dragged in the baby, the gifts, the flowers, and the balloons, and you've collapsed in the nearest chair. As you look around these familiar surroundings, now full of baby stuff, breast pads, and car seats, you suddenly realize . . . you're a parent! And you have a baby who's looking to you for all the answers on what to do next.

It's never too soon to set the tone for your own style of parenting. Are you going to be scheduled or flexible? Strict or lenient? While most likely you'll find your style evolving over time, some decisions — like where the baby will sleep, and whether you're going to keep the baby on a schedule or feed on demand — are made very early in your parenting career.

In this chapter, we help you through the exciting but sometimes frightening first weeks alone with your baby, and we address some of the common breastfeeding questions and issues that arise. For more ideas on how to become the parent you want to be, check out *Parenting For Dummies* by Sandra Harding Gookin and Dan Gookin (Wiley).

Leaving the Hospital: Reentering Real Life

Perhaps you pictured your arrival at home as triumphant, with you carrying your picture-perfect baby, your partner proudly snapping pictures, and adoring family and friends gazing lovingly at you.

Reality may be more like this: The baby is screaming as you pull up in front of the house. You and your partner have argued for the last three miles about whether you should stop the car and take the baby out of the car seat because she has slipped sideways. Your parents rush out of the house, snatch the baby out of your arms, and leave you — an emotional, exhausted, milk-leaking wreck — crying on the sidewalk. Your sister's 2-year-old is banging all the pots and pans in the kitchen together while his 4-year-old sister shrieks at an impossibly high decibel level.

You may wonder why simply coming home is so exhausting. First of all, just getting out the hospital door with the baby, the gifts, the suitcase, the car seat, and the bill is exhausting. Chances are your clothes don't fit, and your partner brought the wrong baby blanket. The baby's burping funny, and you and your partner are already tired and on each other's nerves. To top things off, your whole family's standing in your driveway. Welcome home!

Requesting some privacy

Chaos is not a good environment for your reentry into real life as a couple and as parents. Your first feeding at home can be tense enough, even if everything goes well. Try very hard to avoid the scenario we just described.

Tell everyone, except maybe your mom or a very close friend, to stay away from your homecoming. If they all come anyway, retreat to your room for a few minutes — and lock the door!

Your first feeding at home should be peaceful. You should not be jumping up to make canapés for your partner's first cousins, and you may not want all eyes watching you, either.

Even if you've been comfortable nursing in front of your family and friends in the hospital, you may want to isolate yourself for the first feeding at home. You need to be relaxed, and you want to connect with the baby at home without feeling like everyone's watching your every move.

If your family's the type that's going to be right there no matter what you say, now is the time to get out your nursing blanket or shawl and settle yourself in the cozy little nursing corner you set up in your living room. Have someone bring you a drink and a snack.

Keeping your focus

When you first get home from the hospital, resist the urge to inspect and clean the whole house. You may immediately focus on the fact that your partner hasn't swept up the dog hair for the last three days, or that the plants need to be watered. Don't look. Just concentrate on you and the baby for now.

As soon as you put your nursing corner to use, you'll realize its flaws. Maybe the table is too far from your chair, or perhaps a TV tray in front of you would be better than an end table. Maybe your footstool is too low or too high. Don't let this distract you from the job at hand; instead, ask your partner to change things around before the next feeding.

Making it through the first night

Before you went into the hospital, you probably decided whether you were going to keep the baby in her own room or in yours. (See the section "Weighing Risks and Benefits of Co-Sleeping" later in this chapter.) Whether the baby's in your room or her own, you can expect to spend a somewhat restless first night. If she's in your room, you may be hypersensitive to every squeak she makes. If she's in the next room, you may spend the night turning up the volume on the baby monitor, thinking you're missing something.

We can *almost* guarantee (*almost* because you may be a really sound sleeper) that you'll hear the baby when she stirs. If you've had a cesarean and are having trouble getting out of bed, put your partner in charge of getting the baby (if she's not in your bed), changing her diaper, and bringing her to you. Then he can go back to sleep while you feed her.

Expect to be woken up for feeding at least twice during the night. If the baby doesn't wake up after four to five hours, you should wake her for a feeding. Later on, you can gladly let her take her long sleep at night, but right now, you're still getting your milk supply established. So don't let her sleep through (not that there's really much chance of that happening).

Settling into a New Routine

You've probably heard the saying, "This is the first day of the rest of your life." At no time is this more true than on the first day at home with your new baby. While everything is exciting (and a bit frightening), you want to start settling into your new routine as soon as possible.

Some families (very few, these days, unless your last name is Rockefeller) have live-in nannies when they first come home from the hospital. Other couples manage to eke out enough for a night nurse to stay for the first few weeks. If you're breastfeeding, you're not going to find a night nurse much help, unless you've hired the last remaining wet nurse (see Chapter 1). You may actually get more benefit by hiring a cleaning person, who can tidy up during the day and keep the dog hairs under control.

Here are some suggestions to help you feel like you've got your days (and nights) under control when you first come home:

- **Get dressed.** While your old pajamas may be more comfortable than your pre-pregnancy jeans, you won't feel too chic answering the door in them. You won't believe how much more pulled together you'll feel if you have on clothes instead of PJs. If this is completely out of the question, wear something that looks like clothes to bed — such as sweats. You'll at least look pulled together, even if you don't feel it.
- **Nap when the baby naps.** Lying down at noon may feel sacrilegious to you, especially if you're a Type A personality. But you can't stay clear-headed if you don't get enough sleep, and your milk production will suffer, too.
- **Realize that the baby is your job.** Don't try to keep up with a million other things, at least not for a few weeks. Don't answer calls from the office, and don't do work at home, unless absolutely necessary. If you're the aforementioned Type A, say it over and over until you believe it: Breastfeeding is a full-time job.

Weighing Risks and Benefits of Co-Sleeping

Co-sleeping is a hot topic in the baby world today. Many people, possibly including your parents, may tell you that co-sleeping is a bad habit to start and that you'll be spoiling your baby, not to mention ruining your sex life. (Chances are your parents won't mention the part about your sex life, but your friends may.)

We're not really sure where the idea of you in your bed, baby in his crib originated. All around the world, babies sleep with their parents, making bonding as important during the night as in the day. Our civilized society, however, has fallen in love with the idea of everything in its place, and this includes sleeping babies.

If you're thinking about asking the baby to join your slumber party, you're not alone. In fact, more than half of all babies end up in their parents' beds, for at least some portion of the night. This is especially true in the first months of life.

TIP

Before you bring baby to bed, make sure that you and your partner are on the same page. Co-sleeping works only if both parents agree that it is the best arrangement. Bringing a new baby home is stressful enough without adding a nightly bedtime battle to the mix.

REMEMBER

Recent studies have found that co-sleeping is good for you and for your baby. Having your baby sleeping with you lying on his back may decrease the possible incidence of Sudden Infant Death Syndrome (SIDS), which we discuss in Chapter 2.

But two sides of the co-sleeping fence exist. One view comes from the U.S. Consumer Product Safety Commission, which performed a study in 1999 that concluded that having babies sleep in adult beds is dangerous. They based this conclusion on fears that a baby could accidentally smother, get caught between the mattress and wall, or be rolled on by a sleeping parent. And there have been cases of babies injured or killed in all of these situations.

However, the incidence of this type of accident is far less than the risk of SIDS. Your baby is actually safer in your bed (under specific conditions) than in his crib alone. This isn't to say that you shouldn't be aware of the potential for injury if your baby sleeps with you. But you can prevent accidents by following some simple steps to make your bed baby-friendly:

- **Have the baby sleep next to you instead of your partner.** Most mothers have a sixth sense when it comes to sleeping with their babies. They have an intense awareness of where the baby is in the bed, even during sleep. In the early weeks and months, other family members and caregivers may not be equipped with this instinct. The best person for the baby to sleep next to is the person most aware of his presence; that would be you.

- **Have the baby sleep between you and a barrier, like a bedrail.** This will prevent him from rolling off the bed. Most times your baby will move toward your warmth, not away from it, but set up your bed just in case he decides to wander.

  If you must use a wall as a barrier, pack towels or blanket rolls between the wall and bed to prevent the baby from slipping in this crevice. Bedrails covered with meshing are better than those with slats, which could entrap the baby's head, arms, or legs. Make sure the baby can't get caught between the mesh and mattress.

- **Never, never leave your baby unattended in an adult bed.**
- **Never place the baby on a water bed.** The "wavy" surface could trap and suffocate the baby. Also, your baby needs to be up where he can breathe fresh air, not lying in a depressed surface where he may be breathing exhaled air. Doing so could cause your baby's respirations to become depressed due to breathing in too much carbon dioxide.
- **Always place the baby on his back.**
- **Do not use large pillows and comforters around the baby's head or as a cover.** Don't lay the baby on top of the pillow either; make sure he's on a firm surface. Softer surfaces could cause suffocation.
- **Use the biggest bed that you can, preferably a queen or king size.** This gives everyone a little moving room.

Following are a few more suggestions to make co-sleeping as safe and comfortable as possible for everyone involved:

- **Don't sleep with the baby if you're taking medication to help you sleep.** Whether you're using a sedative or something as seemingly benign as Tylenol PM, your awareness of your baby may be altered.
- **If you're suffering from sleep deprivation, get some nights of regular sound sleep by yourself before bringing the baby into your bed.** Your awareness of your baby's position could be affected by sleep deprivation. In the early months of your baby's life, sleep deprivation is very normal; don't be afraid to admit that you're experiencing it.
- **If you're very overweight, consider using a bassinet or a *side car* (a three-sided crib that lines up next to your bed).** Obesity can cause *sleep apnea* (periods of interrupted breathing), which causes sleep disturbances and may alter your awareness of the baby. Also, if you have large, pendulous breasts or abdominal rolls, you could suffocate the baby.

- **Don't attempt to fall asleep on the sofa with your baby.** He could get wedged between you and the back of the sofa and be buried in the cushion.
- **Don't wear lingerie with strings longer than 8 inches.** Your baby could get caught in them. The same goes for jewelry such as necklaces.
- **Don't overheat or overdress your baby.** You're already giving him extra heat from your body closeness.
- **Don't put older siblings in bed with baby.** Brothers and sisters may be excited about the new addition, but they don't belong in the same bed.

If you make the decision to try co-sleeping, following are just some of the benefits you may experience:

REMEMBER

- **Co-sleeping can strengthen the bond between mother and baby.** There's nothing better than hearing your baby breathing and smelling his sweet body in the night.
- **Breastfeeding is easier when you're co-sleeping.** When your baby cries, you pretty much just need to undo the clasp on your nursing bra. Your baby is already in place, ready to go.
- **You'll actually get more sleep.** Instead of waking to a screaming baby, you'll wake to a stirring baby who easily attaches to the breast. After feeding on one side, you can hand him off to your partner for a diaper change. When he returns, place the baby on the second breast, and you can both fall asleep. Even your partner may get more sleep in the long run.

REMEMBER

Co-sleeping is not for everyone. You and your partner have to be in total agreement about it, or one of you may end up spending a lot of nights on the couch, sulking. If you try it and it doesn't work out, no harm done.

Dealing with a Night Owl

As a new parent, you'll find yourself asking veterans the million-dollar question: "When is my baby going to sleep through the night?" Your coauthor Carol isn't the best person to ask. Nights were tough times in our household. Most of my boys didn't sleep through the night for years — they were definitely night owls. However, this difficulty did eventually pass, and I now find myself with the opposite problem, trying to wake them up!

Newborn babies often have a somewhat mixed-up clock. They may sleep during the day and be wide-eyed and bushy-tailed through a good portion of the night. Although you may find yourself getting upset by this, realize that your new baby has no concept of time. He can't possibly understand why you're thrilled with him at 10 a.m. and not so thrilled at 3 a.m.!

Most babies settle into the routine of night sleeping by about the age of 6 months. But some babies don't master the fine art of sleeping through the night for a long while, even up to two years.

REMEMBER

You actually don't want your new baby to sleep through the night too soon. A newborn's stomach is about the size of a golf ball. Breast milk moves quickly through his stomach, taking only about 90 minutes to digest. Breastfed babies need to take in approximately one-third of their calories during the night.

Recognizing sleep patterns

Most babies who are under 3 months old need 16 hours of sleep in a 24-hour period. That sounds pretty good when you're pregnant, but the reality is those 16 or so hours don't come in very large chunks at first. For an infant, "sleeping through the night" means sleeping for at most a five-hour stretch.

But things do get better! By six months, your baby will probably be sleeping longer at night and taking two naps during the day.

REMEMBER

Babies have different sleep cycles than adults. They have shorter, lighter cycles, waking every three to five hours. This prevents them from falling into deep sleep like an adult.

Research has found that babies who sleep very deeply may be more susceptible to SIDS. When a baby sleeps too deeply, she literally can't wake herself up. So waking up two to three times during the night is normal in a baby under 6 months old and should be viewed as a reassuring sign.

Setting the stage for sleep

Everyone has something to say about handling a night owl. No matter what they say, remember that you and your partner are there at night; other people aren't. You need to do what's right for you. To help you make it through the night, following are a few pointers:

- **Get your baby in the mood for sleep.** Setting the mood isn't just for lovemaking. Get your baby ready for sleep by winding down his day. Stick to activities that help him relax, such as taking a bath, rocking, and cuddling. Set up a nightly routine.
- **Feed the baby right before you go to sleep.** Most times when your baby wakes up, he does so because he's hungry. If you wake him up and feed him before you go to bed, you may have a chance to sleep until his next feeding, three to five hours later.
- **When he does cry at night, try to handle him with the least amount of stimulation.** Low lights and a warm, comfortable area are best. This is not the time to play patty cake! If he needs a diaper change, do it quickly and quietly.
- **Stay calm and collected.** You accomplish more if you don't fret. If you feel yourself becoming upset, try to remove yourself from the situation until you are calmer.
- **Make sure caffeine isn't part of the problem.** Are you taking in more caffeine than you should? This could be passed through the breast milk and make your baby restless. It can also make you edgy. If you think this may be part of the problem, cut your intake down and see if it makes a difference in both of you.
- **Consider co-sleeping.** As we discuss in the previous section, co-sleeping can help with nighttime baby care. You may find it much easier to roll over and feed the baby rather than having to walk to the next room for a feeding session.
- **If your baby becomes fully awake after feeding and a diaper change, try rocking him back to sleep.** The trick is not to put him down until you know that he is fully asleep. This can be checked very simply. Pick up his arm. Is it limp, or does he jerk it back into position? If he responds by dropping it back into his lap, you're probably safe to lie him down.
- **Consider the simple things first.** Is he too hot or too cold? Is a bright light coming in from the street? Is he hungry? (If three or four hours have passed since the last feeding, he probably is.) Does he have a wet diaper?
- **Check the baby's temperature.** Does he feel warm or cold to the touch? If he does, take his temperature. Sick babies are usually restless. Very young babies, less than 3 months old, don't usually run fevers when they're sick. Their temperature may be lower than normal when they're ill.
- **Be proactive about teething discomfort.** In spite of what many family members and even physicians may tell you, your baby reacts when he's cutting teeth. If you know he's teething, try some infant acetaminophen, such as Tylenol, before bedtime.

- **Try just being in the room without picking him up.** Sometimes just your presence is enough to reassure your baby that everything is okay. On the flip side, your baby may become furious if you enter the room and don't pick him up. It won't take you long to figure out which type your baby is!
- **If you know he is not hungry, wet, or in discomfort, try just letting him cry.** This may be difficult, especially the first time. If he hasn't settled down after ten minutes, pick him up. Many a parent has sat outside the nursery and cried listening to her wailing baby. We survived this time, and so will you!

Knowing If You're Nursing Enough

If your baby eats every hour for an hour, you'll probably suspect that he's nursing too much. But what if the opposite is true, and you have to wake him up every five hours to eat? You may be tempted to pat yourself on the back for your baby's wonderful sense of timing, even though you know in your heart he should be eating more. How much is too much — or too little — when it comes to breastfeeding in the first few weeks at home?

Going with the flow versus setting schedules

Imagine yourself at a party, reaching for your third handful of nuts. The hostess shakes her head, slaps your hand, and says, "You can't possibly be hungry, you've eaten half a can of nuts already."

Are you always starving when you eat? Do you put food in your mouth only when you absolutely need to eat? If you're like most of us, the answer is no. Sometimes, you eat because you need something else, like comfort, or you want to fill some need you can't even explain.

Feeding on demand

WARNING!

Imposing a nursing schedule on a newborn may result in some of her needs not being met. For one thing, breast milk is digested quickly — much more quickly than formula. So while it may seem as if your baby can't possibly be hungry an hour or two after her last feeding, the truth is that she can be. Don't you sometimes dig through the freezer for ice cream an hour after you finish dinner?

Also, an infant has few comfort resources when something seems not quite right in her world. *You* are her primary comfort resource!

She may not be hungry when she starts rooting, looking for a nipple. She may just need a little comfort.

Another reason to avoid imposing a strict nursing schedule on your baby is that her nutritional needs aren't always the same. When your baby goes through a growth spurt, she may need to nurse much more often than she normally does. Growth spurts usually occur when your baby is 2 to 3 weeks old, again when she is 6 weeks old, and around the age of 6 months. You may notice your baby wanting to nurse frequently for two or three days. The best way to handle growth spurts is to let the baby nurse as often as she needs; she'll soon settle back into her established nursing pattern.

TIP

Don't wait until your baby cries to feed her. Watch for early signs of hunger, such as turning her head as if looking for a nipple, putting her fist in her mouth, or making sucking motions.

Dealing with naysayers

Unfortunately, some people may give you a hard time about letting the baby — not the clock — decide when it's time to eat. That's because four-hour scheduling was all the rage in baby care 30 years or so ago. Try to remember this when someone accuses you of "raising a little tyrant." They don't really mean this. Honest. They're genuinely concerned about you and the baby, so explain to them (nicely!) that your doctor advised you to feed on demand.

Even better, print out the following short list of what the baby learns when no one listens to her cries:

- She learns that her feelings of hunger aren't important.
- She learns that it doesn't do any good to ask for help.
- She learns that she doesn't know what she really needs.

Looking forward

Rest assured that as the baby gets older, she won't always want to nurse when she's unhappy. Maybe she'll respond positively to a change of scenery, a little attention, a position change, or a diaper change. Chances are you'll get her on a nursing schedule in a few months, but in the first few weeks, listen to her needs.

You may feel like little more than a milk machine in your first weeks at home. That's alright, because being a milk machine means you have to be available and close to your baby most of the day and night. That's how you spin the connections that bind you together for a lifetime, and it's how you begin to know who your baby is.

You may wonder how you'll ever manage to clean the kitchen if you're always on demand. This is where a baby sling comes in handy (see Chapter 5). Nursing while walking is impossible at first; neither you nor the baby will be quite good enough at latching and staying latched. But after a few weeks, when you've got nursing technique under control, you can move around while the baby nurses. Don't carry this mobility to extremes, though! The whole idea of nursing is to spend time with your baby, not to dispense milk while pushing potato peels down the garbage disposal.

In your first few weeks at home, let your baby set the schedule. If you feel like you're meeting yourself coming and going at Mom's Milk Bar, remind yourself that this too shall pass. In fact, it passes all too quickly, and soon you'll be looking back on these newborn days (and nights) with a sense of nostalgia. We promise.

Monitoring the baby's intake

Some of you may be obsessed with knowing how much milk the baby's getting, no matter how often we tell you not to worry about it. That's the seductive draw of bottle feeding; you know, without a doubt, how much milk the baby's getting at each feeding.

If you are really concerned that you're not making enough milk, the following sections explain ways to ensure that you are. Some require mere observation; others require a good-natured pediatrician and an accurate scale.

Weighing the baby

If you're really, *really* concerned about your milk supply, you can weigh the baby before and after a feeding to see how much he took in. This requires a precise scale (not your bathroom scale, which varies up to 5 pounds, depending on whether you lean forward or backward when you stand on it). You'll need a scale that weighs in ounces as well as pounds, because your baby's certainly not drinking a pound of milk at a time.

Most pediatricians have very accurate scales, and if you ask nicely, yours may let you come in and weigh the baby, then nurse the baby, then weigh the baby again. Keep in mind that you can't change the baby's clothes or diaper between weighings; everything has to be exactly the same so that the only variable is the breast milk.

Unless your baby has not regained his birth weight after two weeks, you don't need to be preoccupied with how much he's getting at each feeding. If he's gaining well, he's eating enough. You can buy a baby scale that weighs in ounces if you just have to know, but after a day or two you'll probably get bored with weighing.

TIP

Any time you feel that the baby doesn't seem satisfied, or that she shows symptoms of dehydration (see the following section), take her to the pediatrician's office for a weight check. This doesn't mean you're obsessive; it means you're an observant parent.

WARNING!

Checking for dehydration

A dehydrated baby shows some obvious signs. A baby who is severely dehydrated:

- **Is lethargic.** A dehydrated baby lies still and shows little interest in eating or anything else.
- **Has skin that "tents" when you pinch it.** Rather than springing back, dehydrated skin remains somewhat folded after you pinch it.
- **Has a sunken fontanelle.** The *fontanelle* is the soft spot on the top of the baby's head. If he's dehydrated, the fontanelle may actually be somewhat sunken.
- **Has dull, sunken eyes and a slightly dry mouth.**
- **Has fewer wet diapers than normal.** Most newborns urinate frequently, up to ten times a day. Today's disposable diapers are so absorbent that you may not notice a decrease in wetness at first. If you're concerned that the baby may be dehydrated, use a cloth diaper so you can be sure he's urinating enough.

Counting dirty diapers

Newborns often pass stool every time they eat. (The good news is that breastfed babies have slightly more fragrant diapers than bottle-fed babies!) The typical newborn breastfed baby has:

- Between 3 and 12 stools a day
- Stools that are soft, seedy, or curdy
- Yellowish to brownish-greenish stools

As breastfed babies get older, they tend to have less frequent but still soft stools. Stool patterns often change at around 6 weeks of age, when the baby may have one stool each day, or may have a stool every three to four days. As babies get older, they become more efficient at using more of your milk, so they create less waste. Constipation is rarely a problem for the breastfed baby.

Involving Dad from the Start

The baby's first weeks at home can be stressful for both parents. Yes, you have hormones to contend with, but think of your partner: He has you, in all your hormonal glory, *and* a baby to adjust to.

Even the dad who excelled at backrubs and pep talks through labor and the first days of breastfeeding may become unsure of his role after he's home. He may wonder where he fits into the parenting act that, so far, looks like a one-woman show.

You may have to help him figure out what's in his job description. So, in addition to everything else you're adjusting to, you may need to help your partner find his parenting niche. The following suggestions can help a cautious dad become a first-class caretaker:

- **Babies love to be held.** Skin-to-skin contact provides body heat and fulfills a physical need to be close to another person.
- **Fathers are great scrubber-uppers at bath time.** Let dad be the bath expert. You may even find that he's less nervous about handling a wet, slippery baby than you are.
- **Changing diapers is a great way to make body contact.** Be fair: Don't make dad the poopy diaper king! But your partner can certainly take on the role of getting the baby ready for nursing during the night by changing her diaper. Make sure you both know that this is his job, though, or he may snore peacefully through the feeding and wonder why you're hitting him in the head with a pillow the next morning!

Carol's postpartum flood

I will never forget this episode that occurred after my first son was born. I was home from the hospital, thinking life was back to normal. I thought I could do everything: take care of the baby, clean the house, run the vacuum . . . you name it. All of a sudden, I felt a huge "swoosh," and a big clot passed. I could feel my heart start pounding in my chest.

I ran to the phone and called my OB, fearing that I was hemorrhaging. Instead, I discovered that I was just doing too much too soon. My doctor ordered me to lie down and rest. The bleeding slowed down shortly after I did. Mother Nature definitely has a way of demonstrating that your body has limits!

Many great books deal with the experience of becoming a dad. These two may help you through the doldrums of new fatherhood:

- *Rookie Dad* by Susan Fox (Silhouette Books). This book suggests exercises and games to help dads bond with their new babies. Because men tend to be more physical, this gives dads ideas to help them relate to their babies in fun, active ways.
- *The New Father: A Dad's Guide to the First Year* by Armin A. Brott (Abbeville Press). The title says it all. Every guy could use a guide to help with the ups and downs of baby's first year.

Numerous Web sites also offer new dads information, including these two:

- /http://babyparenting.about.com//cs/focusondad/ This Web site has sections on fatherhood, including ideas for handling its ups and downs.
- www.babycenter.com. This Web site has specific sections on helping dad understand his breastfeeding partner.

Getting Your Body Back

What goes up usually comes down. This should apply to your pregnancy weight gain and body changes. *Some* pounds (never as many as we'd like, but *some*) drop off before you even go home from the hospital. But don't expect to leave the hospital in your pre-pregnancy jeans — it just isn't going to happen! What should you expect? After delivery, your body immediately starts to work itself back into shape. The process may take longer than you'd like, but rest assured: You'll be back to your old self long before the baby leaves for college!

Here are some of the biggest changes you experience postpartum:

- **Your uterus *involutes,* meaning it shrinks back to almost its pre-pregnancy size.** This takes approximately six weeks and starts happening as soon as you put your baby on the breast after delivery. Right after delivery, the top of your uterus can be felt around your navel. By 10 to 12 days after delivery, you won't be able to feel the top of your uterus.

  Your uterus shrinks whether or not you breastfeed, but it occurs more rapidly if you nurse (see Chapter 2). Remember, breastfeeding can help get you out of your mu-mu dress and back to your jeans a lot faster than bottle feeding!

- **Your vagina returns to its normal shape.** Your vagina stretches tremendously during delivery, becoming a tunnel-like structure leading to the uterus as the baby is born. Performing simple exercises called *Kegels* (see the nearby sidebar "Doing your Kegel exercises") helps tighten your vaginal muscles.
- **You shed your extra blood volume.** Increased blood volume, plus extra water retention, is what makes your face look puffy and your hands and feet swollen before delivery. You start shedding this extra blood volume through increased urination soon after delivery.
- **Abdominal muscles, stretched during pregnancy, return to almost a pre-pregnancy state.** Abdominal exercises help.
- **Your breasts change, whether you're breastfeeding or not.**
- **Vaginal bleeding, called *lochia,* changes during the first six weeks after delivery.** Initially your lochia is bright red. This bleeding can be very heavy and contain clots in the first 12 to 24 hours. Gradually it decreases, changing to a pink color and finally to a yellow-white discharge. Lochia consists of blood and uterine lining that your body is shedding. As the blood vessels in your uterus clamp down (due to hormone changes and breastfeeding), your lochia decreases.

WARNING! If you experience heavy vaginal bleeding more than six weeks after delivery, call your doctor. Keep in mind that if you're very active when you go home, your lochia may change from a pinkish discharge to bright red bleeding. But continued passing of clots or bright red blood can mean a piece of the placenta is still in your uterus, or that you've developed an infection.

TIP

Doing your Kegel exercises

Doctors and nurses may tell you to "do your Kegels" to tighten your vaginal muscles and help prevent incontinence (leaking urine) after childbirth. "Doing your Kegels" simply means tightening the muscles of your pelvic floor four to five times in a row, four to five times a day.

To locate your pelvic floor muscles, try to stop urination midstream. The muscles that are required to stop your urine are the same muscles you need to tighten after delivery.

Coping with the Wet T-Shirt Look

You can recognize a brand-new mom by the round wet circles on her T-shirt. Leaking breasts are a common occurrence when you first get out of the hospital, because your hormone levels are high and your body reacts to any and all stimuli, possibly including the baby on the Pampers box.

Preparing for leaks

There are varying degrees of leaking, ranging from needing a shirt change every couple of hours (even if you're wearing breast pads in your bra) to hardly leaking at all. The first-time breastfeeder probably won't be lucky enough to experience the latter. Women who have nursed previously, on the other hand, may have already conditioned the let-down reflex (see Chapter 6) to some extent.

During the early weeks of breastfeeding, try to consider your wet T-shirt look a proud sign of motherhood. Leaking breasts are a release valve so you don't become engorged and develop a breast infection. They may also remind you that feeding time is near. Have patience; your body will adjust your breast milk supply and demand.

REMEMBER

If the thought of doing carpool duty while dripping milk on the leather seats has you alarmed, relax. This too shall pass, and in the meantime you can stock up on breast pads to help you through. Most women find their let-down reflex is more predictable after six to ten weeks. When your body learns to control your let-down, you may worry that your milk supply has decreased — it hasn't. When leakage stops, that means everything has finally come together.

TIP

When you first nurse your baby, your opposite breast will probably leak. To deal with this drippy situation:

- Try to collect the leaking milk by placing something like a plastic cup under your breast. Choose something lightweight and easy to prop in that position.
- If you're not wearing a bra, cover your leaking breast with a cloth diaper or other absorbent cloth.
- If you are wearing a bra, place breast pads in the cups to soak up the leaking milk.

Many moms wake up surrounded by a wet nightgown and bed sheets, especially if the baby has slept longer than usual. Because you tend to be aware of your baby, even in your sleep, his stirring may equal an instant wet nightgown!

We're sure you've heard this story from a new mom you know: She's at the supermarket, picking out pears, when she hears a baby cry. Within seconds, the grocery store could turn off its sprinkler system and use her instead. When your milk ejection reflex is not quite controlled, hearing or seeing any baby can set off a fountain. We discuss what you can do to control this in the next section.

Keeping Mt. Vesuvius under control

If your baby is with you and your let-down reflex lets loose, your best option is to nurse him. But if you're out without him or returning to work before your let-down reflex is established, you may need to find other avenues to handle the situation:

- **When you start to feel the tingling that occurs from the milk ejection reflex, cross your arms across your chest.** Essentially, you're giving yourself a big hug. This applies pressure to the breasts and decreases the flow from an uncontrollable let-down.

  Don't do this too often during the early weeks of breastfeeding. When your milk let-down is in the learning stage, leaking actually prevents clogged milk ducts. Also, your let-down helps to regulate your milk supply; disrupting it this early could be counterproductive.

- **If you need to place something in your bra to help absorb the leaking milk, use either a cotton pad or a non-plastic lined breast pad.** Plastic-lined breast pads encourage a moist environment for bacteria to grow. Change pads often when wet.
- **Express milk manually or with a pump.** Doing so gets you over the hump until you can nurse, and it lessens the possibility of engorgement and infection. Save the milk you pump; you can feed it to the baby later if you store it in a sterile container.
- **Use breast shells to collect milk.** This suggestion comes with caveats. Breast shells (see Chapter 5) do collect milk, but you may still have spillage. Shells can also set up an environment that may cause nipple soreness and breast infection. Unless you're able to store the milk immediately after it leaks, don't save it; milk that sits in the shell may grow bacteria.

- **Wear loose fitting, patterned shirts.** Prints camouflage wetness much better than solid materials. Also, always bring an extra shirt or jacket with you; doing so gives you some options if you do leak through breast pads.

Weeping and Wailing: Managing Your Moods

After delivery, you may feel extremely happy and very sad all within the same minute. Trust us: You're normal. For months, including during the labor and delivery, you've been the center of attention; now everyone's focus is squarely on the baby.

In the following sections, we discuss what to expect from the baby blues, as well as how to cope with the much more serious issue of postpartum depression.

Feeling the baby blues

REMEMBER

During the first few weeks of motherhood, feeling down and crying for no reason are perfectly normal. Sixty to eighty percent of new moms have the "baby blues" to some degree. (Keep in mind that baby blues are much different than postpartum depression; we discuss this more serious problem in the next section.) You've been on a hormonal high for nine months. When the levels start crashing down and the reality of your new role as a responsible mom sets in, you have every right to shed a few tears!

The first step to handling baby blues is to accept it as a normal phase of your postpartum period. Your partner, family, and friends should also be aware that you may be irritable, slightly depressed, very emotional, and overly sensitive. Lethargy, occasional sleeplessness, and an increased tendency to worry are also normal — as long as they don't incapacitate you or last too long.

All the books, classes, and friendly information in the world can't prepare you for all your new feelings. Before delivery, you may assume that the baby blues or mild depression happens to other people, not you. But no new mom is really prepared for the lack of sleep, the constant care a baby requires, the engorged breasts, the aching stitches, and the impact of coming off the delivery high. Just thinking of early motherhood is exhausting!

REMEMBER

The most important thing for you and everyone around you to know is that the baby blues are not an illness. In most cases, the symptoms recede as quickly as they come.

The treatment for baby blues is pretty basic. Follow these simple suggestions, and those difficult days should pass quickly:

- **Rest!** Try to sleep when your baby does. Sleep deprivation only makes your blues worse. Many new moms feel overwhelmed by all their new responsibilities.
- **Express yourself.** You'll feel better if you know that you're not in this alone. Your partner and family can help, but you have to let them know what you're feeling, whether you do so through conversation or crying!
- **Limit activities.** This is where your partner comes in. He can help you handle visitors, take phone calls, and set priorities.
- **Take some time for yourself.** Do something you enjoy; it will remind you that life outside the nursery goes on.

Recognizing postpartum depression

You and your partner should be aware that baby blues can advance to postpartum depression in some women. If you have a previous history of depression, or a family history of depression or postpartum depression, you must be aware of this possibility. If your mood isn't improving after approximately two weeks, seek professional help. The first step toward wellness is recognizing that you need some help.

The symptoms of postpartum depression tend to be exaggerated symptoms of the baby blues. They can include crying all day (not just for short periods), experiencing insomnia and/or panic attacks, and lacking interest in yourself or the baby. Or you may be overly anxious or feeling guilty about the baby.

WARNING!

Depression should be taken seriously, because worsening symptoms can lead to danger to yourself or the baby. Without treatment, postpartum depression may become a lengthy, dangerous ordeal.

To treat postpartum depression, you and your partner must first recognize the problem. Next, take the following steps:

TIP

- **Talk to someone.** Share your feelings, whether with a friend, a new mother support group, or a health professional. You may need to speak with a psychologist, counselor, or other medical professional familiar with postpartum depression.

- **Get as much sleep as you can.** Taking care of the baby is more than a full-time job. No one can be up night and day, weeks at a time, without consequences. If you find yourself unable to sleep, talk with a health professional.
- **Reduce your responsibilities.** Don't worry about the house, the clothes, or your previous routine. Ask someone else to take care of these things, or at least to help you. Also ask someone to watch the baby for a half hour or so whenever possible, and allow yourself the chance to do anything you wish — take a nap or a shower, perhaps, or talk to an old friend.
- **Go outside.** Take a walk with the baby if the weather allows, or go for a stroll by yourself when someone else can watch the baby. Breathing fresh air can really help your mental state; it reminds you that life exists outside your four walls.

While these suggestions are helpful, if your situation is severe, you may need a more aggressive treatment, such as medication. Don't feel bad about needing medication if you have postpartum depression; just make sure your medical professionals know that you're a breastfeeding mother before they prescribe medication.

Many antidepressants are safe to take while breastfeeding. Zoloft is currently the medication of choice for breastfeeding moms. Next often prescribed is Paxil. Paxil is also known to have a low transfer rate to the baby; one study showed that Paxil was undetectable in the blood of seven out of eight breastfed babies. See Chapter 3 for more on antidepressants.

TIP

For further information on postpartum depression, contact these organizations:

- National Institute of Mental Health, 301-496-9576
- Depression After Delivery, Inc., 800-944-4773
- Postpartum Education for Parents, 805-564-3888
- National Women's Health Information Center, 800-994-9662

Eating for a Good Milk Supply

Like many women, you may have thought that pregnancy was your ticket to eating anything and everything, including ice cream sundaes. Who wants to watch calories when they're pregnant?

Your coauthor Carol remembers going to the OB's office during pregnancy and refusing to get weighed. I knew that fluid retention wasn't to blame for every pound I was gaining; I was eating everything within reach!

If you pack on lots of extra pounds during pregnancy, don't jump on the next fad diet bandwagon as soon as you deliver. You need to maintain your health while nursing by eating the right amounts — and right kinds — of foods.

Consuming enough calories

While you're pregnant, you should take in about 500 extra calories a day to help your baby grow. When your baby is born, things shouldn't change too much, because those same 500 extra calories are required for your body to make milk. If you don't take in those 500 extra calories, your baby will probably still get adequate milk, but your health may suffer in the process.

You can calculate your caloric needs while breastfeeding by using this simple formula: Multiply your weight by 15, and add 500 to the total. This number of calories should meet your breastfeeding nutritional needs.

For example, multiply 140 pounds by 15 — that's 2,100 calories. Add 500, so you need 2,600 calories to maintain a good milk supply without causing harm to yourself.

Paying attention to nutrition

Many moms find that eating six small meals works better than three meals a day and helps prevent snacking on junk between meals.

Think back to elementary school, when you studied the famous *food pyramid* — the image that shows the elements of a healthy diet. The food pyramid shows the five basic food groups and the amounts you should eat in each group. The pyramid is a good guideline for healthy eating. While breastfeeding, a few more guidelines come into play:

- **Eat fats from the *essential fatty acids* group.** These fats come from nuts, seeds, greens, and fish. Fatty acids are needed for good brain function for you and your baby.

- **Avoid eating *trans fatty acids.*** Trans fatty acids come from processed foods and hydrogenated oils. They are passed through breast milk and interfere with the metabolism of essential fatty acids.
- **Keep taking your prenatal vitamins.** This is especially important if your diet is deficient. Your baby needs vitamins for growth and development.
- **Get plenty of thiamine, folic acid, vitamin B_{12}, and vitamin D.** Other than folic acid, the others are found in animal proteins. Vegetarians should supplement these important vitamins. Folic acid is found in those green leafy vegetables your mom made you eat, as well as in cabbage, broccoli, and Brussels sprouts.
- **Take in plenty of vitamins C and A.** Vitamin C is found in citrus fruits (including orange juice), strawberries, tomatoes, and (surprisingly) potatoes. Vitamin A is found in green and yellow vegetables like broccoli, carrots, and pumpkins.
- **Drink plenty of water, at least eight glasses daily.** If you become dehydrated, your milk production decreases. Have a drink of water when you nurse. Drinking lots of water also helps prevent constipation.
- **Pump iron.** Pregnancy and breastfeeding both deplete your iron stores. Low iron can make you feel tired and lethargic, and you won't have time to feel that way after the baby arrives. Red meat, chicken, fish, whole grain bread, nuts, beans, and leafy green vegetables are all good sources of iron.

REMEMBER

If you decide to start a diet after delivery, wait at least six weeks to help get your milk supply well established and to help your body heal from the delivery. Eat from all the food groups, rather than eliminating one or more. Avoid fad or starvation diets, because these may result in nutritional imbalances in you or the baby.

WARNING!

Stay away from over-the-counter weight loss products, especially products that contain the herb ma huang because they could harm both you and your baby by placing strain on the heart.

If you find yourself losing more than 5 pounds a month, your baby's nutritional status could become compromised. A study done by the *New England Journal of Medicine* found that women who exercised and dieted in moderation lost weight, and their babies continued to develop and grow normally. This is the goal you want to achieve.

Considering How to Supplement

In a perfect world, you wouldn't ever have to supplement your baby's feedings with bottles. If you were always available to nurse the baby for at least the first year of his life, the issue of supplementing would never come up.

However, if you have to go back to work, you want to occasionally go out to dinner without the baby, you become ill and unable to nurse, or you just want a break from nursing for a feeding or two, you need to decide what to supplement with and how to give it.

Pumping milk versus using formula

If you can pump, using breast milk should be your first choice for supplementing. There are two reasons for this:

- **Breast milk is better for your baby than formula.** See Chapter 1 for our discussion of the reasons why.
- **Your breasts work on the principle of supply and demand.** They make as much milk for Tuesday as was removed from them on Monday. So if, on Monday, you give your baby two 8-ounce bottles of formula, you make 16 ounces less milk the next day. Not a good idea if you want to keep up your milk supply.

The problem with using pumped breast milk is that you may have a hard time pumping. If you pump only occasionally, you probably haven't purchased one of the fancy $200 double breast pumps, and the less expensive pumps are less effective (see Chapter 4). You may have to work really hard for a few ounces, because breast pumps just don't have the same sucking power that a nursing baby does. Some women can express only a few drops with the less expensive pumps and may do better with hand pumping.

If you experience this difficulty, and if you don't need to supplement often enough to justify the expense of a fancy breast pump, you may decide to open a can of formula. Doing so won't harm your baby in any way.

Picking the best formula

The shelves of the discount stores are lined with pretty cans of formula, done in soft pastels with adorable bunnies or picture-perfect babies on the labels. Formula companies really know how to appeal to their customers. But your task isn't to pick the prettiest can; you need to pick the formula most like breast milk. Each one says it's just like breast milk, of course, but if you've read Chapter 1 you already know that's not true. So what do you look for?

One consideration is a fairly recent development: In an attempt to make formula that is closer to breast milk, formula manufacturers have added the long-chain fatty acids DHA and ARA to their formulas. DHA and ARA are associated with increased brain function and development.

One disadvantage of using the DHA- and ARA-supplemented formulas is price: They cost about 15 percent more than regular formula. If you're bottle feeding using formula only occasionally, the DHA and ARA supplements aren't a big deal for your baby; she's getting enough in your breast milk.

Most formula manufacturers also offer the option of purchasing soy-based formula, in addition to formula based on cow's milk. For an occasional supplementary bottle, unless your baby has an allergy to cow's milk, you don't need to use soy formula (which is often more expensive).

Avoiding getting baby hooked on the bottle

Nipple confusion (see Chapter 5) is a hot topic among breastfeeding experts. You may be scared by reports of babies refusing to breastfeed after being given even one bottle. But in the real world, many of you will have to give the baby a bottle at some time. And you shouldn't worry that you'll ruin breastfeeding for all time because of it.

Bottle feeding is much easier for your baby than breastfeeding. The milk basically flows constantly from the nipple, and all he has to do is swallow it. Because your baby, like the rest of the human race, will generally take the easy way out of anything, this may seem like a really good deal to him.

Try not to use any bottles for the first three to four weeks, if possible, to ensure that your milk supply is well established. After this time, the baby should make the occasional transition from breast to bottle without difficulty.

If you're going to supplement frequently, use a nipple that's as similar to yours as possible. A good nipple is hard to find. Many of the nipples that look superficially most like yours are the worst at imitating the suck needed to breastfeed. See Chapter 5 for our suggestions on the best nipples for breastfeeding moms.

Don't bottle feed your baby for two feedings in a row. If you're having surgery, or if some other emergency arises, this may be hard to avoid. But whenever possible, breastfeed between bottle feedings so the baby doesn't get too used to bottles. If you have to miss several feedings in a row, ask the caregiver to use a cup or eye dropper to feed him, or to finger feed (see Chapter 9) if possible.

Storing pumped breast milk

Freezing breast milk isn't exactly like slinging leftover pizza slices into a baggie and shoving them to the back of the freezer. Freezing breast milk destroys some of the milk's antibodies (see Chapter 1), so you want to take steps to keep your milk as nutritious as possible.

Choosing containers

Some controversy exists over what type of container you should use to store breast milk. (Are you beginning to get the feeling that there's controversy over everything in breastfeeding? You're right!) Obviously, the container should be sterile if you're storing the milk for any amount of time.

Plastic bottles have some advantages over glass; for example, plastic containers don't break as easily. Also, some white blood cells may stick to the side of glass bottles but not to plastic.

Many breast pumps (see Chapter 5) allow you to pump directly into a plastic bag or bottle for storage, which eliminates the potential for contamination when the milk is poured from one container to another.

Specially designed plastic bags made for milk collection are sterile and are more easily thawed than a hard plastic or glass bottle.

Refrigerating and freezing

You can store breast milk in the refrigerator for five to seven days; keep it toward the back of the refrigerator where the temperature doesn't vary much. You can keep frozen breast milk for four to six months in a regular freezer and up to a year in a deep freezer.

Whether you refrigerate or freeze milk, always label your containers by date and use the oldest ones first.

Chill milk in the refrigerator before freezing it. Freeze breast milk in small amounts, from 2 to 4 ounces, to avoid waste. Whichever containers you use, fill them only to around two-thirds full; the milk expands when frozen, and you don't want containers exploding in your freezer!

Thawing

To thaw breast milk, set the container in a pan of warm water, or run it under warm tap water. Don't put the container directly into boiling water, because the milk may curdle.

Never thaw milk in the microwave; it heats unevenly, and it destroys some of the nutrients. Don't refreeze milk that has been thawed.

Thawed breast milk can vary quite a bit in color, depending on what you ate before you pumped! Don't be surprised if it has a bluish, brownish, or yellowish color. Thawed milk may also separate, with a layer of cream appearing on top of the milk; mix it gently before feeding.

Chapter 8

Coping with Early Breastfeeding Problems

In This Chapter

- Healing nipple problems
- Dealing with mastitis and yeast infections
- Soothing colic
- Handling vomiting and reflux
- Increasing your milk supply
- Giving up nursing

Rarely does a woman breastfeed without experiencing some problem along the way. Most problems, like sore nipples, are easily solved. But others, like reflux, can be complicated to manage.

In this chapter, we discuss some of the challenges that nursing moms encounter most often, and we tell you how to deal with them. We also look at the problem of not producing enough milk — or producing too much! — and the difficulties of handling a baby who doesn't nurse well, no matter what you do.

Soothing Nipple Issues

Nipple problems can make or break breastfeeding. Many women experience soreness in the beginning; after all, your nipples have probably never gotten this much use! Look at possible causes as soon as any soreness develops, so you can try to prevent cracking, bleeding, and scabbing.

Identifying sources of pain

If your nipple begins to get sore, especially at the start of a feeding, the most important thing you can do is make sure your baby is properly latched on. Try placing your index finger on the baby's chin to make sure his lower lip is in the right position. His lower lip should cover more of the areola than his upper lip, and his lips should appear to flange out. See Chapter 6 for a detailed discussion of proper latch-on.

Also review the breastfeeding positions we show you in Chapter 6. In the following section, we remind you of some basic positioning techniques that can prevent the baby from pulling on your nipples and causing damage.

The fungal infection thrush, which we discuss later in this chapter in the section "Sharing Yeast Infections," can also cause nipple pain. Discomfort from thrush occurs throughout the feeding, not just at the beginning, and is often described as a burning sensation. If you suddenly develop this type of discomfort when you had been nursing without pain, chances are you have a yeast infection.

Preventing problems

To prevent nipple damage, remember these basic positioning techniques:

- Hold your baby high, chest-to chest, with his legs even with your other breast for the cradle hold or cross cradle hold. For the football hold, keep your baby's bottom high along your side. If your baby's legs drag down into your lap or to the bottom of the bed or chair, the baby's weight pulls on your nipple.
- Position the baby to face the breast directly so he doesn't have to turn his head to nurse, which pulls on the nipple.
- Remember that your baby's nose should be touching the breast. (Don't worry — he can still breathe!) Do not press down on your breast to keep it away from his nose; doing so pulls the breast out of the baby's mouth slightly, which can cause nipple damage.
- Keep your hand underneath your breast throughout the feeding, at least for the first week or so. Your baby's jaw muscles are not strong enough to hold the weight of the breast in the beginning, and he may slip down onto the nipple as the weight of the breast pushes on his chin.

Also try the following tips:

- Massage your breast before having the baby latch on to help soften the areola and encourage your let-down reflex.
- Don't just pull your baby off the breast when you're done nursing. Use your finger to break the suction so he doesn't cause nipple trauma.
- If you notice that your nipples are starting to get sore, try nursing more frequently but for a shorter duration (10 to 15 minutes instead of a half hour, for example).
- Always pat your nipples to dry them; don't rub.
- Avoid using soaps that can dry out the nipples and ultimately cause cracking or even eczema.
- After a feeding, rub some of your breast milk on each nipple and let it dry. Then apply a coat of a purified lanolin cream, such as Lansinoh (see Chapter 5). However, don't use lanolin-based creams if you have an allergy to wool products.

Coping with soreness

If you develop nipple soreness in spite of your preventive measures, keep doing everything listed in the previous section and add these steps:

- Feed your baby on the side that is less sore, at least until your milk lets down.
- Try different breastfeeding positions. Doing so could help your baby latch on properly.
- Use your finger as a pacifier — rather than your breast — until the soreness decreases, if the baby wants to keep sucking after he's had enough to eat. (You'll know the feeding is finished when you hear long pauses between short bursts of light sucks. If he still wants to suck, offer him your finger.)
- Avoid engorgement. This can be difficult when you have sore nipples; you may feel so much discomfort when the baby latches on that you delay putting the baby to breast. However, after let-down occurs, much of the pain is relieved.
- Pump or hand-express a little milk prior to feeding to soften the areola so the baby can latch on effectively.
- If you're using a breast pump frequently, use a good one. Cheaper pumps can cause breast trauma.

- Dry your nipples after each feeding. Air drying works best. If you can expose them to the sun without getting arrested, that's even better!
- If you use breast pads to absorb milk leaks, make sure they don't have plastic liners, and change them frequently so that bacterial growth doesn't occur.

If soreness progresses to nipple cracking or bleeding, add these measures to your arsenal:

- Continue to nurse, even if your nipples are bleeding; your baby won't be harmed. If your nipples start to scab, soften the scabs with the following two methods:
  - Hand-express some milk and rub the milk on your nipple. Let it dry before putting your bra or clothing on.
  - After you nurse, use a purified lanolin cream such as Lansinoh to encourage healing (see Chapter 5).
- Place ice on your nipples right before nursing, but keep it there only for very short periods so your nipples don't become numb. (Numbness can interfere with let-down.)
- If ice doesn't help you, try a warm compress (a hot wet washcloth) for a few minutes right before you nurse.
- If you're in considerable pain, try hand-expressing or pumping for a day, and feed your baby the expressed milk.
- Use a breast shell (see Chapter 5) to keep pressure off a sore nipple when you're wearing clothing, but use it only for short time periods. Make sure that your bra isn't rubbing against your nipples.
- After you nurse, rinse your nipples with a saline solution. Mix ⅓ teaspoon of table salt in one cup of warm water. You can also buy packaged saline solutions at pharmacies. Spray the solution on the nipple area with a squirt bottle, then pat it off.
- Contact a health professional or lactation consultant if you're not seeing any improvement or if you develop a fever, which could mean a more serious infection. Ask about topical antibiotics, which can be thinly applied. A triple antibiotic like Polysporin (an over-the-counter medication) is better than Neosporin (an antibiotic ointment containing neomycin), which could cause a rash around your baby's mouth. Some recommended topical antibiotics are available by prescription only. Always discuss antibiotic use with your doctor or lactation consultant first.

Using shields for inverted nipples

We hope that by the time you're home after delivery, your inverted nipples (see Chapter 6) have corrected themselves or at least improved enough for the baby to latch on without difficulty. But sometimes the problem persists, and you may become dependent on using aids such as nipple shields (see Chapter 5) to nurse.

If you use nipple shields frequently, your baby may become used to the firmness of the rubber or silicone shield and refuse to nurse without it. This is a situation you want to avoid, because if you continue to use the shield, your breasts may not get adequate stimulation to build and maintain a good milk supply. The baby may also get less milk and not gain weight adequately. You may also be more prone to plugged ducts from incomplete emptying, which can lead to mastitis.

However, you also want your baby to enjoy nursing and trust you. If every nursing without the shield is a frustrating experience for both of you, breastfeeding probably isn't going to last. Using a shield at first and then gradually weaning off may be the only way you can continue breastfeeding.

You may need to start the baby nursing with the shield, to get her to draw the nipple out. In the middle of a feeding, remove her from the breast, take off the shield, and put her back while the nipple is still protruding. If one breast needs the shield and the other doesn't, use the shield only where necessary.

You may find that your baby nurses best without the shield when she's drowsy. Experimenting with different positions may help as well.

Watch your baby's urine output and stools to assure that she's getting enough milk (see Chapter 7). Look for six to eight wet diapers and frequent soft stools, and check her weight at least once a week until she is able to nurse without the shield, or until you establish that she is getting enough milk while nursing with it. Pumping a few times a day can give you extra stimulation to maintain a good milk supply.

If you use a nipple shield, the baby's stimulus to suck is the firm nipple of the shield rather than your breast, which is soft. Don't reinforce this stimulus by offering your baby a pacifier. If the baby needs to suck, let him suck on your finger, which stimulates a suck similar to the breast.

It may take a few weeks to wean a baby off a nipple shield. Be patient, and keep in mind that breastfeeding with the shield is better than not breastfeeding at all.

Developing Mastitis

You don't have to be a nursing mom to develop *mastitis,* a breast inflammation. (Your coauthor Sharon never had mastitis while nursing but developed it in her 40s, about 20 years after she stopped breastfeeding!) However, nursing mothers are more prone to mastitis, because bacteria that cause the inflammation usually enter the breast through cracks or fissures in your nipples.

As many as 1 in 20 nursing moms have at least one bout with mastitis. Mastitis occurs most often in the first month of breastfeeding, but it can occur at any time.

Sometimes the first sign of mastitis is feeling like you've got the flu. You may run a fever (over 100.4° F), have chills, or feel achy or ill. Another obvious sign of mastitis is having red, hot, or swollen areas on your breast. Usually only one breast is affected — more often the left than right. The reddened area is frequently the upper outer quadrant, near your armpit.

A plugged duct — when milk becomes clogged in a duct — may feel like a tender lump in your breast, but it differs from mastitis because it's not usually accompanied by a fever or flu-like symptoms. If not treated, a plugged duct can lead to mastitis.

Realizing risk factors

If you're rundown and stressed, or if your immune system isn't functioning properly, you're more likely to develop mastitis. Other risk factors for mastitis are:

- **Incomplete emptying of the breast:** If your baby nurses less on one side than the other, you're more likely to develop mastitis on the side used less often. Milk ducts can become blocked if the baby doesn't remove enough milk from the breast, because the milk sitting in the ducts thickens. Blocked ducts increase the risk of mastitis.
- **Missed feedings:** If you supplement (see Chapter 7), make sure you pump enough to compensate for the missed feeding.

- **Sustained pressure on your breast:** This pressure can be from wearing a too-tight bra, carrying a heavy purse or diaper bag, using a baby carrier, sleeping on your stomach, or sleeping with the baby lying on top of you.
- **Poor latch-on:** If the baby isn't properly positioned, she won't empty the milk ducts thoroughly.
- **History of breast surgery or trauma:** Women with this type of history may be prone to developing blocked ducts and mastitis. Women with *fibrocystic breasts* (breasts that contain cysts) may also have this problem.
- **Sudden weaning:** If you stop breastfeeding suddenly, you're more likely to develop blocked ducts. If you have to wean suddenly, pump your milk until you can gradually decrease the supply of milk you're making.
- **Yeast infections:** If your baby has *thrush* (a yeast infection in the mouth, which we discuss in the section "Sharing Yeast Infections"), or if you have a yeast infection, it can lead to mastitis.

Treating the infection

If you experience the common symptoms of mastitis, see your doctor. Most likely, she'll prescribe antibiotics. You should feel better and see an improvement in the breast within 48 hours after starting the prescription; if you don't, call your doctor because you may need a different antibiotic. Make sure you finish all the medication, or the infection may return — and it may be worse than it was initially.

TECHNICAL STUFF

The bacteria most frequently responsible for mastitis is *staphylococcus.* The antibiotics most commonly prescribed by doctors for mastitis are Augmentin and Erythromycin.

TIP

You can take pain relievers such as ibuprofen or acetaminophen as needed. Alternating hot and cold packs may also help relieve the discomfort. Gently massaging the affected area can increase blood flow and loosen plugs in the ducts.

Following are other helpful steps to take:

- **Drink lots of fluid.** Staying hydrated helps you feel better and recover faster. This is especially important if you run a high fever.

- **Get lots of rest.** Remember that you're sick. You need to lie down as much as possible. Doing so helps your immune system fight off the infection.
- **Go braless, or wear a loose-fitting bra.** Put as little pressure as possible on the breasts.
- **Nurse in different positions.** Vary the holds you use while nursing, so that all the ducts get thoroughly emptied.

Continuing to nurse

If you have mastitis, you should continue to breastfeed. Otherwise, the infection could turn into an *abscess,* an isolated pocket of pus that would need to be drained surgically.

If possible, start each feeding with the affected breast, to make certain the ducts are being drained completely. You may find this too painful; if you do, start with the unaffected side and switch after your milk lets down. Nursing is usually more comfortable after letdown occurs.

Some babies may refuse to nurse on the affected side because the milk tastes more salty than normal due to the inflammation. If that's the case, you'll have to thoroughly pump the affected side to make sure the infection doesn't worsen.

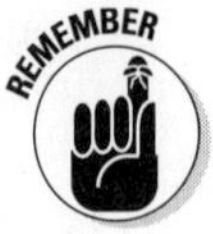

Nursing with mastitis is not dangerous for the baby. Either the bacteria that caused the infection came from the baby's mouth to begin with, or you passed the bacteria on before you realized you had the infection. Continuing to nurse ensures that the baby benefits from the antibodies you're developing to fight the bacteria.

Having mastitis more than once

Some women are prone to mastitis, developing it several times. This is not only frustrating and debilitating, but it may also make you question whether breastfeeding is a good thing for you to do.

If this happens to you, you need to look carefully for the cause. Consider the following:

- **Are you finishing the complete course of antibiotics?** Many people stop taking antibiotics as soon as they start feeling better, figuring they don't need them anymore. This allows more resistant and stronger strains of bacteria to infect you again. Make sure you finish all your medication!

- **Are you putting pressure on your breasts?** Is your bra too tight, or are you doing some sort of repetitive movement that is compressing your breast tissue — an exercise, or something like shoveling snow? Do you sleep on your stomach?
- **Are you allowing the baby to nurse until finished?** Don't feed for a limited time, such as five minutes on each side. This can result in plugged ducts because not enough milk is being removed. Also, vary the position at each feeding, to make sure all areas of the breast are being emptied.
- **Are you rundown?** Make sure you're eating well and resting enough and that you aren't anemic. Keep taking your prenatal vitamins to help supply nutrients you may be missing. Don't try to be superwoman, maintaining five carpools and two PTA positions, as well as spackling the bathroom and refinishing the deck, while nursing with one hand. Sit down and enjoy the experience!

Sharing Yeast Infections

Perhaps you've experienced a vaginal yeast infection — the incredibly itchy, cheesy white growth you can get from taking antibiotics or wearing nylon underwear. When you're nursing, yeast can grow on your nipples or in your baby's mouth, causing problems for both of you.

Realizing the origins of candida

All of us carry some forms of microorganisms on our skin. *Candida,* or yeast, is a fungus carried by half the population. Normally, microorganisms such as candida cause no problems at all. However, if the normal balance between good and bad microorganisms in your body is upset, the harmless yeast fungus can overgrow, causing symptoms such as painful red skin, itching, and a white appearance.

Yeast usually flourishes for one of two reasons: Either the good bacteria that keep problem-causing organisms like yeast under control are destroyed (as is the case when you take antibiotics), or an area that is usually fairly dry becomes more moist than normal. Yeast thrives in dark, warm, moist areas — you can have a yeast infection in your vagina, under your breasts, in the baby's diaper area or mouth, or even under your fingernails!

The recent invention of antibacterial soaps, which kill both good and bad germs, may contribute to the spread of yeast. Wearing wet breast pads for extended times can also give candida a nice warm growth area, especially because the fungus grows well in the sugar found in breast milk.

Yeast reproduces itself very quickly and can survive on dry surfaces. It's notoriously hard to get rid of and can infect every member of your family.

Treating thrush in your baby

Babies can acquire yeast infections simply by being born; many pregnant women have yeast infections from increased hormone levels, changes in vaginal pH (acidity), or (dare we say it) increased weight. The weight itself doesn't cause a yeast infection, but an increased number of crevices and folds of skin can provide the dark, moist environment yeast loves. The baby picks up the fungus on his maiden voyage, and from that point on, the two of you may pass it back and forth.

Thrush generally affects babies in one of two ways: as a mouth infection called *oral thrush,* or as a diaper rash. Both are uncomfortable, and oral thrush can interfere with nursing.

Oral thrush usually shows up as white patches inside the baby's mouth, including on the tongue. If you wipe the white area off, you can see reddened, irritated skin underneath. The baby may refuse to nurse, or nurse only a short time before crying. He may be especially gassy (a side effect of yeast). Before the patches show up, you may notice that the baby's saliva and the insides of his cheeks have what's been described as a *pearly* appearance.

The baby may or may not have yeast in the diaper area at the same time. Diaper rash is especially common if the baby is heavy; yeast grows in the moist crevices. Instead of white spots you may see a very bright red, bumpy rash; the affected skin may be cracked and oozing clear fluid and blood.

Oral thrush is usually treated with Nystatin oral suspension, a liquid applied with a cotton swab to the entire inside of the baby's mouth. Nystatin, available by prescription, works best on contact rather than by taking it orally.

If you use Nystatin, pour the liquid into a small cup; don't dip the cotton swab directly into the bottle, especially if you dip the swab several times to paint all the areas. Discard the swabs after use; don't reuse them, or you'll reinfect the area.

· Apply Nystatin after a feeding. The usual dose is four times a day, and you continue treatment for two weeks after all of the symptoms are gone.

Candida in the diaper area is treated with Nystatin cream, which is applied to the entire diaper area four times a day for two weeks. Make sure you complete the treatment, or the yeast may return.

REMEMBER

Both you and your baby need to be treated any time one of you has a yeast infection so you don't keep passing it back and forth to each other. Yeast is very tenacious! Be sure to ask both your obstetrician and the baby's pediatrician for medication to treat both of you. Your partner can also develop a yeast infection on the head of his penis; he may need to be treated as well.

Battling your own yeast infections

You may have a yeast infection and not even know it. With all the discomforts of late pregnancy, a yeast infection may go unnoticed.

REMEMBER

You probably associate yeast with vaginal infections, but yeast can grow anywhere the conditions are right. Pregnancy can foster yeast growth for several reasons: You may develop extra folds of skin under your enlarged abdomen and breasts; you may experience increased perspiration; and your hormone levels spike. Even your chocolate cravings can contribute to the problem, because yeast thrives in a sugar-laden environment!

If you receive antibiotics after a cesarean section, you can easily develop a yeast infection, because killing off the good bacteria with the bad allows yeast to overgrow. You can infect your nipple with yeast by touching another yeasty area, such as your vagina, and then your nipple, or the baby can infect you with thrush from his mouth.

Yeast on your nipples may not be visible at all; your first symptom may be sharp, stabbing pain in the nipple. Sometimes infected nipples crack, itch, burn, or turn bright red. You may even experience shooting pains in the breast.

TIP

If your nipples are infected, your first treatment should be to always wash your hands before touching them. Also, rinse your nipples after each feeding, using either plain water or a vinegar solution made with a tablespoon of vinegar per cup of water. This changes the pH of your skin to make it less hospitable for the yeast to grow.

To cure the fungus, first try a local treatment. After each feeding, apply an antifungal cream to your nipples and areola. Gently wipe off any excess if you can still see it before the next feeding. Some of the common topical antifungal medication brand names are Monistat, Nystatin, and Lotrimin.

You can also try a 1 percent solution of Gentian violet twice a day for three to four days. (Dilute one part Gentian violet to one part water that has been boiled and cooled.) Gentian violet is available in most pharmacies over the counter, but you may have to ask the pharmacist for it. Use a cotton ball or swab to apply it to your nipple and areola. Use caution, though, because it can stain your clothes purple. Cover your nipples with breast pads to prevent bra stains.

TIP

You can also use Gentian violet to treat thrush in the baby's mouth, but be sure to dilute it with two parts water. Apply it to all of the surfaces in the baby's mouth, and use it for no more than three days; continued use may irritate the baby's mucous membranes. Apply some Lansinoh cream around the baby's mouth to keep the Gentian violet from staining her skin.

If topical solutions don't work, you may need to take a pill called Diflucan. Your doctor can prescribe this medication; you'll need a two-week course to make sure the yeast is eradicated. Also, be sure to talk to your lactation consultant. She may have additional information on how to help you treat thrush.

A vaginal or skin yeast infection is treated in the same way, trying topical medications first and then using Diflucan if they don't work.

Knowing When Crying Becomes Colic

Do you recognize this baby? He's sleeping peacefully in his infant seat as you stir the spaghetti sauce for dinner. Suddenly, he wakes up, draws his knees up to his chest, and begins to howl. You try feeding him, rocking him, carrying him in the sling, putting him in the swing, singing to him, jiggling him up and down, and he just cries. And cries. By the time your partner walks in, two hours later, you and the baby are both sobbing. You shove the baby at him, pour the burned spaghetti sauce down the disposal, and collapse in a heap on the nearest chair.

The first time this happens, you may chalk it up to a bad day. By the fourth or fifth day in a row, your worst suspicions are confirmed. Your baby has colic.

Recognizing the signs

Distinguishing a crying infant from a colicky infant isn't difficult. Both babies are trying to tell you something, but with the crying baby, you can usually figure out what it is. A colicky baby is just as confused as you are, uncertain about why he's feeling this way.

The word *colic* comes from the Greek word *kolikos,* which translates roughly into "colon." Colic has long been thought to be a gastrointestinal problem. Unfortunately, no one is really sure what colic is, or why it happens. One thing that everyone involved knows is it can bring parents as well as babies to tears.

Colic attacks start early, at around 2 weeks old. Colic occurs in about 20 percent of babies, occurring equally in boys and girls, whether breastfed or bottle-fed. It generally reaches a peak at around 6 weeks but may continue until 4 months of age. The worst part of this early infancy condition is that there's no known cause and no specific treatment. This is what makes a colicky baby so frustrating.

Colic seems to occur most often in firstborns. Perhaps that's due to first-time parents being nervous about their parenting skills. We can attest that parenting skills become more fine-tuned with each baby, resulting in calmer, more relaxed parents. But beware: Even if your first three babies are angels, the fourth one may have colic. (Your coauthor Sharon knows from experience!)

As quickly as it comes, colic can disappear, or the good days may slowly replace the bad ones. However it ends, by the time it goes away, everyone in your household will be exhausted, frazzled, and praying that your baby will soon go off to college.

REMEMBER

Colic-type symptoms occasionally can indicate a more serious problem. Notify your pediatrician if your baby develops colic to rule out any potential serious conditions that the colic symptoms could camouflage.

Avoiding foods that upset baby

Sometimes what you eat can aggravate colic. If you suspect this may be the case, experiment with eliminating certain foods from your diet to see if the colic improves.

Linking colic and cow's milk

If your baby's colic is worsened by what you eat, cow's milk is the most likely culprit. Gas can form inside his bowel from the protein in the cow's milk, causing cramping, diarrhea, abdominal pain, or vomiting.

Sensitivity to cow's milk doesn't happen overnight. It usually takes about two to three weeks before a colicky reaction shows up.

To test for cow's milk sensitivity, completely eliminate dairy products from your diet for at least two weeks. It will take that long to clear your system. If dairy products are the culprit, you'll see a much happier baby within four to five days. If you don't see an improvement in a week or so, dairy is probably not the culprit.

If you do see an improvement, try reintroducing dairy products into your diet slowly. Start with processed forms of milk products, such as hard cheeses like cheddar or Swiss. The more processed the product, the easier it will be for your baby to digest. If cheese doesn't seem to upset him, next try softer dairy products, such as cottage cheese, ice cream, and yogurt. The last thing you want to reintroduce is milk. If, at any point, your baby's horror movie personality reappears, back off all dairy products and try again in three to four weeks.

REMEMBER

People of Asian, African, or Hispanic descent have a higher chance of being lactose intolerant. You may be surprised to find that you feel better yourself when you lower your dairy intake.

If you're a real dairy lover and feel withdrawal symptoms, try soy or rice milk instead of cow's milk. Use non-dairy creamers. Think sorbet instead of ice cream. You don't need to drink milk to make milk!

TIP

If you're giving supplemental formula, use soy-based formula if cow's milk in your diet causes problems for your baby.

Diagnosing other diet issues

Some foods — such as cabbage, broccoli, and beans — have a reputation for causing intestinal problems or for giving your milk a flavor that the baby may refuse. But not every nursing mom has the exact same experience. Spicy foods and foods that give you gas may cause your baby to have an upset stomach. Then again, they may not!

Before dismissing things like corned beef and cabbage permanently from your diet, try them one at a time. Doing so can help you figure out whether your baby reacts negatively when you eat them.

Another common culprit is caffeine, which can make you and your baby more restless and irritable. Try to limit yourself to two caffeinated drinks per day.

Watch out for foods that you or your partner are allergic to, because allergies sometimes run in families. In addition to cow's milk, common allergic foods include peanuts, eggs, wheat products, soy, citrus foods, corn, and fish. An allergy could cause colic symptoms, or it could take the form of asthma, diarrhea, or eczema. Babies exposed to allergens at an early age are more likely to develop allergic reactions to them later in life.

Soothing a colicky baby

Despite your friends' and family members' opinions, no hard and fast remedies for colic exist. Some techniques work for one baby and not another. Experiment with these suggestions until you find something that helps!

- **Hold him.** Babies love to be held. Some also like to be tightly wrapped (swaddled) in a blanket. Try holding your colicky baby in an upright position, which helps if the symptoms of colic are a result of reflux (which we discuss in the next section).

  You may also try the colic hold (see Figure 8-1), which puts pressure on the baby's abdomen and can help ease the pressure from intestinal gas.

- **Move it!** Most babies love movement, but make sure that you're not overstimulating him. Move him in a gentle rocking, rolling motion — don't take him on a roller coaster ride! Try walking him, putting him in a baby swing, rocking him in a chair, going for a ride in the car, or taking him for a walk in a stroller.

- **Make some noise.** Many babies like background noise, such as a vacuum or clothes dryer. Try putting her in her baby seat, securely fastened, and placing it on top of the dryer. (You'll have to stand right there to make sure she doesn't vibrate off the machine, though!) One of our friends swore by the vacuum cleaner; she ran it day and night.

Running water also is soothing; you can buy CDs with running water sounds, if you're trying to keep the water bill down! Other CDs reproduce the sounds the baby heard in the womb, which may help her calm down.

Also, try singing or humming to your baby — your voice may be the most soothing sound of all.

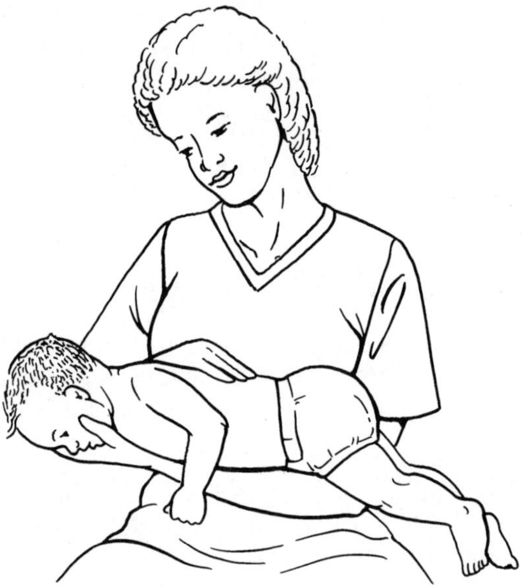

Figure 8-1: Positioning the baby in a colic hold may help ease distress and calm him down.

- **Get (the baby) naked.** Some babies don't like to be swaddled — they actually feel better when their clothes are removed. Just make sure the room is warm.
- **Keep calm.** Overstimulation with noise, lights, and conversation may make your baby feel worse. Signs of overstimulation include spitting up, hiccups, and yawning.
- **Make sure you're not part of the problem.** Avoid stimulants such as coffee, tea, and other caffeinated beverages. Evaluate your diet to be sure something you're eating isn't causing the baby discomfort.
- **Warm his belly.** Sometimes warmth on the baby's abdomen brings comfort. You can place a hot water bottle (filled with *warm* water, never hot) on his abdomen; wrap it in a soft cloth — never place it directly on his skin. Remember that the baby's skin is much more sensitive than yours. Test the water temperature on a delicate area, such as the inside of your wrist.

- **Consider medications.** Years ago, doctors recommended using sedatives and even barbiturates, such as Paragoric, to calm a colicky baby. These medications put the baby to sleep but didn't address the cause of the problem. Today, some doctors recommend using anti-gas agents (such as Mylicon drops) and anti-spasmodic medications. Medications don't always help, but they may be worth a try — ask your pediatrician.
- **Know your limits.** Some babies are very sensitive to their surroundings. If you get upset, your baby may get upset, too. Know when you've had enough. When Dad comes home, you may need to hand her over for a while. If your partner isn't available, get someone else to help you. Even a short break can improve your state of mind. Stepping away could also prevent the possibility of hurting your baby. A screaming baby can be overwhelming. Don't be afraid to admit it.

Nursing through colic

If your baby is experiencing colic, keep the following in mind:

- **Nursing from both breasts at each feeding may result in the baby getting too much foremilk and not enough hindmilk.** The *hindmilk* — the creamier milk that appears after the baby has been eating for several minutes — has a high fat content that is needed to satisfy her hunger. If the baby doesn't get the hindmilk, she needs to nurse more often. This means she takes in more foremilk, which contains more sugar. The sugar load, without the fat to balance it, can cause gas and explosive bowel movements.

  TIP: If your baby's distress seems to be accompanied by loose green bowel movements, she may be getting too much foremilk. Try letting her nurse as long as she wants on one breast, so she gets enough hindmilk to keep her satiated longer. When she nurses again, start on the opposite side, and repeat the process.
- **Your baby may be allergic to substances in your diet.** Most times the allergy is to cow's milk (see "Linking colic and cow's milk" earlier in the chapter).
- **An overactive let-down reflex can cause colic-type symptoms due to frustration in the baby.** We discuss this later in the chapter, in the section "Having Too Much of a Good Thing."

Colic-type symptoms are not a reason to give up breastfeeding. Chances are that your baby's symptoms would worsen if you switched to formula. Colic symptoms should resolve by four to six months. And just think: In the years that follow, you can share stories of these trying times with your teenager. He'll get a good laugh, and so will you!

Dealing with Vomiting and Reflux

Some babies vomit, and some babies *vomit.* Your coauthor Sharon's life would have been a lot easier when her fourth son was throwing up on every surface in the house if doctors had known what they know now about reflux.

Not all babies who spit up have reflux. Studies show that as many as half of all babies spit up daily between the ages of 1 and 3 months. (This is no secret to parents; hardly a mother alive doesn't have telltale yellow stains on the shoulders of nearly every shirt she owns.) By six or seven months, only 20 percent of babies are still daily vomiters, and the number decreases to 5 percent by one year.

Spitting up after feedings is normal. Usually the amount is small, and the milk sort of rolls out of the baby's mouth. This is the kind of spitting up that burp cloths were invented for.

A baby spits up after feedings for several reasons:

- **She swallowed air during the feeding.** This is most common when you have a forceful let-down reflex and the baby has to swallow a large amount of milk quickly.
- **The baby nurses frequently, and you have a large supply of milk.** If your baby is a comfort nurser, she may simply be taking in more milk than her stomach can hold. The excess may be spit up.
- **She may be sensitive to something in your diet.** Some babies vomit if you eat a large amount of an allergenic food, such as dairy products.

Spitting up is not a problem for most babies. They gain weight, cry a normal amount, and leave yellow stains on clothing. And then there's reflux.

Diagnosing reflux

Gastroesophageal reflux disease (GERD), commonly called *reflux,* is a problem found in infants and adults alike. It occurs when the ring of muscle found at the top of the stomach, where the stomach meets the esophagus, doesn't close properly (see Figure 8-2).

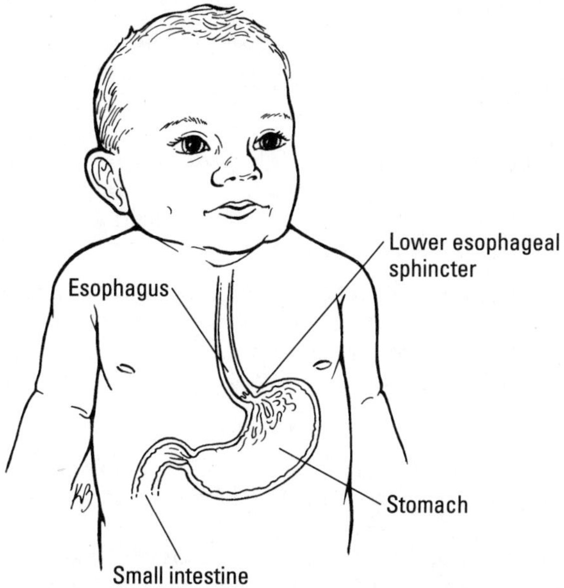

Figure 8-2: Reflux is caused by improper closure of the muscle at the meeting point of the esophagus and stomach.

Here's how reflux works: Milk moves from the stomach back into the esophagus, along with acid from the stomach. (Adults experience this as heartburn — the pain is caused by the acid irritating the lining of the esophagus.) The milk and acid can be aspirated into the baby's lungs, causing respiratory problems as well as pain.

Babies with reflux vomit, cry, refuse to nurse, sound hoarse, wheeze, gag, have apnea, wake up crying, and may be slow to gain weight. Breast milk is better for babies with reflux because it irritates esophageal tissue less than formula, and it leaves the stomach faster so it has less time to back up into the esophagus.

Most babies with GERD are diagnosed according to their symptoms rather than through medical procedures. If necessary, reflux can be diagnosed by medical procedures such as an upper GI series, where the baby is fed a barium solution that can be seen on an x-ray. Acid levels in the baby's throat can also be measured using a pH probe.

Treating reflux with simple methods

Sometimes simple methods for treating reflux have good results, and you can avoid medications. Try these methods first if you suspect your baby has reflux:

- **Feed your baby in an upright position.** Keep the baby's head higher than his stomach. Using the football hold (see Chapter 6) or using a baby sling may help you hold him more upright. Gravity can help the milk stay down.
- **Keep the baby upright after feeding for at least 30 minutes.** Keep her in the baby sling or in an infant seat. If you use an infant seat, make sure she's not bent in a position that puts too much pressure on her abdomen.
- **Make sure you get the burps up.** As tempting as it is to lie a sleeping baby down without burping her first, you'll probably pay later when the burp brings with it half the last feeding and some irritating acid to boot.
- **Express milk first if you have a heavy let-down.** Nurse for a minute to encourage your let-down reflex, and then take your baby off the breast and "mop up" the first forceful amounts of breast milk. This prevents her from having to gulp and swallow large amounts of air.
- **Keep the baby away from cigarette smoke.** Secondhand smoke can aggravate reflux.
- **Experiment.** Some babies do better if they nurse on one side at each feeding. This encourages them to take in more of the calorie-laden hindmilk, rather than needing larger amounts of foremilk to satisfy their hunger. Some do better with small frequent feedings, others with larger feedings further apart.
- **Keep the baby calm after feedings.** Most parents know this, but visitors may not! Right after a feeding isn't the best time to toss her in the air and tickle her from head to toe.

Medicating reflux babies

If the methods in the previous section fail, or help only a little, you may need to go to your pediatrician for drugs. (By this time, you may need drugs yourself!) Esophageal damage from reflux can be treated effectively by several different categories of medication.

TIP

Most medication used for reflux falls into one of the following categories: antacids, acid blockers, acid inhibitors, anti-ulcer medications, and drugs that affect *motility* — movement of food through the stomach.

- Antacids neutralize acid in the stomach, which decreases the harm done to the esophagus. The frequency of reflux won't decrease. Mylanta and Maalox are antacids. Antacids should not be used for extended time periods because they contain aluminum; they may also cause diarrhea and, in high doses, may cause *rickets,* a thinning of the bones.
- Medications such as Mylicon or Gavescon lessen intestinal gas.
- Xantac, Tagamet, and Pepcid are acid inhibitors and blockers that decrease the production of acid in the stomach. Like antacids, they don't decrease the frequency of reflux, just the damage and pain from the acid entering the esophagus. These medications may cause drowsiness.
- Carafate, an anti-ulcer medication, coats the stomach with a foam-like layer that allows it to heal.
- Reglan increases motility in the stomach, as does erythromycin, an antibiotic. These medications move milk through the stomach more quickly, leaving less to be vomited. Long-term use of Reglan may cause stiff or tense muscles and *tardive dyskenesia* — unusual muscle movements or twitches. These side effects are rare. Reglan may also increase seizure activity in babies with a seizure disorder.

WARNING!

Because many of these medications react with each other, your baby's doctor must be aware of all medications being given to your baby, including over-the-counter medications.

Surgically treating reflux

In severe cases, reflux is treated with a surgical procedure called *Nissen fundoplication.* This procedure is done under general anesthesia, so it should be considered only if all other methods of controlling reflux have failed. The top part of the baby's stomach is wrapped around the lower part of the esophagus so that food can get into the stomach but can't get back out as easily.

Living with reflux: Sharon's story

In retrospect, I can say with great confidence that my fourth son, Benjamin, had reflux. He was a crying, scrawny, vomiting breastfed baby. Only another parent of a baby with reflux can understand what it's like to have a baby who cries all the time. *All* the time: all day, all night. Our next-door neighbors commented on it when Benjamin was 8 months old and we had the windows open. Nothing helped. He was frequently sick; when he was admitted to the hospital with a virus, his doctor referred to him in an admitting note as a "frail-looking infant who has been somewhat sickly his entire life." What an understatement.

He vomited frequently until he was 15 months old. All our rugs were permanently stained when he started to crawl. We spent night after night rocking him. His doctor had no suggestions and no answers, except that he'd outgrow it eventually. He also recommended trying hypoallergenic formulas instead of breastfeeding, which didn't help at all and probably worsened things.

Benjamin did outgrow it and became a delightful, happy child. But the misery he, and we, went through would have been greatly alleviated if reflux had been treated in infants in the '70s as it is now.

No matter what treatment your baby requires for reflux, the good news is that all but a tiny percentage of babies outgrow reflux problems by the time they're 18 months old.

Realizing complications of reflux

Over 90 percent of babies with reflux outgrow it; those who don't may need surgery (see the sidebar nearby "Surgically treating reflux"). Most babies have no long-term effects from reflux.

A few babies with reflux experience recurrent pneumonia, which results in long-term lung damage. A small number develop *strictures,* or narrowing in the esophagus, which may need to be surgically enlarged.

Increasing a Low Milk Supply

Some moms don't make enough milk to completely supply their babies' needs. If your baby isn't gaining enough weight despite frequent nursing, your doctor may prescribe medication to increase your milk supply, or a lactation consultant may suggest taking herbs such as fenugreek.

These remedies have both positive and negative effects and should be weighed carefully. None of them should be taken until you've eliminated poor latch-on, ineffective sucking, or infrequent nursing as possible reasons for decreased milk supply.

Taking prescription medications

If your milk supply is low, your doctor may recommend taking either Reglan or Motilium.

Reglan

Reglan, a drug that can be used to treat reflux, is also used to increase milk supply. Reglan (generic name *metocloramide*) is a pill that you take three or four times a day for a week; you then reduce its frequency of use for the next week. Reglan increases your secretion of *prolactin,* the hormone responsible for milk production.

You should see results within two to four days of starting Reglan. You must continue nursing and/or pumping frequently to make sure your milk supply increases.

Reglan has some potentially serious side effects. You shouldn't take it if you have asthma or a seizure disorder, because Reglan may worsen both of these problems. Also avoid Reglan if you have high blood pressure or intestinal problems, such as bleeding or obstruction. Reglan can also worsen depression.

In very rare cases, people taking Reglan have developed *tardive dyskenesia,* a neuromuscular problem. This disorder causes unusual muscle twitches or movements or lack of coordination. Call your doctor immediately and stop taking Reglan if this occurs.

More common side effects of Reglan are drowsiness, headache, and diarrhea. You should take Reglan for no more than a few weeks.

Motilium

Motilium isn't readily available in the United States, because it isn't yet FDA approved, but some pharmacies *compound* it (create it in-house rather than purchasing it in pill form). This is perfectly legal; you just need a doctor's prescription. Like Reglan, Motilium (generic name *domperidone*) increases milk production by increasing the hormone prolactin.

You take Motilium three to four times a day for up to eight weeks. It has fewer side effects than Reglan; most common are headache, dry mouth, and abdominal cramping. Positive results are usually seen within three to four days of starting the medication.

Using herbs to increase milk supply

Many lactation consultants suggest the use of herbs, such as fenugreek, to increase milk production. Fenugreek, which is used largely as a seasoning for food in Middle Eastern countries, is a very safe herbal supplement. Many mothers have good success using fenugreek to help increase their milk supply, and it is often used prior to trying Reglan or Motilium.

Fenugreek needs to be taken in fairly high doses — six to twelve pills a day divided into three doses — to have a positive effect. Most mothers notice an improvement in their milk supply within two to three days. This herb is also used to flavor maple syrup products, and taking large amounts will make you, your milk, and your baby smell like a walking maple syrup factory. In some cases, this has resulted in babies being mistakenly diagnosed with Maple Syrup Urine Disease, a serious metabolic disorder. Make sure your baby's doctor knows you're using fenugreek!

WARNING!

Fenugreek, like most herbs, is not without side effects and absolutely should not be used in some circumstances. Don't use it if you are pregnant, because it can cause uterine contractions. Don't use it if you have asthma, because it could worsen your condition. Fenugreek can also cause low blood sugar and changes in heart and blood pressure. Because it's related to the peanut family (one of the most commonly known allergens), it can also cause allergic reactions in you or the baby.

Other herbs often recommended are Blessed Thistle, fennel, and alfalfa. Blessed Thistle is probably safe in small amounts, although no formal studies have shown any real benefit from taking it. This is true for alfalfa and fennel as well.

REMEMBER

Herbal manufacturers are not well regulated, and many people have suffered adverse reactions from taking over-the-counter herbal preparations in recent years. Be very careful about taking any type of herb!

Having Too Much of a Good Thing

Two problems some breastfeeding moms experience are hyperactive let-down and *hyperlactation,* or an overabundant milk supply.

Hyperactive let-down

Most women experience hyperactive let-down — having too much milk coming down too fast — for the first few days after delivery. But for some women, the problem persists.

How do you know you have a hyperactive let-down reflex? Your baby latches on and begins to nurse, then pulls off coughing and sputtering to catch his breath. While the baby is off the breast, you may see streams of milk spraying forcefully from your nipple. Your other breast may be leaking copiously at the same time.

If you have hyperactive let-down, try expressing some milk first to get beyond the initial forceful flow of milk, then put the baby on the breast. This prevents the baby from gulping in air, which can cause gas. Also, use gravity to your advantage: Try reclining after the baby gets latched on to help slow down the flow of milk.

Hyperlactation

If breast milk is good, then a lot of breast milk is better, right? Not necessarily. There is such a thing as having too much milk, and it can cause problems just as having too little milk can.

Why is overabundant milk supply a problem? When you have too much milk, the baby gets full on the large amount of foremilk. If the baby eats a large amount of foremilk, which is high in sugar, he may become gassy and colicky, passing frequent watery green stools. Your nipple may be white or creased at the end of the feeding, from his efforts to slow down the copious flow. He may also stop drinking before he gets the hindmilk, which contains more fat and keeps him satisfied longer between feedings.

To allow the baby to get to the hindmilk, you may need to feed him on the same breast — and only one breast — for two or more feedings. In other words, if you feed him on the left breast at 2 a.m., you give him the left breast again at 5 a.m. This helps empty the breast so he gets to the hindmilk without becoming full on foremilk. It also helps concentrate the milk supply by decreasing stimulation to the other breast for a period of time.

If the other breast becomes engorged or uncomfortably full, express just enough milk to ease the pressure, so as not to stimulate more milk production on that side.

WARNING! Moms with hyperlactation have a higher chance of developing plugged ducts or mastitis. Watch for the signs we describe earlier in the chapter.

If you really have a lot of extra milk, consider doing something wonderful for someone else. Contact a milk bank (see Chapter 9) to see if you can donate your excess to a baby who needs it.

Feeling Like a Failure

All babies aren't easy to nurse; some seem to fight breastfeeding, pulling away from the breast, fighting against being held in a nursing position, and making their mothers feel rejected, as if the baby somehow doesn't like them or their milk.

If you have a baby like this, we empathize. But we also want to reassure you that you're not being rejected by your baby in any way. Not every breastfeeding story has a happy ending, and most of the time, it isn't anyone's fault.

Giving your baby a break

Women choose to breastfeed for many reasons. The main reason, for most of you, is because you know it's the best thing to do for the baby. You invest a lot of time preparing yourself for life with him, and when he doesn't nurse well, you can feel personally rejected.

Unfortunately, the baby isn't aware of your expectations. He doesn't have the advantage of picking up this book and reading about "what to do when you're hungry, what to do when you don't feel like nursing, what to do when your mom's not holding you comfortably."

REMEMBER Your baby doesn't choose to be a difficult nurser. He doesn't have a preconceived idea of what he's going to do when he arrives at your home. Many new moms think that their babies should know how to breastfeed because it's as natural as the sun in the sky. This is not true. Babies learn how to nurse with your help and direction.

Giving yourself a break

When breastfeeding doesn't go well, no one is to blame. Following are a few things to remember if you struggle with breastfeeding:

- If you nurse your baby for a week, and you decide to bottle feed after that, you've given your baby a great gift.
- You can only guide your baby; you can't make him nurse. Don't be physically aggressive in your attempt to put him on the breast.
- Believe it or not, your baby really isn't behaving this way to drive you crazy!
- Wherever you can get the job done is fine. It could be your bed or your bath. Use trial and error to find the right place to nurse.
- Help is available. Ask for help from your lactation consultant, a La Leche League representative, or your pediatrician.
- Your instincts are usually right — follow them.
- A mom who is exhausted cannot nurse well, so be sure to get some rest. Until breastfeeding is established, get someone else to handle the running of the household.
- Monitoring your own nutrition is crucial (see Chapter 7). If you don't eat or drink enough, you'll have a milk production problem. You need energy and calories to make milk.
- If you're feeling like a failure at breastfeeding, you could easily be experiencing the baby blues, or even the much more serious postpartum depression. See Chapter 7 for information on both.

Making the decision to wean

Most moms go through a difficult time if they decide to stop breastfeeding because of difficulties. Only time heals these wounds.

No matter how old your baby is when you wean, you may go through a grieving stage, which can be overwhelming. More than likely, you've been trying for weeks to nurse your baby — sometimes successfully, sometimes not. When you finally reach the decision to stop, you may feel a tremendous loss.

Only after you realize that your relationship with your baby hasn't changed (except perhaps to improve because you've removed a daily struggle) will you feel better. Until you reach that point, don't doubt your mothering skills because you decided not to continue with breastfeeding. Mothering is so much bigger than this. You're so much more to your baby than a source of nutrition.

Listening to your baby's signals: Carol's difficult nurser

Jonathan is my second son, and he is my living example of "listening to your baby's signals." He breastfed well in the hospital, but after a few weeks, Jonathan's personality was starting to evolve, and nursing wasn't going well. I tried everyone's suggestions, which ran the gamut from putting a little sugar on the nipple to getting into a bathtub to nurse him in a quiet environment. Everyone's intentions were good, but I was still facing a baby who fought nursing, cuddling, and closeness. After six weeks, I decided that bottle feeding was going to be best for the entire family. It was a difficult decision, and I felt guilt and a sense of loss.

As time passed, I saw that Jonathan behaved the same way with a bottle. He didn't like to be held close. I had to hold his bottle outward into the room, rather than pointed to my chest. Perhaps this was his problem with nursing. He was telling me something, but I wasn't listening!

Jonathan grew into a wonderful young man who is probably my most sensitive son, loving but still "hands off." He's proof that personalities develop early!

Chapter 9

Breastfeeding in Special Circumstances

In This Chapter

- Breastfeeding a premature baby
- Feeding twins or triplets
- Nursing a baby with health problems
- Choosing to nurse an adopted baby
- Breastfeeding through illness and surgery
- Banking milk

Sometimes pregnancy and breastfeeding don't go as planned. You may deliver prematurely, deliver twins or triplets, or have a baby with health problems. Each of these situations complicates nursing.

Even after nursing is established, things can go wrong; you or the baby may get sick, or one of you may need surgery. You may need to use banked breast milk. Or, on the brighter side, you may want to donate breast milk to a milk bank, or to breastfeed your newly adopted baby. In this chapter, we look at breastfeeding under all kinds of special conditions.

Nursing a Preemie

Giving birth prematurely can be such a shock that breastfeeding may be the last thing on your mind. But breast milk can help protect *preemies* (premature babies) from the infections they commonly experience. You may not be able to nurse your baby physically at first, if he's unable to take feedings because he's on oxygen or not strong enough to suck well. However, you can pump milk in order to establish your milk supply for when the baby comes home, and that pumped milk can be tube-fed to your baby as soon as he's able to receive feedings.

If your baby is born early, the milk you produce is different than the milk you would produce if the baby were born full-term. Premature milk contains more protein, iron, sodium, and chloride. It's easily digestible, so your baby uses fewer calories to break it down — calories he needs to grow. The milk is also richer in factors that help your baby's immune system mature.

Like full-term breast milk, premature breast milk contains antibodies to protect your baby from infection. Studies have shown that babies fed breast milk are three times less likely than bottle-fed babies to contract *Necrotizing Enterocolitis,* or NEC, a bowel infection that affects 5 to 12 percent of all preemies and has a death rate of 20 to 40 percent.

Breast milk also decreases the chance of eye damage, common to babies born prematurely. This may be due to the presence of DHA, a fatty acid found in breast milk.

Keeping up your supply

Staff members in neonatal intensive care units (NICUs) are usually well aware of the value of breast milk for preemies and do everything they can to help you establish your supply and keep it going while your baby is hospitalized. Keep the following in mind if you find yourself needing to pump milk for a preemie:

- Most hospitals have (or can find for you) commercial grade electric breast pumps (see Chapter 5). If your baby is premature, your insurance may pay for the pump. To establish your milk supply and keep it up for weeks or even months, you need a commercial pump that can pump both breasts at one time.
- The NICU usually supplies you with small bags or bottles for collecting your milk. These have labels so you can write down the date and your name; you don't want your milk getting mixed up with anyone else's in the hospital freezer! You'll need to freeze any milk not being used within a day or two; if your baby isn't ready for feedings yet, you can build up a frozen supply for when he's able to feed.

  If you freeze milk, don't overfill the containers. Milk expands as it freezes, and you don't want to blow the top off your carefully saved liquid gold.

TIP

- Fresh is better than frozen milk; frozen milk loses some of its nutrients. After your baby starts to take tube feedings, fresh milk can be used each day; most NICUs have a refrigerator to store that day's milk. If they don't, buy a cooler and keep it at the nurses' station or at the baby's bed side. Put your name on it in big, bright letters so it doesn't get lost!
- You need to pump eight to twelve times a day to establish your milk supply. Two medications, Reglan and Motilium, can be helpful if your milk supply drops after five or six weeks of pumping without actually nursing. (See Chapter 8 for more about these medications.)

If your delivery hospital can't meet all of your baby's needs, he may be taken to a different hospital for care. In this situation, you may find yourself exhausted, visiting the baby as soon as you're released while trying to take care of yourself and possibly your other children. This type of stress, along with concern for the baby, can put a real dent in your milk supply. Don't let pumping fall by the wayside! Take your pump with you when you visit the baby, and sit in a quiet room somewhere and pump for 20 minutes. (Most NICUs have quiet rooms for nursing moms.)

If your baby is very tiny or very ill, pumping to keep up your milk supply may sometimes seem like a waste of time. Feeling this way is normal; don't feel guilty about it. If you pump more milk than your baby will ever be able to drink, consider donating some to a breast milk bank (which we discuss later in this chapter in the sidebar "Banking breast milk").

REMEMBER

Not every new mom can maintain her milk supply for months just through pumping, so don't feel guilty if you can't. Take pride in the fact that you did the best you could for your baby.

Breastfeeding in the NICU

Some preemies are able to nurse fairly soon after birth. If your baby is 33 or so weeks at the time of delivery (a normal pregnancy lasts 40 weeks), you may be able to breastfeed as soon as the baby's breathing stabilizes. This may happen in a day or a week.

TIP

Some preemies do well nursing with the help of a preemie-sized nipple shield. The shield helps keep the breast in the baby's mouth with less energy expenditure than breastfeeding without the shield. You still need to pump to maintain an adequate milk supply, and you'll need to wean the baby off the nipple shield as she grows stronger and can handle breastfeeding without it.

Your coauthor Sharon nursed two preemies in the NICU — one born at 33 weeks and one at 35 weeks. My 35-weeker had trouble breathing and had to be transported (during a major Ohio blizzard, no less) to a larger hospital. A few days later he was sent back to our local hospital. I went to see him a few times a day for feedings, and I took pumped breast milk in for the remaining feedings. We had no trouble at all establishing breastfeeding when he was discharged two weeks later.

My 33-weeker was also hospitalized for two weeks. Because he was almost an hour away and I had two other small children, I could visit him only once a day. Again, I pumped and eventually breastfed him once a day. We had no trouble establishing breastfeeding full-time when he came home.

In both cases, the hospitals involved were very supportive of breastfeeding. They supplied a separate room for nursing moms, encouraged frequent visits, and observed to make sure breastfeeding was going well before the baby was discharged.

WARNING! Some hospitals don't have the space for separate nursing rooms; you may find yourself separated from the hubbub of the nursery by a flimsy screen. Nothing is less conducive to let-down than to hear the NICU staff working on a sick baby on the other side of the screen. Beg for a private room, even if you have to use the nursing administrator's room after hours.

Tube- or finger-feeding breast milk

Long before your preemie can suck on a nipple, he can be fed breast milk through a *nasogastric tube,* which goes through the nose directly into the baby's stomach. Studies have shown that breast milk decreases the chance of infection and diarrhea no matter how it's given, so try to have a supply of breast milk ready as soon as your baby can tolerate any type of feeding.

TIP If your baby's going to be in the hospital only a short time and you want to avoid nipple confusion (see Chapter 5), ask if the nurses are willing to try finger-feeding the baby. This isn't as disgusting as it sounds: The baby isn't actually eating off the nurse's finger, but sucking milk through a tube attached to her finger.

With finger feeding, a tube runs from the milk supply to the feeder's finger. The baby can suck on the feeder's finger, and the milk flows into the baby's mouth. You need to keep the pad of your finger facing upward, to stimulate the same kind of suck the baby will use to breastfeed. This process is time-consuming, and some hospital staff members won't have the time or patience for it. However, they may be willing to let you try it.

Preterm babies can also be fed by cup or spoon, although this too is very time-consuming. Some studies show that cup-feeding is less stressing physically to preemies than bottle feeding. If you use a cup or spoon, be sure to give the baby milk slowly; don't pour it into the baby's mouth!

If you have difficulty keeping your milk supply up through pumping, you can still breastfeed by using a lactation aid (which we discuss in the section "Using lactation aids" later in this chapter). You supply formula or pumped breast milk through a tube taped to your nipple; the baby's sucking stimulates your milk production while he receives nutrition through the tube.

Fortifying breast milk

Human breast milk contains 20 calories per ounce; formulas made for premature babies contain 24 calories per ounce. To help your baby gain weight faster by increasing the calorie count of breast milk, some NICUs add a human milk fortifier to breast milk. In addition to calories, fortifiers may also add phosphorus, sodium, and calcium, which may be low in preterm breast milk.

The problem with fortifiers is that they're based on cow's milk and may trigger allergic reactions. Talk to your baby's doctor about whether the benefits outweigh the risks of adding fortifiers to your breast milk.

Another way to increase the caloric count of your breast milk is to save the *hindmilk* — the milk produced at the end of a feeding — separately from the foremilk. Hindmilk is higher in calories than foremilk. If you're concerned about your baby's weight gain, ask her doctor about the possibility of feeding mostly hindmilk.

Bringing your preemie home

Most hospitals discharge preemies when they weigh less than 5 pounds, as long as they're doing well. Studies have shown that babies gain weight faster and are healthier at home.

You may find that your preemie doesn't cry when she's hungry. Watch for signs that she's ready to eat; she may mouth her fist or turn her head while moving her hand toward her face. Try to feed her before she starts crying; crying uses calories she needs to devote to growing.

Handling Twin Nursers (or More!)

Can you breastfeed twins? Of course you can — you have two breasts! What about triplets, quads, or more? Obviously, the more babies you have, the less likely that you'll be able to breastfeed all of them without supplementing with bottles.

If you have twins, you should be able to breastfeed without supplementation. If your twins are premature — and many are — the information in the previous section can give you some ideas on breastfeeding a preemie or two.

If you're able to breastfeed your twins right after delivery, you may wonder if you should start feeding both at the same time or each one separately. For scheduling purposes, you'll probably find it easier to feed both at the same time; otherwise, you may feel as if you're breastfeeding 24 hours a day. However, you may want to nurse them separately at first to make sure they're both latching on properly and nursing well.

Positioning two babies at once

If you deliver more than one baby, a twin breastfeeding pillow is probably the best investment you can make. The pillows, which are C- or U-shaped, allow you to position two babies for feeding at one time. (See Chapter 5 for more about breastfeeding pillows.)

You can place the babies so that their legs cross over each other, in the cradle hold, as shown Figure 9-1a. Many twin moms find the football hold, as shown in Figure 9-1b, to be the easiest way to feed both babies at one time. Or you can face both babies in the same direction so that one baby's head is resting on the body of the other.

Trying to latch two babies on at the same time can be a real challenge. You get A on, and B falls off the pillow. You pick B back up, and A comes off the breast. A kicks B in the face, and they both come off, so you start all over. Don't expect this to go well right off the bat; you all are learning, and the learning curve with two is going to be steeper than it is with just one.

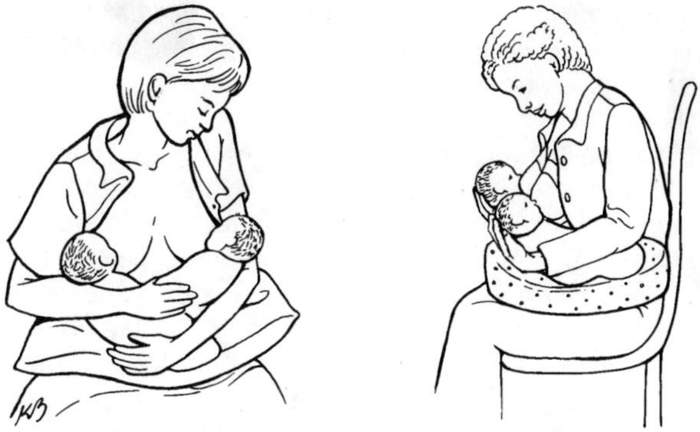

a. b.

Figure 9-1: Twins can be positioned in a variety of ways for simultaneous feedings.

Deciding when and where to feed

If you decide to feed both babies at the same time, you probably want to schedule feedings based on the hungrier of the two babies. Make sure you alternate sides, so that you don't end up lopsided from one baby drinking more than the other.

Consider changing sides daily rather than with each feeding. Even when we were feeding one baby at a time, we got confused about which side we started and finished on!

You may want to keep a notebook of who's eating when, especially if the babies aren't on the same schedule. You don't want to be feeding one baby twice and skipping the other altogether! If your twins are identical, find some way to tell them apart until you get to know them better. Put something distinctive on one that won't come off, like a little ankle bracelet. (If you do something like nail polish on one, make sure you hide the nail polish so your 2-year-old doesn't come down one morning and color all the toes on both babies. It may be years before you figure out which one is really Tommy and which one is Timmy!)

When you're doing a lot of night feedings, consider keeping the babies in your room and feeding them in bed with you. On the other hand, if your partner's a light sleeper, he may be totally unable to sleep because of the nightly activity. You may find it easier to put a cot in the babies' room to sleep on if that's the case.

If you plan on nursing twins, organize your nursing areas ahead of time. You'll need several nursing "stations" set up, one on each floor if you have a multi-story house. You need to be prepared, when the babies come home, to make nursing your full-time job for a while. Help is almost essential.

One of the best things about breastfeeding, especially with twins, is that it forces you to sit down. You may be able to walk around nursing one baby while making dinner, but you'll find it impossible to do with two. So sit down. Spend some time getting to know your babies as individuals. You may find that your babies' nursing styles, like their personalities, are quite different. Perhaps one nurses with a single-minded seriousness while the other looks around, smiles, and lets milk dribble out of the corner of her mouth. Nursing your twins provides you with ample opportunity to get to know them.

When your twins get a little older and cut down on their feedings, you may want to feed them separately. As the babies grow, they may kick each other or entertain each other so much that they're not concentrating on eating if you feed them together. Feeding them separately also gives you some one-on-one time with each baby.

Seeking advice

If at all possible, attend Mothers of Twins meetings as soon as you're able to comb your hair and get dressed. No one can give better suggestions than people who've been through it. You may actually want to become acquainted with other parents of multiples before you deliver. The rate of multiple births has increased greatly with the use of fertility drugs, so most medium-sized towns have their share of twins and triplets, as well as parents' groups.

You're bound to have problems and questions when nursing two or more babies, so find a lactation consultant you trust and tattoo her number on your wrist. Better yet, put her on speed dial. You may get to know her so well that you end up inviting her to the babies' first birthday party!

Feeding triplets or more

If you have triplets or more, you'll probably need to use supplementation to meet their needs. The babies may be born prematurely and come home from the hospital at different times. This means you may find yourself pumping for one baby and nursing the other two, or vice versa.

Your body tries to make as much milk as your babies demand. Frequent nursing, especially in the beginning, helps ensure a good supply for the babies. Be sure to keep up with your body's own requirements by eating well and drinking lots of fluid.

REMEMBER

Any amount of breast milk is better than none at all, especially for preemies. Don't decide not to breastfeed just because you can't supply all of the babies' nutrition.

Many parents of multiples find that their babies are more adaptable than singletons; this adaptability is probably born of necessity! You may find your triplets much more able to adapt to a combination of breast and bottle feedings. They may also be more agreeable to having their schedules manipulated, so that all of them are on the same schedule at first.

TIP

If you have triplets or more and have people coming in to help with their feedings, a schedule book is a necessity. You may need to paste schedule sheets on the kitchen cabinets so everyone can chart feedings easily, and you can ensure that no one's being missed.

Breastfeeding a Baby with Physical Problems

We all pray and hope for the perfect baby. The thought of your child being born with something wrong is hard to comprehend, but birth defects can and do occur.

When you're first faced with the care of a baby who has physical problems, you may think that breastfeeding is out of the question. However, for the reasons we discuss in Chapter 2, breast milk is the best food possible for a baby with health problems. In the sections that follow, we talk about several common birth defects and their effects on your baby's ability to breastfeed.

Cardiac problems

Babies with cardiac problems may have a hard time nursing because of their physical weakness. Cardiac problems don't automatically mean you won't be able to breastfeed, but you need to evaluate what's best for your baby.

A *congenital cardiac defect* occurs during early pregnancy and can take the form of a hole between the chambers of the heart, an abnormally sized heart, or an abnormally shaped heart. Cardiac defects can occur if you contract a virus like German measles while you're pregnant, or if you take certain medications in the first three months of pregnancy, such as lithium (for bipolar disorder) or retinoids (for severe cystic acne). Some congenital heart defects run in families.

Babies with heart defects use a lot of calories just breathing and growing. Your most important task with a cardiac baby is to help her grow, especially if she needs to reach a certain weight before surgery can be performed. Learning how to work with her illness and still accomplish weight gain can be a full-time job. You need to tap into available resources; a Web site that seems particularly thorough is `www.congenitalheartdefects.com`. Your lactation consultant and cardiologist can also work together to help you.

Babies with cardiac problems have difficulties feeding because they breathe quickly, tire easily, and retain fluid. A cardiac baby frequently has to make the decision, "Should I eat or breathe?" As you might guess, she chooses the latter. You may have to pump your breasts and feed the baby from a bottle or a cup because doing so is less exhausting for her. In extreme cases, your baby may need to be fed through a tube in her nose.

If your baby isn't gaining weight because she's burning too many calories, you may need to pump and also add a high-caloric supplement to help her grow. Consider enlisting a dietician, your pediatrician, and your cardiologist to work together to plan your baby's care.

A baby with cardiac problems often needs to gain weight before going into surgery. Following are some suggestions to help your baby gain the weight she needs:

- Allow rest periods for the baby, whether you're breastfeeding or bottle feeding breast milk.
- Give her small, frequent feedings to allow your baby to maintain a steady caloric intake.
- Avoid letting your baby cry. Crying burns calories a cardiac baby can't afford to use.
- Watch for signs that your baby is retaining too much fluid — such as if she isn't having eight wet diapers a day. Your cardiologist will give guidelines specific for your baby.

Having a baby with a cardiac defect is a big challenge. Contact support groups for parents of babies with cardiac problems, either locally or on the Internet, for support and suggestions. Don't feel guilty if you can't breastfeed your baby; you need to make feeding choices based on what's best for your baby.

Breathing problems

Breathing problems can make breastfeeding difficult for your baby. A healthy baby breathes about 40 to 60 times per minute; this gives him enough time to perform other simple functions, such as breastfeeding. When your baby has a problem with his lungs, he tries to compensate by breathing faster, as much as 80 breaths (or more) per minute. Breathing this rapidly makes it hard for him to suck and swallow, and it uses up energy. You may not be able to breastfeed until his breathing slows down to more normal levels.

Some breathing difficulties are temporary, but some are permanent. Some start before the baby is born and continue for a period of time after delivery. Other breathing problems can begin after the baby is discharged from the hospital. Following are some of the most common causes of breathing difficulties:

- Breathing problems may start before a baby is delivered if the baby passes *meconium,* the first bowel movement, before delivery. If the baby takes a breath before he's born, meconium, which is sticky and sometimes even chunky, can cause severe breathing problems. Some babies with meconium aspiration have no problems at all; others have severe breathing problems that last for several days.
- Some babies develop *Transient Tachypnea of the Newborn,* or TTN, after delivery. *Tachypnea* means "fast breathing." This is caused by fluid in the baby's lungs that hasn't yet been absorbed. Babies delivered by cesarean section (see Chapter 6) are more prone to TTN, because babies born vaginally have this fluid squeezed out of their lungs during the delivery process.

  TTN causes the baby to breathe harder and faster because his lungs aren't exchanging air as efficiently as they should, due to the presence of the fluid. This condition is temporary, lasting up to three days.
- Gastroesophageal reflux, or GERD, can also cause breathing difficulties. In babies with GERD, food in the stomach comes back up through the esophagus (see Chapter 8). This can cause breathing problems if the stomach contents enter the lungs through the *trachea* (the breathing tube).

Breastfeeding may not be possible until the baby's breathing problems are under control. During this time, your baby's nutritional needs may have to be met through intravenous fluids or tube feedings (which we discuss earlier in this chapter). If tube feedings are an option, you can pump your breasts and give the milk through the tube, or you can freeze the milk for later use.

Down syndrome

Down syndrome, also called *Trisomy 21,* is one of the most common and recognized chromosomal errors; it affects approximately 1 in 800 babies. Babies with Down syndrome are more frequently born to mothers age 35 and older, but you can have a Down syndrome baby at any age. Mothers of all ages are offered a blood test during pregnancy called a *triple screen,* which determines the risk that the baby has Down syndrome. If you are age 35 or older, your doctor may recommend the following tests in addition to the triple screen:

- **Chorionic villus sampling:** A small piece of placental tissue is checked for abnormal chromosomes.
- **Amniocentesis:** A small amount of amniotic fluid is withdrawn and checked for abnormal chromosomes.

If your baby has Down syndrome, you may be in a state of shock or denial right after delivery. Many misconceptions about Down syndrome exist; you may think your baby can never lead a normal life, or that she'll be severely retarded. This is not necessarily true; many children with Down syndrome live full and happy lives, and with early intervention, many are only mildly retarded.

Unless you find out months in advance that your baby has Down syndrome, your first reactions are likely to be negative. Don't feel guilty about this; it's normal to grieve when faced with this reality. Breastfeeding may help you bond with your baby while coming to grips with her condition.

Breastfeeding a baby with Down syndrome can be difficult, due to the baby's likely physical characteristics. Most babies with Down syndrome have large tongues and small jaws, which can make latch-on difficult. They also have poor muscle tone and are somewhat "floppy"; they may have an uncoordinated suck and difficulty swallowing. Babies with Down syndrome are also often placid, sleepy, and not very demanding when it comes to feeding time. Last of all, they tire easily. All these factors add up to a real challenge for breastfeeding.

Nonetheless, breastfeeding is very beneficial for a baby with Down syndrome. Following are just some of the benefits:

- **Breastfeeding may enhance the bonding process.** If you weren't expecting a baby with Down syndrome, breastfeeding may help you overcome any initial negative feelings.
- **Breastfeeding improves mouth and tongue coordination and aids in speech development.** Because of their large tongues and small jaws, children with Down syndrome are prone to speech problems.
- **Breastfeeding is more work for the baby.** Babies with Down syndrome often have poor muscle tone and a weak suck; breastfeeding helps develop muscle tone.
- **Breastfeeding increases intelligence, even if only by a few points.** Your baby will have some degree of retardation; breastfeeding can help her develop her full potential.
- **Breastfeeding protects against infection.** Babies with Down syndrome have underdeveloped immune systems and are prone to infections.
- **Breastfeeding provides tactile stimulation.** To develop their full potential, babies with Down syndrome need extra stimulation.
- **Breastfeeding helps prevent constipation.** Babies with Down syndrome are prone to constipation due to their sluggish intestines.
- **Breastfeeding decreases ear infections.** Due to facial malformations, babies with Down syndrome often have ear infections.
- **Breastfeeding helps prevent dental problems.** Babies with Down syndrome often have trouble with their teeth.

You need to be both patient and aggressive to establish nursing. Your baby may not wake up and cry to eat, so watch her closely for signs that she's hungry. As soon as she stirs, try feeding her. Attempt to feed every three hours or so around the clock.

TIP

You may need to wake your baby thoroughly before eating. Try removing her diaper, placing her skin-to-skin with you, or sitting her up in your lap. She may stay awake longer if you feed her using a modified football hold instead of a cradle position. The cross cradle position may also work well, because it gives you more control over her weak neck. See Chapter 6 for illustrations of these breastfeeding positions.

Babies with Down syndrome often arch their backs when you hold them. Hold the baby so that she's flexed at the waist to help prevent this. If she's prone to choking, you may need to feed her in a sitting position — the modified football hold works well.

A lactation consultant can help you get the baby properly latched on. You may need to help the baby open her jaw wide enough to nurse; you can do this by pulling down on her chin with your finger.

Many babies with Down syndrome also have heart or respiratory problems. See the preceding sections for advice on handling babies with these problems.

No one plans to have a baby with Down syndrome. Your first reaction may be that your world has been shattered. Although you may feel that way, your baby will not. She'll come to you as a newborn looking for the comfort of her mother. Responding to her needs as you would to those of any other child helps you move on to acceptance of your baby as a unique and treasured individual.

Cleft lip or palate

Having a baby born with a cleft lip or palate can be a terrible shock. Few deformities scare parents more, especially if the cleft is complete on both the lip and palate. You may wonder how on earth your baby will ever look normal, or how he'll ever be able to eat.

Surgery for clefts usually begins early, at age 3 months or sooner. Your baby may need several surgeries to repair both the lip and palate. An excellent Web site for parents of babies with cleft lips and palates is `www.widesmiles.org`. The site contains lots of practical information, as well as many before and after pictures of babies with clefts. You'll come away feeling much better about your child's future after looking at these pictures and reading the stories.

Although the term *cleft palate* is used by lay people to mean any type of lip deformity, different types of clefts exist, and they affect breastfeeding differently. A cleft lip can extend partially or completely up to the nose and can affect one side of the mouth (*unilateral*) or both (*bilateral*). A baby with a cleft lip may or may not have a cleft palate, and a baby with a normal-appearing lip can have a cleft palate.

If your baby has a unilateral cleft lip, you probably will be able to breastfeed without too much trouble. If he has a cleft palate, you may be able to breastfeed if the cleft is narrow and affects only the soft palate.

Bilateral clefts make breastfeeding difficult because they interfere with a good seal around the breast. If they're extensive, they make sucking very difficult; you may need to pump your milk and use a special bottle that you squeeze to get milk into the baby's mouth.

REMEMBER

Despite the difficulties, breast milk can be quite valuable for a baby with any type of cleft. For one thing, these babies are very prone to ear infections and to irritation from milk dribbling out their noses. Breast milk helps reduce the risk of ear infection (see Chapter 2) and is less irritating to the fragile nasal tissues than formula.

As we discuss in Chapter 2, breast milk also helps build up the baby's immune system. Any baby with a cleft will have some sort of surgery — that's a given. Breast milk can help him better withstand the stress of surgery at such a young age.

TIP

You can breastfeed using a supplemental feeding system, which can be set up to drip milk into the baby's mouth without a lot of sucking effort. Even if the baby can't suck at all, you can pump breast milk and give the baby the immunologic benefits of breast milk.

As Figure 9-2 shows, you may be able to nurse best by having the cleft lip closest to your breast; this decreases the amount of air the baby sucks in and gives a better seal. If the cleft is small, you can block it with your finger to accomplish the same thing.

TIP

Most babies with a cleft do best when fed in an upright position. The football hold, modified so that the baby is in a semi-sitting position, may work well for you (see Chapter 6).

If you nurse exclusively, keep a close eye on the baby's weight and be aware of the signs of dehydration, which we detail in Chapter 7.

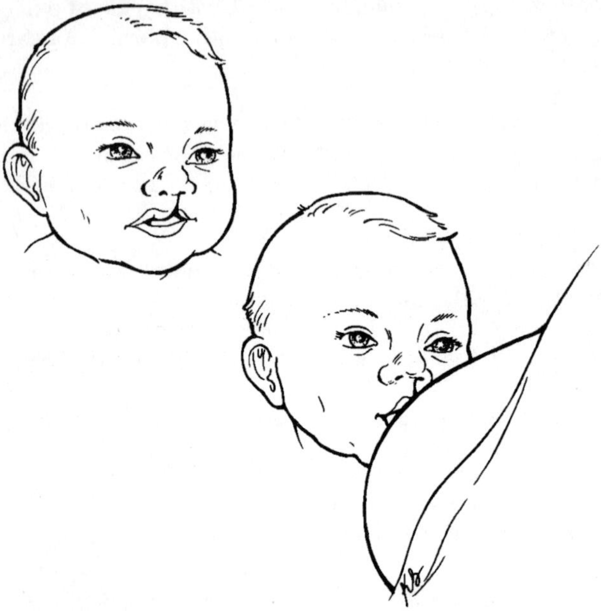

Figure 9-2: Positioning the baby so his cleft is next to your breast may help him latch on.

Short frenulum (tongue tie)

The *frenulum* is the piece of tissue that connects your tongue to the bottom of your mouth. In most people, the frenulum is pretty far back on the tongue. If a baby's frenulum is shorter than normal and attaches very close to the tip of the tongue, the doctor may say he's *tongue tied* — or he may use the scientific term *ankyloglossia,* which is likely to scare you to death.

A short frenulum prevents the baby from extending his tongue past the lower gums to cup the underside of the breast. The baby may have a hard time latching on, resulting in inadequate feeding (as well as sore nipples for you).

TIP

You can tell if your baby has a short frenulum by watching his tongue when he cries. He won't be able to stick his tongue out past his teeth, and when he cries, the tip of his tongue may look heart-shaped (see Figure 9-3).

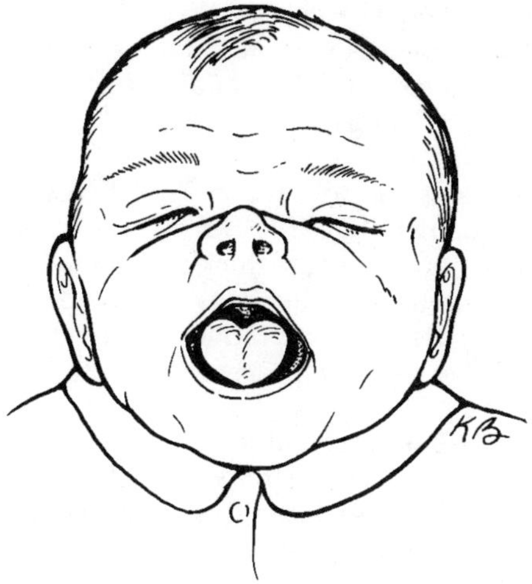

Figure 9-3: The tongue of a baby with a short frenulum looks heart-shaped when he cries.

Having a short frenulum clipped is somewhat controversial. The clipping itself is quite easy and fast; it can be done with a local anesthetic, with minimal blood loss. However, some doctors feel that cutting the frenulum may leave scarring that will cause more problems than the original short membrane.

If the baby's frenulum is attached to the very end of his tongue, most doctors will cut it, because the baby could have speech problems due to his inability to move his tongue around. If the frenulum is only somewhat shorter than normal, many pediatricians take a wait-and-see approach. As your baby grows and his teeth come in, the frenulum becomes less prominent and the difficulty may lessen.

TIP

If your baby has trouble staying latched on, makes a clicking noise when nursing, or isn't gaining weight well, you may want to have his frenulum clipped. Often pediatricians refuse to do this procedure and refer you to an ear, nose, and throat specialist.

Cystic fibrosis

A few decades ago, cystic fibrosis (CF) was a death sentence. Today, that's not the case. However, a child with CF will be chronically ill, and the strain of raising that child can be enormous. Many support groups for parents of CF children exist, because more than 30,000 Americans have the disease. Some states now require a blood test to identify babies with CF right after birth, so treatment can begin before too much lung damage occurs.

CF is a recessive gene disease; both parents must carry the gene and pass it on for the baby to have CF. The disease causes mucus, bile, and pancreatic fluids to become thick and sticky. Because of this, CF causes severe damage to the lungs and the digestive tract. Babies with CF are also deficient in enzymes needed to digest food properly; failure to thrive can be an early sign of CF.

Parents of a baby with CF may also notice that the baby tastes salty when they kiss her; this is due to CF changing the composition of fluids in the body. Babies with CF sweat more than other babies and can easily become dehydrated.

A baby with CF can be *pancreatic sufficient* or *pancreatic insufficient.* Breastfed babies who are pancreatic sufficient often won't be diagnosed until they start eating solid foods — around six months — because breast milk contains enzymes that aid digestion. Most babies with CF in the United States are pancreatic insufficient. These babies may be diagnosed at birth when they fail to pass *meconium,* their first stool. This results in an intestinal blockage. They may have severe respiratory distress due to the mucus collection in their lungs.

REMEMBER

Babies with CF need intensive, chronic care. A few years ago, doctors recommended that these babies not be breastfed, because they need high-calorie intake to grow. However, doctors now recommend that you do breastfed a baby with CF, because breast milk is more easily digested than formula. Often, additional enzymes are given to aid in digestion.

Your baby may need supplemental vitamins as well as a high caloric intake. Make sure your own nutritional and hydration needs are met (see Chapter 7) so that your baby gets the milk he needs.

Most babies with CF require physical therapy and lung drainage treatments to keep the mucus moving so it can be suctioned or coughed out of the lungs. Because this is a rigorous schedule for you as well as the baby, you need to keep your energy levels up with good nutrition.

Breastfeeding has the following benefits for a baby with CF:

- Breast milk is easily digestible and contains the enzyme *lipase.* Lipase breaks breast milk down into smaller curds, which decreases the possibility of an intestinal blockage.

- Human milk contains vitamins and minerals in forms that can be more easily absorbed than those in formula.
- Breast milk promotes healthy, normal *flora,* the good bacteria that keep your digestive tract in balance. This is particularly good for babies with CF because they frequently are given antibiotics due to their susceptibility to infection. Antibiotics destroy normal flora in the body.
- Human milk decreases respiratory and intestinal infections and also decreases inflammation and allergic reactions.

Metabolic disorders

Metabolic disorders are abnormalities in the body's chemistry. Many metabolic diseases are inherited, and babies can be tested for them right after birth. States have different regulations for testing newborns for metabolic disease. If your baby is born at home, your midwife may also do the testing or may send you to your doctor's office to have it done.

PKU

PKU stands for *phenylketonuria.* Babies with PKU are missing an enzyme that breaks down a protein called *phenylalanine* ("phe" for short). When phe accumulates in the body rather than being broken down, it can cause severe brain damage. In the United States, one out of 12,000 to 15,000 babies is born with PKU each year.

Babies with PKU are often fair-haired with blue eyes. They appear normal at birth, before the phe levels have built up. By the time they reach a year of age, if they haven't been on a phe-restricted diet, most are severely retarded. They may have a musty odor, seizures, poor growth, and undeveloped muscle tone.

Until a few years ago, doctors believed that babies with PKU absolutely could not breastfeed, because breast milk contains phe. (although a smaller percentage of phe than regular formula). Some doctors now suggest that you can partially breastfeed a baby with PKU, although it requires close recordkeeping and more frequent blood tests for your baby.

Even children with PKU need some phe in their diets. The trick is to make sure that all the phe required comes from breast milk; you'll need to supplement with phe-free formulas such as Phenex or Phenylac. Supplementation is required, because your baby can't receive all his calories from breastfeeding.

A diet of only breast milk for a baby with PKU will result in dangerously high phe levels. You must monitor your baby's levels and balance his phe-free formula intake with his breast milk intake very carefully under your doctor's care. If you aren't willing to keep very close track of your baby's intake and his PKU levels, you should not breastfeed!

Classic galactosemia

Babies with classic galactosemia have inherited the gene for galactosemia from both parents. Babies with galactosemia are missing the enzyme that breaks *galactose,* a simple sugar, down into glucose. Without this enzyme, galactose builds up in the body and causes brain damage, liver and kidney damage, and cataracts. Galactosemia occurs in 1 in 50,000 births.

Babies with classic galactosemia can't be fed *any* breast milk or regular formula; they must be fed a galactose-free formula such as Nutramigen.

Duarte's galactosemia

Babies with a variant of galactosemia called *Duarte's galactosemia* have inherited the galactosemia gene from one parent and a variant called Duarte's galactosemia from the other. These babies have a diminished ability to break down galactose; they have about 25 to 50 percent of normal enzyme activity.

Some doctors believe that babies with Duarte's can be safely breastfed; others restrict galactose in the diet for the first year. If you want to breastfeed, you need to be under the care of a doctor specializing in the treatment of Duarte's galactosemia. Your baby may need close monitoring and frequent blood tests to make sure his galactose levels aren't too high.

Nursing an Adopted Baby

You may think this is a no-brainer; of course you can't breastfeed an adopted baby! But the truth is you *can* breastfeed an adopted baby. How much of the baby's milk supply you're able to provide depends on the circumstances; in most cases, you need to supplement breastfeeding with formula or breast milk from a milk bank.

Establishing a milk supply

Unless you've recently delivered a baby or been pregnant, your body isn't producing enough of the hormones necessary for lactation — oxytocin and prolactin (see Chapter 1). However, nipple stimulation is the essential part of milk production.

Using a breast pump on a regular basis, beginning well in advance of adoption, may help stimulate your body to begin milk production. For example, some adoptive moms have found that using a hospital grade pump six to eight times a day for several weeks before their babies arrived helped establish their milk supply. But others have had different experiences and say the pump wasn't nearly as helpful as the baby's actual suckling. These moms recommend just nursing the baby when she arrives and using a lactation aid until your milk comes in (see the next section).

Establishing your milk supply is easier if you've breastfed before, because your body knows what to do. To boost the amount of milk you produce, you may consider taking a medication such as Reglan (see Chapter 7), although you must consider the side effects.

TIP

If you've never nursed, you may find it worthwhile to try pumping for several weeks before your baby arrives. A few weeks may pass before you see even a few drops of milk, and you may not be able to pump more than a few ounces a day before your baby arrives. However, any amount of breast milk is good for the baby, and so is the closeness that comes with breastfeeding.

Using lactation aids

Your milk supply develops in response both to stimulation and hormones. Taking certain medications can boost your hormone levels, while having the baby suck helps to stimulate your breasts. But most babies won't keep sucking if they're not getting any milk. That's where supplemental nursing systems come into play.

You can make your own supplemental nursing system using a syringe and a piece of tubing, or you can buy a commercial system. If you need to supplement a large supply of milk, you probably want to invest in a commercial system.

The two best-known commercial systems are Lact-Aid, made by Lact-Aid International, and Supplemental Nursing System (SNS) by

Medela. With both systems, a milk container is suspended from a cord around your neck. Thin tubes lead from the container to your nipples. As the baby sucks, milk is drawn through the tube into his mouth, so he gets nourishment even if your breasts aren't producing any milk.

The systems differ somewhat, and you (or your baby!) may like one more than the other. Following is some information about each system, so you can compare before you buy.

The Lact-Aid system

- Dispenses the supplement from a plastic collapsible bag, which holds 4.5 ounces
- Has only one tube (so you have to switch tubing when you switch sides), which comes in only one size
- Lies fairly flat (so it hides well under clothing)
- Can be difficult to assemble
- Can be held upside down (called a *gravity feed*) if you need it to flow faster because your baby has a weak suck
- Can be used lying down

The Supplemental Nursing System

- Has a rigid plastic bottle that holds 5 ounces of supplement
- Has two tubes (available in three different sizes), so you can switch sides easily
- Is visible under clothing and also makes a gurgling noise
- Is easy to assemble
- Uses gravity feed, so you can't nurse while lying down

TIP

A kit containing the feeding system costs around $50. You should have either a spare kit or replacement parts for the main components in case something breaks, and you have a screaming baby to feed!

The container shouldn't be held higher than the baby's head; normally it rests between your breasts. The milk should be sucked through the tube; it shouldn't flow constantly into the baby's mouth, unless the baby has problems sucking.

Many Internet specialty stores sell either Lact-Aid or the SNS; just type either name into your favorite search engine. Lact-Aid

International and Medela both have Web sites of their own, with more information on their products; go to www.lact-aid.com or www.medela.com.

Nursing When You're Sick

Not too many years ago, if you became sick, the first words out of your doctor's mouth would have been, "You have to stop breastfeeding." Most doctors now realize that, under most circumstances, you don't need to stop nursing when you're sick.

Research has shown that breastfeeding while you're sick with a minor illness doesn't hurt your baby, but rather the opposite; it may help him fight off the bacteria or virus that's making you sick. If your doctor advises you to stop nursing due to an illness, seek a second opinion before making your decision.

However, breastfeeding through an illness isn't always the best choice. More serious illnesses may require that you stop nursing until you are well. Infections such as Strep A can be devastating to a newborn. In some cases, your baby may require preventive antibiotics through the non-nursing period. Always talk with your doctor about your specific situation before deciding whether to continue nursing while you're sick.

Working through a minor illness

You can generally continue breastfeeding if you experience a minor illness, such as a common cold, sore throat, cough, urinary tract infection, stomach virus, stomach upset from food poisoning, or mastitis (which we discuss in Chapter 8). You can take most medications prescribed for these illnesses without harming your baby, although you should always make sure your doctor knows that you're breastfeeding.

To keep your milk supply strong while you're sick, do the following:

- **Rest.** Take your baby to bed with you. Leave the running of the house to someone else. Your primary job is to take care of yourself and your baby.
- **Drink plenty of liquids.** If you have a fever, vomiting, or diarrhea, you could become dehydrated. Remember that some drugs, like antihistamines, tend to decrease your milk supply and make your baby drowsy. Watch for these symptoms if your doctor prescribes antihistamines or if you're taking over-the-counter drugs such as Benadryl.

- **Reduce your fever with acetaminophen or ibuprofen.** Make sure that your ibuprofen dose doesn't exceed 400mg, and avoid extra-strength formulas, which contain higher medication doses.
- **Take antibiotics prescribed by your doctor.** Make sure she knows you're breastfeeding. Antibiotics are needed only if you have a bacterial infection; they won't help the common cold.
- **Relieve gastrointestinal symptoms with antacids.** Products that are safe to use include Mylanta, Maalox, Tums, Mylicon, DiGel, Alka Seltzer, Rolaids, and Pepto-Bismol.
- **For nausea and vomiting, take Benadryl, Emetrol, or Dramamine, which are safe for your baby.** Watch for drowsiness as a side effect in your baby. Try taking these medications after nursing, not right before.
- **To combat diarrhea, take Donnagel, Diasorb, Kaopectate, or Pepto-Bismol.**
- **Make sure your cold and cough medications are limited to one ingredient only.** This way, you can ensure that you aren't taking a second medication that isn't safe for your baby. Avoid extended relief medications — ones that promote 8 or even 24 hours of relief. They can have a greater impact on your milk supply because their effectiveness lasts longer.
- **Relieve a sore throat with preparations such as Cepacol lozenges, NICE, or Vicks lozenges, which contain menthol or benzocaine.** Avoid lozenges and sprays that contain phenol or hexylresorcinols; examples include Cepastat, Listerine and Sucrets lozenges, and Vicks Chloraseptic Sore Throat Spray. A simple warm water and salt mixture to gargle with may work just as well as over-the-counter products; so may drinking something warm or simply turning on a humidifier!

Responding to criticism

TIP

Some well-meaning person (like your mother) may ask, "Why are you still nursing? You're going to make your baby sick." We know the value of having ammunition in times like these, so here are some helpful responses:

- By the time you start feeling like you just want to go to bed and sleep until next year, your baby has already been exposed to the virus affecting you. Stopping breastfeeding at that point does the baby no good.

- When the baby gets exposed to your virus, breastfeeding actually puts him one step ahead of you. Your breast milk provides him with the same antibodies that you are producing to fight your flu. If your baby does catch the bug, he'll already have some antibodies to fight against it.

If your baby catches your illness, most likely he'll have a lesser version of it. Many times, everyone in the family except for the breastfed baby gets sick.

REMEMBER

An ounce of prevention is worth a pound of cure. Illnesses are usually transmitted through skin and secretion (nose and mouth) contact. Wash your hands before handling your baby, especially if you feel a cold coming on. And, obviously, you should avoid sneezing and coughing in your baby's face!

Maintaining your milk supply

If your illness is severe, or if it requires you to take a medication that is not safe for your baby, keep up your milk supply while you feed your baby a supplement. Pump about every three hours, even if that's the last thing you feel like doing! (Be aware that even with pumping, you may experience a temporary drop in milk supply after being sick.) After you pump, discard the pumped milk.

As soon as you're healthy, or as soon as you've finished your entire round of medication, you can get back to breastfeeding. With good stimulation from the baby, your milk supply should pick up and be back at your pre-illness levels in no time.

REMEMBER

You won't be sick forever! If your milk supply does decrease due to poor stimulation and dehydration, be patient. With continued stimulation from the baby and additional pumping, your levels should be back to normal in a week or so. You'll probably find your baby nursing more frequently if your supply has dropped; frequent nursing brings the supply back up to satisfy the baby's demand.

Feeding a Sick Baby

Sooner or later, your baby will get sick. Often, sick babies don't want to eat; they want comfort. Fortunately, many babies use nursing not only as a nutritional source, but as a comfort source, too. So your breastfed baby may keep her fluid and nutritional intake up, even when she's sick. Because babies can easily become dehydrated, this is a real plus of breastfeeding. (Another bonus is that antibodies in breast milk can help her fight the infection.)

But not every baby behaves the same way, and you may find that yours simply doesn't want to eat while she's sick. If that's the case, read on for advice.

Encouraging your baby to nurse

Most likely, your baby's first illness will be something simple, like a cold. If she has a stuffy nose, she may push away from the breast and refuse to eat. If she has a hard time nursing, try the following:

- **Hold her in an upright position.** The football hold (see Chapter 6) is good for keeping her head elevated. You can also try the *Australian position,* where you lie down and the baby lies on top of your breasts.
- **Keep her nose clear with saline nose drops.** Place a few drops in her nose, keeping her head lower than her body. After a few minutes, suction her nose with a bulb syringe. Remember, your baby breathes through her nose. If she can't breathe, she can't nurse. Try to clear your baby's nose before she nurses, not after. If you try this after she eats, she is probably going to vomit what you just fed her.
- **Keep a humidifier in the room.** Also, if your baby is really congested, try nursing her in the bathroom after running a hot shower. The moist, warm air helps her breathe more easily.
- **If your baby develops a fever, call her doctor.** She may need an antibiotic. Babies under 3 months rarely run fevers.
- **If your baby develops an ear infection, try to breastfeed frequently — at least once an hour.** An ear infection may make it painful for her to breastfeed. If you find that she just isn't interested in nursing, keep your supply up by pumping your breasts. If she's nursing for only a short period, pump after she nurses. If she still refuses to nurse after a day or so, contact your pediatrician.
- **Try feeding her expressed milk in a cup, spoon, dropper, or syringe.** You can also freeze your milk until it's slushy and feed it to her with a spoon. This is particularly good if your baby has a sore throat.

REMEMBER

Contrary to the old wives' tale, milk does not increase mucus in your baby's nose and chest.

Can I nurse through infertility treatments?

If you needed fertility treatment to get pregnant with your baby, you may be torn between the desire to nurse your baby and the need to begin treatment again so that you can have another baby before too much time passes.

Or you may be hoping to get pregnant again but haven't had a period since your baby was born. Spontaneous ovulation may not occur while you're exclusively breastfeeding, even in normally fertile women. When you introduce supplements and nurse less frequently, you'll most likely begin to ovulate again. But if you don't, you may find yourself knocking on your doctor's door, looking for help in becoming pregnant again.

Clomid is a pill commonly given to induce ovulation in women who aren't ovulating normally. If you're breastfeeding, do not take Clomid because:

- Clomid passes through your breast milk and can affect the baby.
- Clomid may reduce your milk supply.
- Clomid has caused reproductive tract disorders in rats.

The same warning holds true for injectable stimulating medications called *gonadotropins.* In the clinic where we work, mothers are advised to stop breastfeeding before starting any type of fertility injections, including lupron and gonadotropins, because the effects of these drugs on infants aren't well studied, and the drugs do pass through the breast milk.

Dealing with diarrhea

Diarrhea is less common in breastfed babies than bottle-fed babies because breast milk contains antibodies that help prevent bacteria from attacking the intestines. If your baby does develop diarrhea, breastfeeding is the best way to get fluids into him.

The definition of diarrhea is 12 or more stools in a day. These stools are usually loose and watery. They may smell foul and can even contain blood and mucus due to irritation in the intestines. Many times vomiting accompanies a diarrhea-type virus.

Notify your pediatrician if your baby has diarrhea for 24 hours or more, especially if your baby is under 3 months old. Infants can become dangerously dehydrated quickly. (See Chapter 7 for more on recognizing dehydration.)

Breast milk has a high water content, so nursing helps prevent dehydration. Breast milk is also easily and quickly digested. Even if the baby vomits shortly after a feeding, some milk is already out of his stomach and on its way to provide nutritional and fluid value.

To help keep the baby hydrated during diarrhea, try the following:

- Offer frequent, short feedings, at least every hour.
- Ask your doctor if the baby needs an electrolyte solution like Pedialyte. This would be needed only if the diarrhea were severe. Usually breast milk provides all the fluids and nutrition your baby needs.

Needing Surgery

If either your baby or you need surgery while you're still breastfeeding, you may wonder if you can continue to nurse. Only you and your doctor can make that decision. However, if the surgery is not an emergency event, you may have time to do some planning that can increase your odds of returning to breastfeeding.

Surgery on mom

Many a nursing mom has been faced with the need for surgery. This can be a difficult time emotionally and physically, but you can take steps that will help you continue to nurse.

TIP

One of the most important things to do is make sure that you have plenty of help available when you get home from the hospital. Recuperating from surgery and breastfeeding your baby are more than enough to do in the first weeks during your recovery.

Investigating hospital policies

Before you're admitted to the hospital, find out what nursing arrangements the hospital allows:

- **Inquire about the hospital policy on nursing babies staying with their mothers after surgery.** If the hospital employs a lactation consultant, call her first. If it doesn't have one, try a patient representative, who should be knowledgeable about the hospital's regulations. Policies can range from allowing the baby to stay 24 hours a day to allowing the baby in only for feedings.

- **If the hospital allows rooming in, plan on having another person with you to take care of the baby when you are resting.** Supplies for the baby will probably not be provided. You may want to ask if a private room can be provided and what the additional cost will be. Your insurance may not pay for the added expense.
- **If rooming in is not allowed, ask if the baby can be brought in and out for feedings.** This may be difficult for the person doing the transporting, but with luck it will last only a short time. Check on the hours when the baby could be brought in to you. If the baby can't come to you, perhaps you can go to a hospital lounge to nurse the baby after you're feeling better.
- **Find out if the baby can be with you in the hospital unit where you will be moved after surgery.** If not, ask if you can be moved to a floor such as pediatrics or maternity.

You may be concerned with bringing your baby into the hospital environment. But if you're in a private room, your baby will not be in the main stream of viruses and bacteria. He probably is exposed to just as many germs when he's at the mall with you.

Storing milk and preparing your baby for change

Even if the hospital will allow you to keep your baby with you, pump and freeze several bottles of milk prior to your hospital admission. This way, if you're not up to feeding your baby right after surgery, someone else can feed him your breast milk.

REMEMBER

If possible, introduce your baby to an alternate feeding method before surgery. Use a small flexible cup, syringe, medicine dropper, or spoon if your baby is less than 6 weeks old and you're concerned about nipple confusion (see Chapter 5). If your baby is older and is a well-established breastfeeder, you should have no problem introducing a bottle.

TIP

Don't be surprised if your baby won't take a bottle from you. He associates your smell with breastfeeding and may become upset if you offer him a bottle. Have your partner or someone else give the bottle. If your baby is 4 to 6 months or older, you may be more successful trying a cup.

Arranging to pump

If you cannot bring your baby into the hospital for feedings, you need to pump to maintain your milk supply. You may need the assistance of a nurse or lactation consultant. Try to maintain the same schedule you were on when feeding your baby. Find out if a freezer or refrigerator is available so you can store the pumped milk.

Prior to surgery, notify your anesthesiologist that you are a breastfeeding mom. Most general anesthesia medications clear your system quickly and cannot be detected within seven hours. A good rule to use is that anesthesia medication is out of your system when you are awake and alert. Remember, we're saying "awake and alert," not "just barely awake enough to open your eyes"!

Try to breastfeed right before you go into surgery. Then be prepared to pump and dump your breast milk within four hours after surgery.

Taking medications

Don't be afraid to take pain medication after your surgery; see Chapter 6 for details about breastfeeding while taking pain medication. Your baby receives only a small dose of medication in your milk, which shouldn't affect him. (On the other hand, if you're in considerable discomfort, your let-down could be affected.)

If you need any other medications, such as antibiotics, talk with your pediatrician or lactation consultant to find out what's safe or not safe for the baby.

Surgery on baby

The anxiety you feel prior to having surgery yourself is minimal compared to the anxiety you feel preparing for your baby to have surgery, no matter how minor. The more you know what to expect, the better you'll handle this difficult time. Get as much information as possible from your pediatrician and the surgeon, and let them know that you want to resume breastfeeding as soon as possible.

Withholding food

Whether your baby is having a simple outpatient procedure or open heart surgery, you need to prepare her in pretty much the same way. For a period of time before surgery (as well as after), she won't be allowed to have any food. This prevents the aspiration of fluid into her lungs in case she vomits during or right after the surgery.

Although withholding the breast from your baby will be difficult for both of you, your baby's safety depends on it. Try getting someone else to hold the baby during this time period, because she associates you with eating and may become frustrated if you don't feed her. If you're holding her, avoid the cradle hold, especially if this is your usual nursing position. Also try to keep her interested in her surroundings, walking her around in an upright position.

Banking breast milk

Breast milk has literally saved the lives of some babies. Premature babies, babies with severe allergies, and babies with metabolic deficiencies and other health conditions can benefit from *breast milk banks* — places that store donated breast milk.

Adopted babies and adults who undergo liver transplants also benefit from donated breast milk. You may be interested in donating excess milk to a milk bank, or you may find yourself in need of a milk bank if your baby needs more breast milk than you can supply.

The cost to purchase donated breast milk is around $2.50 an ounce (shipped). Your insurance company may pay for breast milk if it's medically necessary. Breast milk from established centers is pasteurized; pasteurization destroys the HIV and CMV viruses.

Milk donors are tested for diseases such as HIV, HTLV, Hepatitis B and C, and syphilis before their milk is accepted. Donors are also required not to smoke, drink, or take certain medications, herbs, or any types of illegal substances. Certain medications, such as insulin, thyroid replacement medication, and low-dose progestin birth control pills, are acceptable. Donors are not paid for donating milk.

Your doctor must write a prescription for you to obtain donated breast milk. Frozen breast milk can be shipped anywhere.

If you want to donate breast milk, you'll need to be tested for infectious disease and be medically cleared. You'll be given detailed instructions on how to collect and ship your milk.

Only six milk banks are associated with the Human Milk Banking Association of North America, which was started in 1985. This organization's purpose is to review and revise guidelines for milk banking; share information with the medical community; encourage breast milk research; and act as a clearinghouse for milk banks.

The locations and phone numbers of these six milk banks are:

- Lactation Center and Mothers' Milk Bank: Raleigh, N.C.; 919-350-8599
- Mothers' Milk Bank at Austin: Austin, TX.; 512-494-0800
- Mothers' Milk Bank P/SL Medical Center: Denver, CO.; 303-869-1888
- Mothers' Milk Bank: Newark, DE.; 302-733-2340
- Mothers' Milk Bank: Vancouver, Canada; 604-875-2282
- Mothers' Milk Bank Valley Medical Center: San Jose, CA.; 408-998-4550

Be certain to follow the guidelines that your baby's doctor gives you. Current guidelines state that the baby should complete her last breastfeeding four hours before surgery. This is because breast milk is easily digested and out of the stomach very quickly. With formula, no food is allowed for eight hours before surgery.

Keeping your milk supply strong

Before and during your baby's surgery, pump at the times when you would normally be feeding her. If your baby is a newborn when she needs surgery and your milk hasn't come in, try to express your *colostrum* (the first milk), even if you don't think much is coming out. Save the colostrum and feed it to the baby as soon as she can take it, possibly with a spoon or syringe.

After surgery, in most cases, your baby will be able to resume nursing when she's awake enough to drink liquids. Many babies, even veteran nursers, aren't too interested in nursing right after surgery. Disinterest can be caused by residual anesthesia medications in her system or by discomfort. Be patient; she'll come around. If you think she's uncomfortable, ask the nurse if the doctor ordered something for pain. Even infant acetaminophen (Tylenol) could be enough to make her more comfortable.

Part III

Growing with Your Baby

The 5th Wave By Rich Tennant

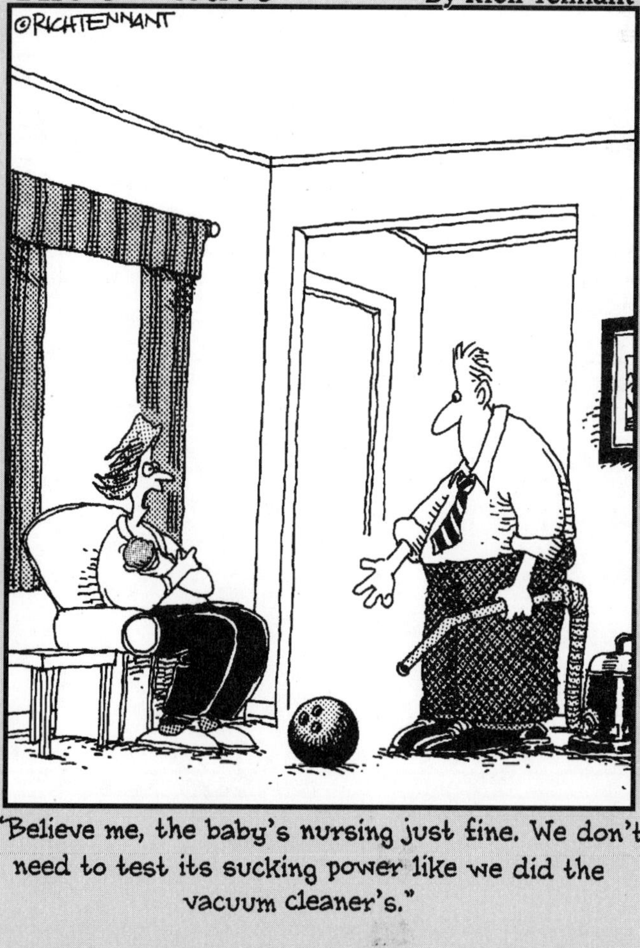

"Believe me, the baby's nursing just fine. We don't need to test its sucking power like we did the vacuum cleaner's."

In this part . . .

When you've got breastfeeding down pat, your work as a new parent is just beginning. To ensure your long-term success, you need to first ensure that your relationship with your partner is strong despite your new stresses. You also want to know what to expect from breastfeeding as your baby gets older, as well as when to consider weaning. This part addresses all these issues.

Chapter 10

Breastfeeding Through Different Ages and Stages

In This Chapter

- Knowing what to expect as your baby grows
- Introducing solid foods
- Relying on pacifiers — or not
- Curbing the biting habit
- Moving the baby into the nursery

Turn around and blink, and your new baby is starting to smile. Look away for an instant, and he's crawling, then walking, then running! Every age has its delights (and its drawbacks).

In this chapter, we look at how breastfeeding changes as your baby grows. We help you anticipate some of the milestones of babyhood, such as introducing solid foods and vitamin supplements, moving the baby to his own room, and curing a biter of a painful habit. We also give you suggestions on how to have fun during feedings. You'll spend hours together nursing — make the most of them!

Growing and Changing

Part of the joy — and fear — of parenting is knowing that your baby is constantly changing. During pregnancy, obviously your focus is on figuring out what to do when the hospital nurse first hands you that little bundle who needs to be held and fed and rocked and changed. We cover that information in detail in Chapter 6, and we show you how to breastfeed your newborn at home in Chapter 7.

But that little bundle gets bigger very quickly. For a month-by-month breakdown of what to expect from your baby during the first year of life, check out *Parenting For Dummies.* In the following sections, we cover what changes to expect as you nurse throughout your baby's first year and beyond.

Three to six months old

In no time at all, the newborn who did little but eat and sleep metamorphoses into a social butterfly. Starting at around 3 months, he's keenly aware of his surroundings; he peers intently into your face, plays with his toes, and even plays with your breasts as he nurses. He's becoming a person.

You are changing, too; you handle him with confidence, and you've become an efficient milk machine. At the three-month mark, you'll be producing about 30 to 36 ounces of milk a day.

Together, you've survived late nights, cracked nipples, and inconsolable crying spells — both yours and his! Finally, you and your baby are in sync, and his growth is a daily reminder of your success.

Sleeping longer

As your baby cruises down the highway of life, you'll see daily — sometimes hourly! — changes. One thing you should notice — usually with great joy — is a change in his schedule. By 3 to 4 months old, he usually drops one of his night feedings. Before you get all excited, at this age the definition of "sleeping through the night" means a six- to seven-hour stretch. Not too many babies sleep for 12 hours straight.

TIP: If you're lucky enough to have a 7 p.m. to 7 a.m. sleeper, we encourage you to nurse more often during the day. You need this stimulation to keep your milk supply at a good level, and he still needs to nurse seven to eight times a day to gain well.

REMEMBER: Your baby should gain about a half an ounce to an ounce a day for the first three to four months. If he doesn't, observe his behavior (and yours) during the day. Is he sucking his fingers or fist? Is he fidgeting? Are you trying to introduce a pacifier when it may be better to offer your breast? (We discuss pacifier use later in this chapter.) Babies do talk to us — with time and experience, you discover how to listen.

Developing a breast preference

Usually by the age of 3 months, even the slow, sleepy nurser turns into a Grand Prix champion. Your well-established let-down reflex and his vigorous sucking technique mean he can get all that he needs in five to seven minutes flat, and he may be interested in nursing only on one breast.

Some babies develop a definite preference for one breast over the other. Although we encourage you to attempt to feed him from both breasts, you may find yourself fighting City Hall. If you have a "one breaster," try these suggestions:

TIP

- **Offer the least preferred breast first.** This may work best if the baby is sleepy and if the room is dark so he doesn't have his usual visual cues.
- **Change breasts midstream.** If your baby refuses to start with his unfavorite, put him on the preferred breast first. After he nurses an adequate amount (notice when he starts to slow down his sucking), try to casually slide him over to the other side.
- **Don't push the issue if he's uncooperative.** If you try to force him to nurse from the side he doesn't prefer, he may start refusing to nurse on either side! You risk decreasing your milk supply on the side he prefers.
- **Attempt to maintain your milk supply by pumping the less preferred side.** The hope is that he will eventually return to nursing on both breasts.
- **Watch your own preferences.** Without realizing it, you may have your own breast preference. Often this is tied to your left-or right-handedness. Are you always holding the phone in your left hand so the baby is more often held on your right arm? Try nursing without stirring the mashed potatoes or talking to your mom on the phone.

Going through growth spurts

REMEMBER

Babies have growth spurts around the ages of 3 weeks, 6 weeks, and 3 months. Growth spurts can cause a temporary feeding frenzy, where your baby may nurse almost constantly. This continues for three or four days, until the supply catches up to the demand. Resist the urge to supplement; he's trying to increase the supply by more frequent nursing, and supplementing defeats this effort.

Six to nine months old

Somewhere between the ages of 6 and 9 months, two important milestones occur:

- **The development of mobility.** Sometime during these three months, most babies begin to move. They may roll, crawl, or creep; a few even begin to walk.
- **The introduction of solid foods.** Most pediatricians recommend starting solids around 6 months.

Both events can interfere with breastfeeding. We discuss solid foods later in this chapter, in the section “Introducing Solid Foods.”

Discovering mobility

When your baby becomes mobile (or at least is able to spend time upright in an Exersaucer), he may become impatient with breastfeeding. Some babies don’t want to take time out from their day to lie around breastfeeding. Others welcome the snuggle time.

If your baby is the impatient type, you may need to introduce some new nursing activities to keep him interested enough to eat well. For instance, you may offer something sparkly he can look at or hold only when nursing, like a piece of jewelry. Or nursing time can be your singing or reading time.

Your baby’s newfound mobility may be even more of a problem if you introduce him to a sippy cup or offer him bottles of juice around the same time. He’ll realize quickly that he can eat on the run, and he may prefer doing so to sitting quietly and nursing.

Make sure nursing comes before his solid food or juice, so he’s hungry enough to nurse well.

Getting distracted during feedings

Babies between 6 and 9 months old are very social and easily distracted. If you have other children, the baby may be more interested in watching his big brother make faces than in eating.

Feeding the baby away from your other children may help, but chances are you won’t always be able to keep the 3-year-old out of the room while you nurse. Try to feed the baby when your other children are occupied, such as when they’re eating lunch or watching a special TV show. Put your nursing chair in a spot where you can keep an eye on your other children, but the baby can’t!

Your 6-month-old can easily empty your breast in ten minutes or less. Don’t try to keep him nursing longer when he’s ready to get down and get going, or else he may become frustrated with nursing.

When he's done, let him down. If he wants more nursing time, give it to him. Don't let nursing be your first battle of wills; most parents will tell you that you're very likely to lose this type of battle!

Changing schedules

Your 6- to 9-month-old should nurse three to four times a day. He may still want to nurse at night as well, especially if he sleeps in your bed, and you're easily accessible. (We discuss moving the baby out of your bed later in the chapter, in the section "Moving Baby Out of Your Room.") Remember to breastfeed before offering your baby solids or juice. At least 75 percent of his nutrition should still be coming from breast milk at this point.

Happy birthday! One year old

Many people assume that breastfeeding is over the minute your baby turns 1. After all, pediatricians in the United States recommend breastfeeding for at least a year. People often miss the *at least* part and assume that everyone stops at a year.

If you're a fervent breastfeeder, no doubt you have every intention of nursing for longer. But what if you're an average breastfeeder? The assumption that you'll stop nursing at a year may be making you uncomfortable. You're enjoying nursing. The baby's enjoying it. So why are other people making you feel guilty about it?

Understanding the one-year recommendation

The recommendation to nurse for the first year of your baby's life makes sense for several reasons:

- **At the one-year mark, the risk of your baby experiencing an allergy to cow's milk is fairly low.** That means you can probably go straight from breast milk to cow's milk, without needing to introduce the baby to formula. However, if you have a family history of allergies, you may want to stay away from cow's milk even past the one-year mark.
- **Most 1-year-olds can drink from a cup.** If you nurse for a year, you can probably bypass bottles as well.
- **Many babies start to self-wean at around a year.** However, others are nursing as much as ever, including needing a night feeding. (This is especially true if you're co-sleeping.)
- **By a year of age, your baby needs solid foods for a complete diet.** Breast milk alone won't be adequate. But breast milk in addition to solid food provides great nutrition as well as continued immune benefits.

Making your own decision

No two moms or babies are alike. Your 1-year-old may not nurse much at all, except for a few sucks at bedtime. Your neighbor's baby may run to her all day long, pulling at her shirt and making sucking noises. Both children are normal; they're just different!

You and your neighbor are different as well. You may miss nursing terribly and wish your baby would stay with it a while longer. Your neighbor may be tired of having her nipples poked and twisted and wish this would end, already. Both of you are normal, too!

Most of the time, the outside world is openly approving of breast-feeding — up to a point. When your child is walking and nursing, your public approval rating will drop. This sends some moms into the nursing underground; they just don't tell anyone they're still nursing. Only you know what's comfortable for you. If you and your baby still enjoy nursing and don't want to stop, don't!

Toddlers: One to two years old

Toddlers walk and talk, and many continue to nurse. This can lead to interesting situations when you're in public.

Finding your comfort level

Imagine pushing your cart through the grocery store when your toddler grabs the neck of your shirt, shoves her hand down your bra, and announces in a piercing tone easily heard over the canned music that she wants "booby." Or she picks up your shirt and sticks her head under it while you're waiting in the checkout line.

You may be perfectly comfortable with this. Then again, you may not. Even moms who are happy to still be nursing a toddler often aren't sure about handling the public demands for booby, nips, num nums, or whatever code name your child uses.

Picking a code word you can live with is essential, but to get your child to use the word, you need to start using it early on. If you say "Do you want to nurse?" six times a day for twelve months, you can assume your baby will say "want to nurse!" when that's what she wants. So if you want to use "num nums" or some other code word, use it consistently early on.

You may feel comfortable with public nursing, or you may want to establish limits, such as nursing only in the house, the car, or the bed — not in the convenience store. You need to be consistent to help your child understand this.

Dealing with breast attachment

Toddlers often develop attachments to blankets or other lovey things. If you're still co-sleeping (see Chapter 7), your child may use your breasts as an all-night milk bar or as a comfort object. Some women don't mind having their nipples twisted all night; others find that the constant fiddling drives them wild. If it bothers you to be touched and prodded in the night, try putting your child on the other side of your partner, where you're not so easily accessible.

Some toddlers become very attached to their moms' breasts, hugging them, burying their faces in them, and fingering the nipples. If you're the type of person who likes a lot of personal space, this may bother you. It may especially bother you in front of your husband's best friend or your great uncle. Again, you need to set limits on how much touching and twiddling is acceptable.

Even toddlers understand limits when they're consistent and enforced. If you're conflicted about nursing in public or during the night, your child will pick up on your hesitation and will test the limits in those situations. Sometimes parents are afraid to set limits, thinking that their children won't love them as much, or that their children should have rights. Children do have rights, but so do parents. We always told our children that our family was not a democracy. If you believe that your child should have an equal say in every decision, he'll make sure he gets it!

Continuing the nursing routine

Physically nursing toddlers isn't difficult. You're old pros by this time, and she knows not to bite you. (We discuss biting later in this chapter in the section "Nipping the Biting Habit".) The difficulties are usually more socially oriented, or issues of your own personal space being invaded by the hand up your shirt. Whatever you and your child are comfortable with is right for you. You may find a book called *Mothering Your Nursing Toddler,* written by Norma Bumgarner and published by La Leche League, very helpful.

Two years old and up

Are you hiding in the closet to nurse? Many women in the United States whose children are over age 2 are closet nursers; even their moms or best friends may not know that they're still breastfeeding.

Dealing with criticism

Despite increased support for nursing in general, many women who are still nursing at this point feel public censure for "not letting your child grow up" or "making him a sissy." Studies have shown that these criticisms are totally false; children who nurse past the age of 2 are often more secure and self-assured than children who don't.

In many parts of the world, breastfeeding ends between ages 2 and 4. Of course, in many of these areas, sanitation is poor, and breastfeeding is the best way to keep children alive. Breastfeeding is also somewhat of a deterrent to another pregnancy, though not a reliable one (see Chapter 19).

Some moms nursing older children have actually been accused of child abuse and threatened with visits from Child Protective Services. If you start to feel like you're the only parent in the world nursing an older child, call or visit La Leche League or another breastfeeding organization. This type of organization can help you feel more confident that your decision isn't at all strange, and can help you in the unlikely case that you receive a threat of this type. (See Chapter 15 for more on the legalities of breastfeeding.)

Knowing how often to nurse

If you're still nursing your 2- or 3-year-old, make sure your child is getting an adequate diet; at this point, breast milk shouldn't be his main source of nutrition. Many nursing children at this age nurse only for short times and for comfort, not for the nutrition. Others are regular morning and night nursers. (If your child still sleeps in your bed, the morning and night nursing relationship is easier to maintain.)

Most moms of kids this age can go for long stretches without nursing and not develop engorgement or other problems. This makes it easier to go back to work and still carry on a nursing relationship.

Older children are usually able to understand limits on breastfeeding, such as "We don't nurse in the store" or "We don't nurse at grandma's house." Your 3- or 4-year-old will also be able to tell you how much he enjoys nursing and what it means to him, and sometimes you may find his devotion to your breasts a little overwhelming! As with nursing a toddler, you make the rules about handling your breasts and talking about them!

How long to continue nursing is your decision. If you want to continue past society's idea of when nursing should end, you can find plenty of support if you search the Internet or participate in a breastfeeding organization.

Introducing Solid Foods

Is your baby able to sit up in a high chair and use his thumb and finger to pick up small objects, like Cheerios? Is he grabbing for your food or intently watching you chew on a T-bone? If so, then he may be ready to start solid foods.

Pediatricians generally recommend adding solid foods or juice to a baby's diet around the age of 6 months, but the exact age should depend on when your baby shows signs of interest. As we discuss earlier in this chapter, breast milk should still be your baby's main source of nutrition at 6 months.

REMEMBER

As you begin to introduce other foods into your baby's diet, be sure to always nurse first, then offer foods. If you offer foods first, your baby may not want to nurse, or may not nurse as much, and your milk supply may be affected.

Despite what you may read elsewhere, your baby's first solids don't have to be cereal or vegetables, and they don't have to be commercial baby foods. Many doctors and writers recommend starting the baby on bland foods initially, such as cereals; the theory behind this is that if you start out with sweet foods, like fruits, the baby will expect all his food to be sweet. But breast milk tastes sweet, so the baby is already conditioned to expect a sweet taste in his food. Start with whatever seems right to you.

Very ripe mashed bananas are a great first food. If you want to add cereal, rice cereal is the most digestible. You can mix cereal with water, breast milk, or juice.

REMEMBER

To check for allergic reactions, introduce one new food, and then wait a few days before introducing another. If a certain food causes a rash, fussiness, diarrhea, or vomiting, eliminate it for now. Your baby's gut may be slow to mature, and she may be able to handle foods later that upset her now. Expect to see bits of food in the baby's stool; this is perfectly normal. If her stool is red, think of beets, not blood!

WARNING!

Do not give a baby under the age of 1 pure honey or cow's milk. If your family has a high incidence of allergies, avoid nuts, fish, and eggs until age 2 or so.

When you start introducing solid foods, they shouldn't immediately become your baby's main source of nutrition. Give yourself and your baby time to adjust. You're setting the tone for eating patterns for the rest of your child's life. Don't make eating solids a battle; if he's not interested, try again in a few weeks.

One wonderful thing about breastfed babies is that their taste buds are more adventurous, because breast milk is flavored by what you eat. Bring on the avocados!

Adding Vitamin Supplements

In our society, we have a pill for everything, or so it seems. The trend a few years ago was to supplement breastfed babies with prescription vitamins. Doctors feared that breastfed babies wouldn't receive the necessary vitamins and minerals from breast milk.

Times have changed, and many doctors no longer prescribe a full complement of vitamins for breastfed babies. But certain vitamins are still supplemented, such as vitamin D; breast milk contains some vitamin D, but not enough. We discuss recommended supplements in the upcoming section "Giving baby a boost."

Eating right for baby's health

Doctors now believe — because research proves — that a breastfed baby doesn't need supplemental vitamins if the mother is in a good nutritional state. You need to be sure you're eating a healthy diet, especially if you're a vegetarian. (See Chapter 4 for more about breastfeeding while eating a vegetarian diet.)

If your diet is deficient, you may need supplementation. Obviously, we encourage you to try to eat better, but we all know that eating healthy can be a challenge, especially if you're on the go all day. (Even in fast food restaurants, healthy food choices are available in the form of salads and broiled chicken, but somehow the smell of fire-grilled burgers often wins out!) To boost your nutritional intake, continue to take your prenatal vitamins while you breastfeed.

Giving baby a boost

In certain circumstances, vitamin supplements may be a good idea for your baby. The American Academy of Pediatrics (AAP) has set these guidelines:

- If your baby has a low birth weight (less than 3.3 pounds), AAP recommends supplementing your breast milk with vitamins. At this weight your baby probably cannot breastfeed exclusively due to a weak suck reflex. Supplements are added to your pumped breast milk and fed to him through a tube.

  At this point in his life, your baby needs additional minerals and vitamins to grow. After he has gained weight and is breastfeeding exclusively, your breast milk will provide him with all the vitamins he needs.

- If you and your baby are dark-skinned, you need more exposure to the sun than someone who is fair-skinned to receive an adequate amount of vitamin D. A dark-skinned baby needs three to six times more sun exposure than a fair-skinned baby to produce the same amount of vitamin D. If your baby doesn't spend at least 30 minutes a week in the sun (wearing only a diaper), he isn't getting the proper amount of vitamin D. Babies who are completely covered with clothing don't get adequate exposure to the sun.

  Your baby needs to get vitamin D both from your breast milk and from the sun. If either supply is deficient, he could be at risk for vitamin D deficiency. To prevent the possibility of a vitamin D deficiency, the AAP recommends that all babies be given a minimum of 200 IU (*international units*) of vitamin D daily starting from the first two months of life.

  Vitamin D, which actually isn't a vitamin at all but a steroid hormone, is vital in the prevention of *rickets,* a softening of the bones that causes the leg bones to bow.

  Vitamin D and calcium go hand in hand. Vitamin D helps you absorb calcium, so both are needed for healthy bone growth in your baby. Fish oils, liver, and egg yolks all contain vitamin D.

- A healthy baby has enough iron stores to last for about the first six months of life. After that, he should receive iron either through solid foods or supplementation. A premature infant usually requires iron supplementation after two months.

- Fluoride helps protect teeth. If your water contains less than 0.3 ppm (parts per million) of fluoride, pediatricians often recommend a supplement of 0.25 milligrams a day starting at 6 months of age. A word of caution: Fluoride supplements can make your baby gassy.

  To find out if your water contains the recommended amount, call your local water company. If you use bottled water, call the bottling company. If you have well water, it doesn't contain fluoride. Your pediatrician can decide whether to use fluoride supplements based on your specific situation.

Although research has shown that a breastfed baby can get all other necessary vitamins and minerals from breast milk, many pediatricians would rather be safe than sorry and recommend a multivitamin supplement anyway. If your baby doesn't react well to this supplement, talk with the doctor about her reasons for prescribing it. Most babies put up a fight about taking these supplements — they don't taste very good!

Using a Pacifier

You've seen her in the store: the mom with a ribbon of pacifiers around her neck and two or three more falling out of her purse. Before you became a mom yourself, perhaps you sniffed with disapproval at 3- and 4-year-olds talking around the pacifiers hanging out of their mouths, like old men with cigars. Perhaps you vowed that your children would never be pacifier addicts. One thing to know about parenthood: Never say never!

Babies react to pacifiers in different ways. Some babies, breastfed or bottle-fed, take to pacifiers like fish to water and hang onto them for years. Others spit them out immediately.

REMEMBER

You don't want to introduce pacifiers too early in your baby's life because the use of the pacifier may decrease his nursing time. Decreasing nursing time decreases your milk supply. You especially don't want this to happen during the first six weeks when your supply is being established. Babies cry for many reasons, and while the pacifier may stop his crying, it may not solve the problem of why he's crying. Try not to introduce pacifiers until your breastfeeding is well-established. Before that, if your baby needs extra sucking time, nurse more.

Some babies really have a strong need to suck, so strong that you can't possibly nurse them often enough. If you have this type of baby, try to direct him to his fist to suck on rather than the pacifier, which can fall out of his mouth and frustrate him. (Of course, at a young age, he may not be able to find his fist easily either, because he really doesn't understand that it's attached to him.)

After the first few months, you learn to understand your baby's cues and know why he's crying. When your milk supply is well-established, when your baby is gaining weight like a champ, and when you can "read" your baby's needs, using a pacifier probably won't create any problems — at least not until you try to take it away a few years down the road.

Nipping the Biting Habit

All babies get teeth; what they do with them is very individualized! Not all nursing babies bite nipples, in spite of what you've heard. However, if you do have a biting bronco, stay calm. Biting is usually short-lived if you handle it properly and promptly.

Getting the teething message

Look for possible causes if your baby starts biting. Often, the baby has a reason to bite during breastfeeding. As we mention numerous times in this book, babies do talk to you. Not listening to them tends to be our problem!

Picture this. Your baby is somewhere between 4 and 6 months old. He's grumpy and whiny, and his crib rail has little teeth marks all over it. Everything you give him goes right to his mouth. He's drooling like Niagara Falls. You see a hint of a tooth bud on his gum when you look inside his mouth. Along with all these telltale signs, you find your baby literally chomping at the bit — and that bit is probably you.

Teething is probably the number one cause of nipple biting. Most times after the baby gets his teeth, this problem resolves itself. Toddlers rarely bite, because they understand the punishment for biting is removal from the breast.

If your baby is teething, try to remedy his discomfort without allowing your nipples to become teething rings. Give him a pain reliever, such as infant acetaminophen or teething gel, before nursing, so he's less likely to look to your nipple for pain relief. Make sure he has plenty of things to bite on between feedings; cold teething rings and iced washcloths work well. Also, try rubbing his gums firmly right before nursing to ease some of the discomfort.

Recognizing other reasons

Teething is the main culprit, but babies do sometimes bite for other reasons. For example, your baby may bite if he's distracted, if he's seeking attention, or if he has a stuffy nose.

Slipping off the breast

As babies get older, they become interested in their surroundings. Many times they slip off the breast, still holding on to the nipple, just to check out what's going on around them. Your baby may try this behavior when he's finished nursing and ready for some playtime. To avoid it, try to move with your baby so he stays latched onto your breast until you're both in a comfortable position to release.

Seeking attention

Some babies will do anything to get your attention, even at a young age. Sometimes that means biting a nipple. Most of the time biting for this reason occurs when you're involved in an activity like talking to someone, cooking dinner, or even just watching TV. Try giving your baby your undivided attention during nursing. Keep her in a quiet room with low light. If possible, keep distractions to a minimum, especially from older siblings.

Breathing through a stuffy nose

A stuffy nose seems like a poor excuse for nipple biting if you don't understand the mechanism of a baby nursing. When a baby breastfeeds, his mouth closes tightly around the nipple and areola. Air moves through his nose. When that airway is blocked, he has to struggle to eat and breathe at the same time. In an attempt to do both, he holds onto the nipple with his teeth and opens his mouth wide enough to get some air. Ouch. You can help the situation by keeping your baby's nasal passages open with a bulb syringe and running a humidifier in his room.

Stopping the biter

Knowing why babies bite doesn't make it hurt any less! Following are a few suggestions for dealing with your little biter:

TIP

- **If he starts to bite, pull him close to you, blocking his nose.** He'll release the nipple so he can breathe. This sounds terrible, but it's quick and effective.
- **Watch for cues that your baby is full.** Observe what your baby does at the end of a feeding. Does his jaw start tightening up? This is usually the time that babies start playing with nipples. When you notice a change in his jaw tension, stick your finger in his mouth. This way you can slip out of his mouth and protect your nipple. If your baby starts to move away from the breast, that could also be a sign that he's about to take a bite.

- **Tell him that biting isn't acceptable.** Although he may not understand the words, the tone of your voice conveys your message. Simply say, "No, don't bite mommy." He'll know that what he is doing is wrong. Don't be loud or forceful; you may scare him and potentially start a nursing strike.
- **If verbal reprimands don't work, use the "three strikes and you're out!" method.** After three warnings, take him off the breast. Don't put him back on until the next feeding. If he hasn't eaten anything yet with this feeding, wait a few minutes and try again. Most babies learn quickly what they need to do.
- **If he does stop biting, praise him.** Babies are no different than the rest of us; they like to be commended!

Moving Baby Out of Your Room

Life is never simple. First you agonize over the decision of having the baby sleep in your room, and then you agonize about when to move her out.

Making a joint decision

This is a decision best made by both you and your partner. If he's ready for some peace and quiet in the night and you're enjoying co-sleeping and don't want to give it up, you'll probably end up spending every night on the floor next to her crib! Some couples are perfectly happy to share their bed with their children well into their toddler years. Others feel the need to move their baby to his own room at a much earlier time.

Many times, exhaustion brings you to the decision to move the baby out. Make sure that you're both of sound mind — in other words, not sleep-deprived — before making the choice. You don't want to confuse your baby by bringing her back to your bed because you finally got some sleep and feel guilty over your decision. If your child still nurses at night, the move to her own room will be difficult at first for her and inconvenient for you.

REMEMBER

When you finally decide to move your baby out into the world, be prepared for some difficult nights. Your baby's used to your presence in the night, and she's not going to take kindly to a crib, no matter how much you paid for it!

Moving step-by-step

You may want to start by moving your baby into a crib in your room, if she's been sleeping in your bed. Put the crib right next to your bed at first, then gradually move it further away. After she gets used to sleeping in the crib, you can move her out the door.

Moving out is easier if you've already introduced your baby to the unfamiliar room you call the nursery. First, try breastfeeding her in the nursery. Then begin putting her in her room for naps, in a portable crib or in her infant seat. After a week or so, try the crib at night. Be prepared for some crying (both yours and hers!). If she protests greatly, try sleeping in the same room with her for a few nights; she may find it more tolerable.

As time goes on, inch your way out of the nursery. If your baby is still not sleeping through the night or starts waking up again because of the new arrangements, be patient. It may be helpful to bring her back to your bed to nurse. Or you may find that nursing her in the nursery rocker reassures her that you're still around.

REMEMBER

These are scary times for your baby. Even in the light of day, she's afraid to be away from mom or dad. The nighttime is even more frightening. Make sure that you leave a nightlight on. After she's out on her own, don't confuse her by occasionally returning her to your bed. Doing so will make the next separation attempt a bigger nightmare for both of you.

Chapter 11

You and Your Spouse: Being a Breastfeeding Couple

In This Chapter

- Looking at breastfeeding through your partner's eyes
- Handling disapproval and jealousy
- Finding ways to involve your partner
- Regaining a sex life

Many breastfeeding books talk about you and your baby as a breastfeeding couple. The only problem with this viewpoint is that it eliminates the person who was originally the other half of your "couple": your partner.

Your partner will inevitably feel a little bit left out when it comes to breastfeeding. You need to remember that you and your partner were a couple long before you and the baby were, and (we hope) you will remain a couple after your baby is grown and gone. In this chapter, we take a look at how your partner fits into your feeding triangle and what to do to keep him feeling needed and involved.

Appreciating a Helpful Partner

Some partners take their role as support person seriously; they bring the baby to you, change him, and put him to sleep after feedings. Others take a hands-off approach to feeding time, feeling that feedings are your domain and that dads don't have a role to play.

If your partner is hands-on, he may become the food police, chasing all your friends and relatives out of the house at feeding time to make sure that nothing interferes with breastfeeding. Or he may become so consumed with making sure the baby's eating enough that he's shoving the baby into your lap at the slightest whimper.

Some new dads are so anxious to help that you may find yourself doing nothing for the baby but breastfeeding, because your partner is doing all the rest.

REMEMBER

Keep in mind that your partner is feeling his way into this unfamiliar role of *parent,* just as you are. If he's overstepping his bounds, tell him so — nicely of, course! If he doesn't want anyone within a ten-mile radius when you breastfeed because "other people distract the baby," encourage him to set up a little nursing nook out of everyone's view but still in the same county!

Usually, the zealous dad is very supportive of breastfeeding but wants to feel he's part of the action, too. Realize that you're lucky to have such a supportive guy, and try to tone down his overprotective tendencies without dampening his enthusiasm.

Dealing with Disapproval

Not all partners are helpful. Some actively try to sabotage breastfeeding, making disparaging comments or putting pressure on you to quit nursing. If your partner makes unsupportive comments, such as saying that the baby isn't gaining enough weight or that breastfeeding is making your breasts sag, you need to discuss why he's saying these things.

REMEMBER

Ideally, you should discuss breastfeeding long before the baby is born so you can be aware of your partner's feelings ahead of time. However, even a partner who seems supportive before the baby is born may behave differently after you deliver. Maybe he didn't realize how much time breastfeeding would take. Perhaps he didn't think he'd be jealous, but he is — not only of your closeness to the baby but of the amount of time the baby requires.

Maybe your partner is feeling pressure from someone in his family, or from his friends. He may be getting a garden of misinformation from other people about breastfeeding — that it means you can't have sex, that you'll gain weight from breastfeeding, or that boys who breastfeed too long turn out to be sissies. Whatever his issues are, you can't address them until you know what they are.

WARNING!

When you're exhausted from being up all night and busy with the baby all day, you may think it's easier to just give in to pressure and stop nursing. But if you regret being forced into weaning, the resentment will cause problems between you down the road.

Even if you don't feel like you have the energy to deal with a conflict, try to discuss the issue from both your viewpoints before giving up on breastfeeding. Maybe your partner doesn't realize that all his little remarks about your weight or the baby's health are chipping away at your confidence. Or maybe he's just trying to find a way to get you to look at him as well as the baby.

If your partner forces you into giving up nursing, he may feel guilty and upset about it later as well, so don't give up easily. This may be the first problem you need to solve as new parents. Make sure it sets the tone for cooperative parenting down the road.

Keeping Your Partner Involved

A dad can bond with his baby in many ways that don't involve food. Following are a few ideas for your partner to get close to the new little person in his life:

TIP

- **Read to the baby.** Most babies are mesmerized by a voice reading to them, and it doesn't have to be a Golden Book either. Listening to dad read the football scores is just as mesmerizing!
- **Let him see you.** Babies love faces, even faces of people who think their chins recede or their noses are crooked. Place your face close to his, about 8 to 10 inches in front of him. He will start associating this face with your voice.
- **Take photos.** Taking pictures is a great way for dad to be part of the action. Make sure that you know how to use the camera too, so that you have lots of dad and baby pictures as well.
- **Purchase a snuggly-type baby holder.** Both you and your partner can use it. Your coauthor Carol found that her husband did most of the holding thanks to the backpack carrier he wore through several babies!

After three or four weeks, when your milk supply is well-established, you may want to pump and have dad do a bottle feeding now and then. You may be surprised at how excited he is to be the one feeding the baby!

Battling the Green-Eyed Monster

If you're like most breastfeeding couples, you made a joint decision to breastfeed your baby. But even with the best of intentions, you may find yourself working through not only the growing pains of breastfeeding, but also your feelings that, on some days, dad is more of a problem than the baby! Even the most supportive dads sometimes feel jealous of the attention the baby gets.

How you handle the green-eyed monster can make or break your breastfeeding experience. As a mom, you'll handle balancing acts between groups of people throughout your life, juggling children, parents, friends, coworkers, and (of course) partners! Part of being a good mom is discovering how to care for a screaming baby and a sulky partner at the same time!

What makes a normally supportive, loving, caring father turn green right before your eyes? Following are a few possibilities and some ideas for dealing with the issues:

- **Your partner may feel insecure about his parenting skills.** New dads often haven't had the advantage of babysitting during teenage years, and many aren't sure which side of the diaper is up when they first meet a newborn. Your partner may interpret your one-woman feeding show as giving you a parenting edge.

  The solution? Don't always look so confident, even if you babysat triplets all through high school. Sometimes mothers come on like gangbusters in their new parenting role, like mother bears fiercely protecting their cubs. This intensity can be overwhelming to your partner. Let your insecurities show a little, so your partner knows he's not the only one in the dark!

  Also, praise him for what he does, even if he puts the diaper on backwards or doesn't do things according to your standards.

- **Your partner may feel like the odd man out in your new family.** He may feel like he has no real role to play. This can be a disadvantage to his developing a relationship with the baby.

  The solution? Give him some real, important tasks to do! He'll soon realize that, just because he can't breastfeed, he can still be a parent. He'll cultivate his own skills as he rocks, reads to, bathes, and dresses the baby. Having an involved partner could spell big relief when you're having a trying day with the baby!

- **Your partner may feel that he's competing with his baby for your time and affection.** He may feel like the baby has come between the two of you. You may be saying, "Oh, that's ridiculous," but hold on. We're not saying that this is true, but rather that this could be his perception.

  The solution? Make time for the two of you, alone. You don't have to have romantic three-hour dinner dates. Five minutes of conversation before you collapse in bed is good when you have a new baby. The expensive dinners can come later; you need to keep talking until then so you have something to say to each other when you finally get a night out alone!

You want and need your partner's support. Start by understanding that his feelings are normal. Try to understand how he's feeling: The two of you have been on your own for some period of time, and now he's competing with an 8-pound, screaming infant.

Your partner doesn't have your hormonal advantage (and probably doesn't want it). He's not feeling attached to the baby when Junior is crying inconsolably, urinating in his face, or vomiting on his designer suit. He's just not emotionally wired for the "baptism by urine" in the same way you are.

You have quite a bit of power here. You can cure your partner or kill him — not literally, of course! What we mean is you can encourage his involvement by having him actively participate in his baby's care, or you can foster this segregation by being Ms. Perfect Superwoman. Let him be the hero once in a while.

Resuming Your Sex Life

Sex usually isn't the first thing you think about after your baby is born, but it may be high on your partner's priority list, especially if you weren't having sex the last few weeks of your pregnancy. If he is in the delivery room when your baby is born and has a bird's-eye view of the delivery, he'll probably understand why having sex the minute you get out of the hospital simply isn't possible. Chances are, though, that he's going to be thinking about having sex as soon as possible, while you may be thinking of having sex sometime in the next decade — maybe.

Getting your breasts into the act

While he may be anxious to have sex, your partner may be nervous about making your breasts part of your sexual relationship. He may be afraid of your new breasts, which are much larger and leakier than your old ones, or he may worry about somehow depriving the baby of milk if he touches your breasts. You may worry that your new breasts aren't attractive to him, or you may not feel like having your breasts touched by anyone except the baby. All these concerns can make your postpartum sex life complicated.

Men and women view most things differently, as the book *Men are from Mars, Women are from Venus* by John Gray (HarperCollins) so aptly points out. Men are used to thinking of breasts as sex objects, period. Women think more like this: Take a simple object, like a baby bottle, and consider the ways it can be used. A bottle could be a vase for flowers in your baby's room, or a container for cotton swabs. This creativity makes it easy for you to feel comfortable with your breasts as feeding tools, as your baby's source of comfort, and also as sex objects. Your partner may have real difficulty with this, and your sex life may hit a wall because of it.

Most men support the decision to breastfeed, but the weeks and months after delivery are stressful even under the best of conditions. In the first few months, your sex life will probably fall victim to exhaustion, sore nipples, uncontrolled let-downs, and reduced libido. You feel "touched out" by the end of the day. This isn't the perfect situation for lovemaking! But sex and breastfeeding can coexist; you just need to work at it.

Recognizing physical changes

Why is something you used to enjoy so difficult after you have a baby? If you don't feel like having sex, you may ask yourself, "Why do I feel this way? Isn't this the person I had a child with, the one I cared about intimately?" At the same time, your partner is wondering, "Why doesn't she want me to touch her? Doesn't she realize that I still love her? Does she still love me?"

Understanding what's going on physically can help you relate better to each other:

- **Breastfeeding can suppress your monthly cycle.** This has its pluses and minuses. On the plus side, it can prevent pregnancy when you're exclusively breastfeeding (see Chapter 16). On the minus side, the lack of the hormone estrogen also decreases vaginal lubrication. Without lubrication, intercourse can be painful. The solution to vaginal dryness is as close as a tube of KY jelly, Astroglide, or Replens.

  TIP: Take time (yes, we know, *what* time!) for foreplay. Getting in the mood helps increase cervical mucus, which is a natural lubricant. Saliva can be used as a lubricant also, but not until after your six-week checkup with your obstetrician, because of the risk of infection if you still aren't completely healed.

- **Decreased estrogen levels can decrease your sex drive.** And hormones aren't the only culprit. Fatigue and stress can also turn off the switch, and early parenthood brings plenty of both.

  TIP: Don't place impossible goals on yourself when it comes to sex. Try cuddling, holding hands, and just plain kissing without worrying about where it's going to lead. Eventually, it will lead to the resumption of your old sex life.

- **Leaking milk is a challenge whether you're in the bakery or the bedroom.** Your let-down reflex will settle down eventually, but until then it can make lovemaking messy. Breast stimulation and orgasm can cause you to leak or even spray milk into your partner's face! Ask him if it bothers him. If it does, try nursing the baby before lovemaking, to decrease the available milk in your breasts. You can also wear a bra or nightgown during lovemaking to contain flying milk.
- **Sensitive breasts can be a problem.** When you start breastfeeding, you may feel like you can't handle any more breast contact than you already have with your baby. Or you may experience decreased sensitivity in your nipples. If your nipples are cracked or your breasts are engorged, you may find being touched painful.

  If you don't want your breasts touched, tell your partner that they're off limits for now, but reassure him that this won't last forever. You may also need to use positions that put less pressure on your breasts; you can always check out the Kama Sutra for some interesting suggestions!

Coping with psychological factors

The physical changes that occur while you breastfeed are easier to understand than the psychological changes. Stress and fatigue are difficult to leave in the hallway outside your bedroom. Yes, your sweet little baby can wreak havoc, but you two can fix it. Talk about what you're comfortable with and what isn't working for you.

TIP

If you wait for lovemaking to occur spontaneously, you may wait forever, especially if the baby's sleeping in your room. You may need to put a "play date" on your calendar for the two of you. Be sure it's just a play date, not a "we've got to have sex because it's been three weeks" date. Don't put pressure on yourselves to have sex on a schedule. Just plan some together time to snuggle on the couch, and see where it leads.

Fearing another pregnancy

REMEMBER

The thought of another pregnancy can keep you from resuming or enjoying your sex life. *Exclusive breastfeeding* (giving your baby no supplemental bottles) can protect against pregnancy, but you'll also find plenty of families whose breastfed children are ten months apart. If you absolutely, positively don't want to get pregnant again yet, use an additional method of birth control. We discuss birth control and planning your next pregnancy in Chapter 16.

Sensual pleasure while breastfeeding

Having sensual feelings while nursing your baby can be unnerving. You may wonder if it isn't a little abnormal to experience sensual pleasure while breastfeeding. In fact, you may feel guilty and even a little perverted, but rest assured that experiencing these sensations is not uncommon.

Breastfeeding releases oxytocin, which causes uterine contractions. Rhythmic uterine contractions are also felt during orgasm. Some women find nipple stimulation alone leads to sensual feelings. If you have this experience, enjoy it, and don't worry that you're abnormal.

Chapter 12

Weaning the Baby

In This Chapter

- Knowing when and why to wean
- Anticipating physical changes
- Needing to wean suddenly
- Weaning to a cup
- Feeling emotional about weaning

Weaning is bittersweet, whenever and however it occurs. You may believe that you're more than ready to wean — until it actually happens. Or perhaps you're not ready at all, but your baby is.

Whether breastfeeding is a joy or a pain, whether it lasts two months or two years, the end of nursing is the end of an era in your baby's life. In this chapter, we discuss how to go about weaning so that it causes the least amount of trauma for both of you.

Getting the Timing Right

Although the American Academy of Pediatrics recommends breastfeeding for at least the first year of life, your baby hasn't read the literature. He may be ready to wean before his first birthday, or he may not be ready for months — or even years! — after.

Avoiding a hasty decision

Certain events or factors may push you to consider weaning before you and the baby are ready. For example:

- You need to return to work.
- You or the baby needs to be hospitalized.
- You develop mastitis (see Chapter 8).

- Your baby starts getting teeth.
- You want to lose weight.
- Your family is pressuring you to wean.
- You're sleep-deprived.
- You want other people to feed the baby once in a while.

We don't believe that you should wean for any of these reasons, unless you truly are ready. Weaning may seem like a quick way to make your life easier, but you may make life more complicated if you wean too early or before you really want to.

We certainly understand that getting through the early months of breastfeeding can be stressful. But don't feel this stress means you must wean the baby. Wait for life to stabilize before making this decision. You may change your mind when the dust settles a bit; if you don't, you'll have an easier time weaning when you're calmer. Also, listen to your baby and let him have a say in the decision. If your baby is fighting against weaning, he may not be ready for it.

Reading your baby's signals

Some babies seem to make the decision to wean themselves well before 12 months, while others are perfectly content to still be nursing at age 2.

As your baby becomes more interested in what is going on around him, he may not seem as interested in quietly nursing as he did in earlier months. Don't take this as a sign that he isn't attached to you anymore! A 6-month-old is naturally attracted to activity around him when he's nursing.

If your baby seems to be weaning before you think he should, evaluate the reasons for his behavior. Some babies go on a "nursing strike" for a short time. Could he be responding to a nursing problem that you're not aware of? If your baby seems to lose interest in nursing, examine recent nursing events. For example:

- Did you scream when he bit your nipple and scare him, so that he's afraid to nurse? (No one can blame you if you did!)
- Did he recently have an ear infection that made it painful for him to nurse?
- Did you recently return to work? Is so, life has certainly become a little harried at your house. Your baby may sense that you're too busy to give him the attention he wants.

Working moms can find their new routine decreasing their milk supply. (See Chapter 13 for more on working and nursing.) If you have difficulties with pumping, you may consider supplementing with formula. But if you continue to supplement, your milk supply will eventually decrease. In reality, you could be starting to wean before you're really ready. Make sure you're not giving formula often enough to significantly decrease your milk supply.

Letting the baby take the lead

If you're considering weaning, let your baby take the lead if possible, because both of you will experience less stress. Don't try to decide in advance when weaning will happen. All babies eventually wean themselves, some earlier and some later.

Weaning starts the very first time you feed your baby a supplemental bottle or offer him solid food. If you look at it this way, you can see that weaning is a slow, gradual process occurring over months, perhaps even years. The change in your baby's nutritional needs is part of his natural development, and it should occur in stages.

If you let your baby lead the way, you'll find that he knows what to do. He'll gradually wean himself, eliminating nursing sessions one at a time because he'd rather eat ravioli or mashed potatoes!

If your baby is a year old or older, you can wean him from breast milk to regular milk, eliminating the need to buy costly formula. Babies who wean after they're a year old usually accept a cup at meal times. And by the time your baby is a year old, you can feel confident that his nutritional needs are being met because he's probably eating a full assortment of foods.

We have to say this one more time: Listen to your baby. He may be ready to give up most of his nursing sessions when he's eating regular foods and is fully engaged in the world around him. But you may find him clinging to his bedtime session with you. This is usually the last one he'll give up.

Breastfeeding is about so much more than food. Your baby may not need you as much for nutrition as he reaches the one-year mark, but he still needs you for comfort and security, especially at night. Even as adults, we develop comfort rituals before sleep: a warm blanket, a glass of warm milk, a good book. Your baby is no different.

Weaning Without (Too Much) Wailing

You can take several steps to make weaning go more smoothly:

- **Give yourself the time to accomplish weaning successfully.** Allow at least several weeks to gradually decrease feedings.
- **Let your baby tell you when he wants to nurse.** Lactation consultants often suggest a "don't offer, don't refuse" approach to weaning an older child. If your baby really wants to nurse, he'll let you know, but don't offer if he doesn't ask.
- **Ask your partner to take care of the baby in circumstances that the baby associates with nursing.** For example, your partner can get the baby ready for bed so the baby learns not to expect a bedtime feeding, or he can feed the baby breakfast.
- **Eliminate the easy feedings first.** Watch for your baby's cues. You may see that he's fine with dropping the after-lunch nursing session but cries to nurse at night.
- **Shorten the time of each feeding.** See how your baby reacts to you saying "that's enough." If he's old enough, try using something like an egg timer. This takes the pressure off you as the bad guy saying he's nursed enough. Instead, the hourglass or clock determines when you're finished nursing.
- **Substitute another comfort measure — such as rocking, reading, or singing — for nursing.** Do these activities in areas that your baby doesn't associate with nursing. If he likes to breastfeed in the family room rocking chair, don't pick that area to read to him, at least not in the early weaning days.
- **Be patient and tolerant.** As with all trying times, this too will pass! Every child eventually weans himself.

Preparing for Physical Changes

If you can wean your baby gradually, your body also undergoes gradual physical changes. Sudden weaning is a different story; we discuss what to expect in the following section.

One change that takes place when you begin weaning is something that only your baby notices. Mother Nature, in her wisdom, gives weaning a helping hand by changing the taste of your milk when nursing decreases. As your milk supply drops off, the sodium content increases, causing the milk to taste salty. Many babies decide they dislike the taste and choose to wean fully as a result.

Other physical changes are much more noticeable to you. For example, the fullness in your breasts decreases as time passes; they start to look smaller and less firm. You may look in the mirror one day and wonder where your chest went! Fear not, because your breasts return to their former size within six months of stopping breastfeeding. Keep in mind that your breasts have already successfully made it through some extreme changes, starting with pregnancy. Weaning is just the final step of getting your body back to its normal shape and size.

When you stop nursing, you may notice for the first time that your breasts show signs of stretching and sagging. Remember that stretching and sagging are common in all women after giving birth, not just those who breastfeed. The fullness in your breasts while you were nursing simply helped to disguise these normal changes.

You may find that months — or even a year — after you wean completely, you can still express a little milk from your nipples. This is not unusual. Make sure that you're not encouraging your breasts to make milk with nipple stimulation during lovemaking. (We discuss sex and breastfeeding in Chapter 11.)

If you continue to produce milk long after weaning, contact your doctor, because you may have a high level of the hormone prolactin. High prolactin levels can interfere with getting pregnant in the future and can usually be corrected with medication.

Weaning Quickly

While we certainly hope you can follow the advice we offer earlier in this chapter about letting your baby take the lead with weaning, we're also realists. We know that life sometimes doesn't let you and your baby take your time with weaning. If you find yourself needing to wean quickly — or responding to your baby's sudden decision to stop nursing — the following sections offer some tips for surviving what could otherwise be an ordeal.

If possible, don't wean your baby totally from the breast until you know that he can tolerate formula without any difficulties. Babies younger than 1 year aren't ready for cow's milk.

Cutting back feedings

If circumstances dictate that you wean quickly, try to take as gradual an approach as possible. Eliminate one feeding each day over several days to allow your milk supply to adjust.

If your breasts feel very full when you start eliminating feedings, express a small amount of milk, but just enough to make you feel comfortable. If you pump your breasts completely, your body assumes you need it to continue producing the same amount of milk, and you delay the physical adjustment to weaning.

Continue the process of omitting one feeding at a time over several days until all feedings are eliminated. Or, if you can continue to nurse at certain times of day — such as at night or in the morning — and eliminate the other feedings.

You should wean gradually even if you've been pumping rather than nursing for several feedings a day. For example, if you've been pumping four times a day, eliminate one pumping session over a 24- to 48-hour period. Do this for several days, until you've eliminated all pumping times, and your breasts don't feel full anymore. Or gradually shorten the amount of time at each pumping session.

Going cold turkey

It doesn't happen often, but sometimes a baby who has been nursing regularly wakes up one day and decides he's done breastfeeding. This can be very upsetting, not only emotionally but physically — your breasts will feel like they're ready to explode.

As we discuss earlier in this chapter, in the "Reading your baby's signals" section, you want to be certain that your baby isn't resisting nursing temporarily as a result of some recent event or change in your lives. Contact your lactation consultant for suggestions if you suspect your baby is on a temporary "nursing strike."

You may worry that the baby is weaning because you're not producing enough milk. If the baby is gaining weight well and doesn't show signs of dehydration (see Chapter 7), he's getting enough milk. Remember to always breastfeed before giving solid food if the baby is less than 1 year old; he needs the milk more than the solids at this point.

If you've run through the list of possible reasons for your baby's behavior and still can't persuade him to nurse, get yourself ready for a quick transition. First, wear a good, supportive bra. Next, take acetaminophen or ibuprofen to alleviate the discomfort you feel and apply cold compresses under your armpits. Make sure you take the ice packs off after about 20 minutes. You may have to express some milk if things get too uncomfortable, but pump as little as possible — just enough to relieve some pressure.

This is also a good time to head back to the produce section for cabbage leaves, which help relieve engorgement when you're weaning just like they do when your milk first comes in. Chill them in the refrigerator and then place them inside your bra, crinkling the leaves or bruising them first to allow the liquid inside to seep out. Change them about every two hours; you can also alternate with ice.

If your baby decides to wean himself abruptly, the experience may be very upsetting for you. No matter what anyone says to try to help, the rejection hurts. Support groups are very helpful during this time (see Chapter 4). Remind yourself often that even if you nursed your baby for one month, you have reason to be proud.

Satisfying an Occasional Nurser

Some babies give up all but one feeding, or they nurse only once every few days. If your breasts are being stimulated, even once a day, they will continue to produce milk for that feeding. However, as the stimulation decreases, you may find the well running dry.

You may find that your toddler comes to you to nurse in times of need. For example, if he feels sick or falls down and hurts himself, he may want to nurse. Nursing can be better than a bandage! Sometimes, when a baby is ill and refusing food, he nurses for comfort. In this case, nursing performs double duty, providing fluid and nutrition as well as comfort.

Occasional nursers may nurse only for a few minutes. They aren't there for a meal, but rather for security and comfort. The nice part about the occasional nurser is that he often asks for the breast at times that you want to be close to him, too. What mom doesn't want to comfort her child when he's hurt or sick?

Introducing a Bottle

If your baby has had a few bottles already, weaning to a bottle shouldn't be a big problem. But if your baby has never had a bottle, he may initially reject it. Babies who've never had a bottle may be put off by the smell or taste of formula; the shape, smell, or taste of the rubber nipple; or the faster flow of the milk.

If your baby is older than 4 weeks, breastfeeding should be established enough to introduce a bottle for an occasional feeding. Introducing a bottle does two things. First, it allows you some freedom if you have to go back to work or if an emergency occurs. Second, it prepares your baby for weaning whenever the time comes. If you don't introduce a bottle early, you may face a baby who adamantly refuses to take a bottle from anyone! If you do introduce a bottle, make sure you don't make it a single event. Give a bottle once or twice a week so he remembers the experience.

TIP

To prevent problems, you may want to initially give the baby pumped breast milk in a bottle, so that the taste and smell of the food itself is familiar. Have someone else give him a bottle at first; if he smells your scent, he may expect to nurse and refuse the cold rubber thing you're trying to put in his mouth. Also make sure you warm the milk if it comes from the refrigerator or freezer.

For a baby who balks at the bottle, try one of the slow-flow nipples that are shaped more like a human nipple (see Chapter 5). Or if your baby has a favorite pacifier, get a nipple that resembles it.

REMEMBER

Introduce a bottle when your baby is happy. Offering a bottle when he's really hungry or sick may upset him. You might breastfeed him on one side and then give him a bottle to finish the feeding. Above all, be patient. It may take some time for the two of you to work through the bottle introduction. Take it as a complement that he likes his mom better than the bottle, and try not to get frustrated!

If he rejects the bottle no matter what's in it or what nipple you use, your course of action depends on his age. If he's too young to wean directly to a cup, you may want to continue nursing for a little while longer. If he's old enough, you may want to wean directly to a cup, bypassing bottles altogether.

Moving Straight to a Cup

A baby 9 months old or older may benefit by being weaned straight to a cup without ever having a bottle. Doing so eliminates the need to wean from the bottle down the road. It also avoids the issue of the baby taking a bottle to bed, which can lead to serious tooth decay. Most babies can start to drink from a cup at around 6 months.

TIP

Start introducing a cup when your baby can sit up and seems interested in holding a cup. Get a colorful cup that holds his attention; sippy cups with handles are easiest for babies to use. Make sure it has a lid, unless you want milk all over the house!

Begin with a little juice or breast milk in the cup, and tip the cup up for him. He'll probably try to suck on the spout at first. Offer the cup once a day or so to start; the object isn't to get him to drink a lot from the cup, just to get him used to it.

After he becomes more familiar with the cup, you can use it instead of a bottle to supplement feedings when you're gone. When the time seems right for weaning, replace the feeding he's least interested in with a cup feeding. He needs to be able to take 4 or more ounces from the cup to substitute it for a nursing session.

Your co-author Sharon's grandson wasn't interested in a sippy cup at all, but he really liked sport bottles with straws. He weaned himself directly to them at 10 months.

Keep in mind that some babies still need sucking time after weaning. Don't be surprised if your breastfed baby starts sucking his thumb or pacifier more often after weaning.

Expecting Emotional Letdown

Weaning can make you depressed for many reasons. The first is physical: Your hormone levels drop and your breasts may be uncomfortable. The second is emotional: You may be concerned about losing the closeness that comes with nursing, or feeling sad that your baby is growing up.

Unless you've had a terrible nursing experience, expect to feel an emotional letdown when you stop breastfeeding. You can prepare for it by weaning slowly, so that your hormones don't drop all of a sudden. You can also prepare by being aware ahead of time that you're likely to feel somewhat depressed.

Sometimes your last breastfeeding slips by without you even being aware of it. Your baby nurses fewer times a day, and then he skips a day altogether. Next thing you know, a week has gone by, and you realize, with a feeling of shock, that he's weaned.

On the other hand, you may be counting the days until your last nursing, crying "Free at last!" Feeling that you are no longer the primary caregiver can be a relief. Don't feel guilty for thinking like this. If you have nursed your baby one month or one year, you've given him a special gift and you should be proud of it.

An amazing connection exists between a mom and baby after breastfeeding is an established routine. With the loss comes an emptiness that needs to be filled in other ways. Be sure your partner plays a part in weaning, not just by helping with feedings but also by actively supporting your decision.

Shedding a few tears when nursing ends is normal; becoming seriously depressed is not. If you find yourself crying constantly, unable to sleep or concentrate, what started as mild depression over weaning may be slipping into serious depression. This depression could be caused by your changing hormone levels; see your doctor if you feel your depression is worsening rather than improving.

Breastfeeding is only one small part of a lifetime of parenting. You and your child will bond just as much over learning to ride a bike, going to soccer games, and doing homework. Look at the end of breastfeeding as a natural progression in your baby's life, and start looking forward to the next stage — potty training, for example. Now *there's* an opportunity to bond!

Part IV

Breastfeeding in the Real World

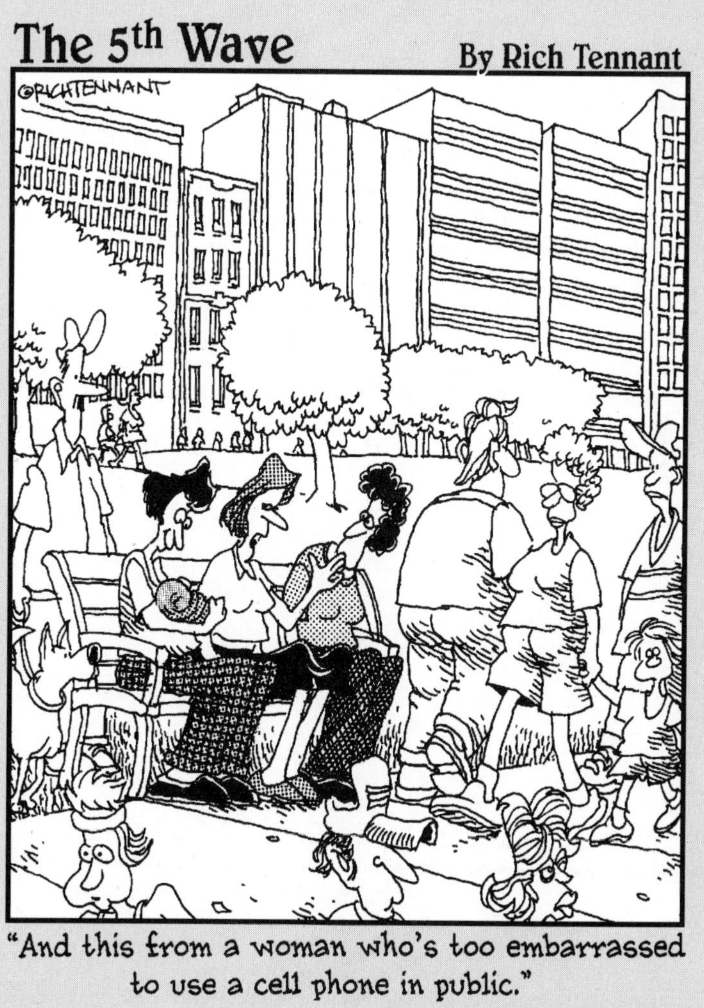

"And this from a woman who's too embarrassed to use a cell phone in public."

In this part . . .

The first few weeks of staying at home with your new baby come to an end all too quickly. Before you know it, you're back to the grocery store, the carpools, and the football games. You need to know how to breastfeed in public and what your rights are when it comes to breastfeeding. You may also be heading back to work, which carries the added stresses of finding the right childcare for your baby and striking a balance between the needs of your employer and your family. As if that weren't enough to deal with, you may already be thinking about giving your baby a sibling! Feeling overwhelmed? The information in this part can help.

Chapter 13

Breastfeeding and the Working Mom

In This Chapter

- Finding time at work to nurse or pump
- Preparing your boss and coworkers
- Sticking to a pumping schedule
- Pumping on business trips
- Balancing working and nursing at home
- Finding a caregiver

Time truly flies after you have a baby; before you know it, maternity leave is over, and you have to go back to work. Whether you're off for six weeks or six months, chances are you'll head back to work feeling conflicted. Can you continue to nurse without your milk supply dropping? What if you start leaking in the middle of an important meeting? Can you pump in a cubicle without becoming the talk of the office?

In this chapter, we help you address all these issues, as well as the question of how to handle business travel. The information in this chapter can give you a head start in figuring out what your life will look like as a working, breastfeeding mom.

Evaluating Your Work Situation

Nursing and working can fit together, but it takes some planning. The ideal time to look at your work situation and consider how it fits with breastfeeding is before your baby is born. Some things to consider are whether you can manage to run home (or to the day-care) at lunch to nurse, and how you can slip away to pump a few times a day.

REMEMBER

The older your baby is when you return to work, the easier time you'll have continuing to breastfeed. Your milk supply will be established, and your baby will probably eat less frequently than she did as a newborn. You'll have mastered the breast pump, as well as the art of let-down (see Chapter 6).

Considering your options

If your company has a nursery on site and you can leave your office a few times a day, you're in breastfeeding heaven. Unfortunately, this kind of setup is the exception rather than the rule.

TIP

If you hire a babysitter to care for your child, you may want to ask her to bring the baby to you a few times a day. If you have an office job where your schedule is predictable, and if you're entitled to two breaks a day plus a lunch hour, this could work well for you.

But say you aren't this lucky — maybe you have a completely unpredictable schedule with little flexibility. Nursing during the day may be out of the question, and even pumping may be difficult. But you do get bathroom breaks, right? You can pump or hand-express at least enough milk to prevent engorgement (see Chapter 6).

TIP

Some states have developed breastfeeding policies requiring companies to provide nursing facilities and specified nursing breaks for new mothers. See Chapter 15 for more on nursing and the law.

Flexing your schedule

If you're really fortunate, you have the freedom to set your own work schedule. But what if you don't? Following are some options to consider:

- **Inquire about job sharing.** Some companies allow an employee to share a job with a coworker, so that two people together do the work of one full-time employee (and split the salary). If you can work four or five hours a day, for example, you may miss only one feeding.
- **Ask if you can work longer hours and fewer days.** For example, would your company allow you to work 4 10-hour days or 3 12-hour days each week? The longer hours may be worth the tradeoff to spend more days at home.

- **Determine if you can you work from home one or more days a week.** Thanks to technology advances, some companies feel comfortable letting employees work from a home office on occasion. You'll still need to hire a babysitter so you can actually get work done, but at least you'll be able to see the baby and nurse when necessary.

Maintaining Your Milk Supply

REMEMBER

Your milk supply is related to demand. If you start nursing less frequently, your milk supply drops. If you plan to ask your baby's caregiver to feed her breast milk from a bottle, you need to pump consistently to keep up your supply. (See more about pumping later in this chapter, in the section "Pumping at Work.") If you're going to ask the caregiver to offer your baby formula instead, and you plan to nurse the baby only a few times a day, a decrease in supply may not be a problem.

TIP

Several weeks before you go back to work, pump as often as you can and freeze everything that you pump. For the last two weeks before you start working, reduce your pumping — perhaps pump and freeze a little after morning feedings, when you tend to have more milk. This should create a good supply of breast milk to use when you first start working, and it helps you become familiar with using a pump. Don't overdo pumping or you may create another problem: an oversupply! This could lead to discomfort when you return to work.

In the last couple of weeks before returning to work, you can also try to adjust your daily routine to what it will be on a workday. Start getting up at about the time that you'll get up for work, allowing extra time for pumping and feeding the baby. Try nursing and pumping at about the times that you will during the workday.

Your baby may adjust to your daytime absence by eating less during the day and more during the evening and nighttime hours. Keep in mind that night feedings are often easier if the baby is in your bed; she can nurse easily, and you'll get more sleep (see Chapter 7).

Talking to Your Boss and Coworkers

TIP

Before you return to work, tell your boss and immediate coworkers that you'll still be breastfeeding. Remember that your coworkers are probably only interested in how your breastfeeding is going to affect *them*. Focus on the positive aspects of breastfeeding as it impacts your work. Explain that breastfed children are healthier, so you won't miss work as often to take your baby to the doctor.

You might remind your boss that the American Academy of Pediatrics recommends that employers assist returning mothers to continue to nurse. (See Chapter 15 for some legal issues related to breastfeeding and work.) Also explain that a positive breastfeeding policy can result in less turnover among women in the company. (A company's commitment to breastfeeding is also a recruiting tool and gives the company a positive image. It's good PR!)

If necessary, offer to pump or nurse only when others are taking breaks or eating lunch, so you won't disrupt the office. Be clear about where and when you'll be pumping. Unless you work alone (or have a very private office), sooner or later your coworkers will figure out what you're doing, even if you don't tell them. The strange noises most pumps make will give you away.

REMEMBER

Most coworkers are no more anxious to barge in on you when you're pumping than you are to have it happen. If you keep them in the loop, that embarrassing situation is much less likely to happen.

As long as your pumping doesn't inconvenience them, most coworkers will be supportive. However, if you dump work on other people because you need to pump every hour, expect resentment. But you should be allowed the same breaks that other people take (such as smokers), and you should be able to utilize part of your lunch hour for pumping or nursing.

Pumping at Work

When you're seriously pumping to keep up your milk supply, you need to invest in a serious pump. See Chapter 5 for our suggestions on breast pumps, and be prepared to rent or purchase an electric pump that can handle both breasts at once.

REMEMBER

Practice with your pump before heading off to work, because pumps can be complicated to use. If your lunch break is only 30 minutes and it takes 15 minutes to get hooked up, you're not going to pump (or eat) much.

Keeping it private (and clean)

If you have an office without a door lock, ask to have one put on, or install a simple hook-and-eye type yourself. If a lock is out of the question, put a sign on your door to let coworkers know that now isn't a good time to bring in the visiting engineers from Tokyo.

Perhaps your job doesn't come with an office at all, in which case you may have to pump in a bathroom. This is certainly possible, though not easy, and definitely not a top choice for cleanliness reasons. Unless you have no other choice, don't pump in the stall; the environment is not very clean. Bring a chair in, and use the sink or a small table to hold all your supplies. Keep in mind that the sink isn't exactly spotless either; always lay down towels or cloths from home before pulling out your supplies.

If you have to pump in a place that's really not clean, you may want to pump and dump. Doing so helps you avoid engorgement and encourages your milk supply, but it avoids endangering your baby with possible contamination. You may also be able to pump in your car, if you can discreetly set up your pump. Park somewhere out of the way to try this, not in the Shop Rite parking lot.

Believe it or not, some pumps can be set up beneath your clothing so you could even pump during a business meeting. But having the boss yell at you about January's sale numbers while your pump whirrs and clicks may interfere with your let-down reflex. Only the rare person can pump nonchalantly in front of the whole shipping department.

Making the process easier

To help with your let-down reflex (see Chapter 6), carry a picture of your baby or an article of clothing, like a hat, that has her smell. Consider making a tape of your baby cooing — or crying!

Make sure to drink lots of fluids throughout the day and to eat well. See Chapter 8 for suggestions on increasing your milk supply if it seems to be dropping.

You can keep pumped milk in the freezer or refrigerator, but make sure you label it so it doesn't end up in a coworker's coffee! If you'd prefer not to use the break room fridge, you can keep the bottles in a cooler that comes with many breast pumps.

Be sure to thoroughly clean your pump after each use, and sterilize the parts according to the manufacturer's instructions.

Dressing for breastfeeding success

Pumping is easier if you wear two-piece outfits, so you can pull up your shirt rather than hiking up your dress. A separate jacket also provides camouflage and gives you an extra layer of protection against leaks.

Wear patterned shirts, if possible, to help hide any leakage, and try every breast pad on the market until you find one that works well for you. (See Chapter 5 for more on breast pads.) Keep an extra shirt at work for those inevitable leaking occasions.

If you start to let down milk at an inopportune time, try crossing your arms across your chest and squeezing. Don't doodle little pictures of the baby or write his name across the January sales reports; thinking about the baby is likely to trigger let-down.

Determining How Much Milk Your Baby Needs

If your baby has never had a bottle, you may not be sure how much she should get at each feeding. One formula says to multiply your baby's weight by 2.5 or 3. The resulting number is how many ounces she needs during one day. For instance, if she weighs 10 pounds, she needs between 25 and 30 ounces a day.

Divide the ounces per day by the number of feedings she normally takes. If our 10-pound baby takes 6 feedings, she needs 4 to 5 ounces at each feeding. If she takes 8 feedings, she needs between 3 and 4 ounces per feeding.

Taking Business Trips

If you have a nanny and an unlimited expense account, traveling with your nursing baby is relatively easy; just take the whole group with you wherever you go. Unfortunately, not too many working moms have that kind of carte blanche with the company's money.

Traveling for even a day means you'll need to pump, both to avoid engorgement and blocked ducts and to maintain your supply. As with pumping at work, make sure you're familiar with your pump before leaving. Check to be certain all the parts are there and that you know how to work them. A pump that comes with a carryall case and a cooler is ideal for traveling.

Before you leave, start pumping after feedings so you have breast milk on hand for the baby to eat. While you're away, try to pump as frequently as you normally feed the baby, even if that means pumping in the middle of the night.

TIP: If you're in the airport and need to pump, check for a family bathroom; these usually have a chair and a changing table that you can lay your supplies on. If you're taking a long flight and know that you'll need to pump, ask to sit in the back of the plane, which is often less crowded. We suggest telling the stewardess what you're doing before you start pumping!

For a trip that lasts a day or two, you'll need to freeze your milk if you want to use it later. (See Chapter 7 for tips on how to freeze milk.) You may need to enlist the hotel staff's help in finding a freezer, because few hotel rooms have them. If you have some flexibility in where you stay, hotels such as AmeriSuites and Extended Stay America have kitchens that feature small freezers. Freeze milk in small bags, make sure you label everything well, and don't forget to take it with you when you leave.

TIP: Breast milk can be shipped home, as long as it's frozen and can be put on dry ice. Some grocery stores sell dry ice; bring something to handle it with, like a glove, because you can't touch it with your bare fingers.

Working at Home

If you work at home, you have an almost ideal setup. We say *almost,* because working at home may be easier or more difficult depending on your baby's ever-changing needs. But at least when your baby is small, you should be able to do computer work or paper work at home while the baby naps.

As the baby grows, working at home without a sitter becomes more difficult. You'll have a hard time sounding professional and businesslike on the phone while you're trying to grab your 1-year-old with your free hand as he careens face-first toward the floor. You'll probably need to hire a sitter for at least a few hours a day so you can get some work done, but at least you'll still be readily available for feedings.

TIP: Following are some of the essentials you need in order to make working at home work for you:

- **Organization and focus.** When you work at home, you're surrounded by distractions, from the dust bunnies on the floor to the crying baby in the next room.
- **A private space away from the main rooms.** Otherwise, every little sound may disturb you.
- **A babysitter who understands that you're working and shouldn't be disturbed for every little thing.** See the next section for more on choosing a sitter.
- **A good answering machine.** It may take a while to convince your mother that working at home is serious business.

Hiring a Caregiver

New moms returning to work after having a baby are definitely not alone. Consider this:

- According to the Bureau of Labor Statistics, 40 percent of women in the workplace are mothers of children under 18.
- Eighty-three percent of new mothers return to work within six months of delivery.
- About 2.3 million people work in the childcare field.

If you've been tearing your hair out interviewing one wildly inappropriate candidate after another, you may be wondering, "If there are 2.3 million people out there taking care of children, why can't I find a good sitter?"

Finding a sitter you feel comfortable leaving your baby with can be a scary and frustrating process. Finding one who fits all your qualifications and also supports your desire to keep breastfeeding is the equivalent of hitting the lottery. The following sections offer some suggestions to help make your search as painless as possible. For more helpful suggestions, check out *Parenting For Dummies* by Sandra Hardin Gookin and Dan Gookin (Wiley).

Finding the right fit

Does your employer have a childcare facility? Could a local commercial childcare provider meet your needs? Is a family member or friend available to care for your baby? We can't give you all the pros and cons on all available options, but we can give you some ideas of what to look for in a caregiver when you're continuing to breastfeed. Childcare centers with cute designs and yards full of plastic play equipment are everywhere, but don't be swayed by colorful toys. A daycare with shabby equipment but fantastic caregivers should win out over a yard full of expensive equipment.

TIP

When you interview potential caregivers, look at the total package and take your time. Make several visits, especially if different workers come in on different days. During your shopping process, take the following issues into account:

- **Is the facility licensed or accredited by the National Association for Family Day Care or National Association for the Education of Young Children?** If so, you can be reassured that it meets certain established standards. If not, that doesn't mean you should automatically eliminate it from your list — only that you need to look a little more closely at it.
- **What's the staff-to-child ratio?** One caretaker to four children is adequate.
- **Are one or two people going to be consistently taking care of your baby?** This situation would be ideal. Having rotating caretakers may make it hard for your baby to develop trust in the person caring for him.
- **Is the building clean, spacious, and safe?** Look at the changing areas, sleeping areas, and play areas (inside and outside). Check out the kitchen, because you'll be providing the facility with pumped breast milk. The milk has to be properly and safely stored until it's used.
- **Is the building set up to take care of young babies and toddlers in separate areas?** This is ideal because toddlers can inadvertently injure small babies. Keeping them separate also keeps your infant healthier, as toddlers are notorious for being germ spreaders.

TIP

Talk at length to both the owner of the facility and the caregivers. Make an appointment so that no one feels rushed. Spend as much time as you need to make an educated decision. Check the credentials of the owner and his/her employees. Prepare a checklist of things to see and ask, so you don't get home and realize you forgot to check out the bathrooms. Make sure the center will meet your baby's needs not only today, but also two years down the road.

REMEMBER

Don't assume that a caregiver working out of her home is better than a commercial daycare center. The most unsafe sitter situation your coauthor Sharon ever ran across was a woman who took care of more than ten children at a time in her basement, with the help of only her daughter.

Following are some additional tips for finding the right place for your child:

- **Look for a facility or caretaker's home that is close to your workplace.** This may allow you to visit your baby at lunch and nurse him. Make sure that the facility has an open door policy.
- **Ask about the facility's sick baby policy.** Find out how *sick* is defined and whether sick children are allowed to stay. You want to avoid extreme situations — either needing to make other arrangements every time your baby has a sniffle or worrying that your child could be in contact with walking pneumonia.
- **Evaluate the owner's opinions of breastfeeding.** Are any other babies at the facility breastfed? Will the staff have any problem feeding your baby your pumped milk? Are the caregivers knowledgeable in the handling and storage of expressed milk? Are they concerned about handling body fluids, and are they going to make a big deal about storing your milk in a separate refrigerator? Will they give you a room to breastfeed in during your lunch hour, if you can arrange this?
- **If the caregivers don't have experience with breastfed babies, find out if they are willing to learn.** This situation means that you must be willing to educate them. Unless you find a caregiver who has breastfed her baby and has a working knowledge of the process, you may need to teach her about breastfeeding and why it's important to you and your baby.
- **Go with your gut feeling.** Visit several different places and follow your intuition. You usually know when you find a good match. No place will be perfect, but if you feel it has the potential to work, it may be the right place for you.

Educating your caregiver

Make sure your caregiver knows how important breastfeeding is to you. She should be aware that the first weeks after you return to work may be difficult, especially if your baby hasn't taken a bottle frequently from other people. If you're considering a person who provides childcare in her home, ask her if she breastfed her children. If she did, chances are she'll be supportive of your decision to continue breastfeeding.

Finding a caregiver who is a nursing advocate is key. Someone supportive of breastfeeding can make the difference between you giving up nursing because of "sitter sabotage" or succeeding with the adjustment of returning to work. (You don't want a caregiver who gives your child a bottle ten minutes before you're due to pick him up at the end of the day.)

By the same token, don't sabotage your sitter by not making your expectations perfectly clear. Tell her what you want done if your baby is hungry and you're just a few minutes away. Explain how you want the milk warmed or what to do if she runs out of expressed milk. Sit down with her and formulate a nursing cooperation plan. If she's good at her job as a caregiver, she will want you to succeed as much as you do.

No matter what type of childcare you choose, make sure that you do a few trial runs before your actual first day of work. Try leaving your baby for a few hours a day. If you have the luxury of gradually easing yourself back to work, do so. This allows both you and the caregiver to feel confident that the baby will eat and settle down without problems. It also gives you the opportunity to see your caregiver in action. Is she the same person you interviewed, caring for your baby the way you thought she would?

Building a solid relationship

The person or facility you choose to care for your child is your stand-in for hours every day. You should share the same values and approach child-rearing the same way. We can't stress enough the importance of really liking the person to whom you entrust your most valuable possession. If you don't see eye to eye with her baby care system, you'll agonize over it the entire time you're at work. This situation won't be good for anyone — not you, not your employer, and definitely not your baby.

You and your child's caregiver both have goals. The caregiver's goal is to make money doing something she enjoys (we hope!). Yours is to have your baby with a caregiver who nurtures him. The only way your childcare relationship will succeed is to make it friendly while still being clear that you're the boss over important decisions concerning your child — including feeding decisions.

Every relationship has some type of conflict. How you handle differences is up to you. Going with your gut feeling is usually a good starting point. If you think you have a good match with your caregiver and things have been going pretty well, don't fret if you start getting the impression that something is bothering her. Get the problem out in the open, where you can deal with it.

Try to be understanding of the caregiver's job; it may not be as easy as you think. If you like this person and the way she treats your baby, resolve issues before they become serious. Try to avoid difficult situations by:

- **Keeping the lines of communication open.** Spend a few minutes every evening talking to the caregiver about how the day went, rather than grabbing the baby and running out.
- **Exercising your empathy.** If the caregiver mentions any struggles with breastfeeding issues, such as thawing milk or feeding the baby more frequently than formula-fed babies she takes care of, acknowledge those struggles even if you can't change them. Most people just want their feelings validated.
- **Reminding her that your time to nurse is short.** Your baby's feeding habits will soon change, and he'll eat less frequently.
- **Letting her know how much you appreciate all she does.** An occasional bouquet of flowers is a great way to say "Thanks!"
- **Trying to make things as easy as possible.** Store frozen breast milk in small breastfeeding bags that thaw and warm quickly. Even better, make up bottles ahead of time so your caregiver only has to warm and feed.
- **Being aware.** See if your baby is content and in good shape when you arrive to pick him up. Is the caregiver ready to pass him off to you in an exhausted state on a regular basis? If this is the case, perhaps you both need to reevaluate the situation.
- **Remembering that there are no perfect caregivers, any more than there are perfect moms or perfect babies.** Undoubtedly you've chosen the best facility or person for the things that are most important to you. You may need to give a little in other areas. So what if they refuse to feed the baby beets because it stains all the bibs red, or if they insinuate that cradle cap means you're not washing the baby's head often enough? You can give him beets on the weekend and write down all their suggestions for dealing with cradle cap if that makes them happy.

Relatively speaking: Using friends or family members

In some ways, using a friend or relative as a babysitter is ideal. After all, the devil you know is better than the devil you don't know, right?

If you use a friend or relative as a sitter, you know what you're in for, which can be good or bad! You may already know that your mom will put three sweaters on the baby if the temperature dips below 80 degrees, or that your Aunt Jane will refuse to take the baby outside if she sees a cloud in the sky. Everyone has idiosyncrasies, and you can usually live with them if they don't actually do any harm.

However, you want to be very clear from the beginning that you're the rule-maker and main caregiver. Grandparents are especially bad about taking a mile when given an inch when it comes to their grandchildren. (Your coauthor Sharon is guilty of this!) If you can't establish — nicely, of course! — that this is your baby and you're going to raise him your way, you may be better off not using a friend or relative to babysit. If you do, you may end up with an ulcer and a sore jaw from grinding your teeth all night long.

Some relatives may insist on babysitting for you for free. This isn't always a good idea, unless you don't mind being held ransom in any number of ways to pay for the "favor" of free babysitting.

Of course, none of these cautions applies to your mother, who is a second cousin to Mother Teresa and obviously the best child raiser in seven continents — after all, look how good you turned out!

Meeting Your Family's Myriad Needs

You may have thought life was tough before you had a baby; you worked all day, made dinner, tried to keep your place clean, spent a little time with your spouse, and took the dog to play Frisbee once in a while. But after the baby arrives, you look back nostalgically on your pre-baby days, wondering what you ever did with such a luxurious amount of free time.

When both you and your partner are working, time is tight. By the time you pick the baby up from the sitter, nurse her, make dinner, clean up, wash a load of clothes, and feed the dog, the evening's over. Never mind such niceties as reading a book, taking a hot bath, or talking to your partner for a few minutes.

Balancing the needs of so many people in such a short time is hard work. At this stage, the baby's needs must come first. Plan on nursing her as soon as you come home, not only to keep your milk supply up but also to reconnect after being apart all day.

Following are some suggestions for keeping your sanity, especially during the first weeks and months after you return to work:

- **Keep meals easy.** Broiled chicken may be boring, but it's simple. And eating take-out a few times a week won't hurt, as long as you seek out reasonably nutritious meals.
- **If your partner gets home before you, ask him to start dinner.** If he does, and his choices tend toward beans and franks, eat them gratefully (as long as they don't give you or the baby gas!). Or have your partner pick up the baby, so you can go straight home.

  TIP

  If you hire a babysitter to care for your baby in your home, she may be willing to start dinner for you. Offer to pay extra if she's willing to take on that responsibility.
- **Keep your clothing purchases simple.** Wear things that require little or no ironing; avoid silk and linen. If money isn't an issue, take your clothes to the dry cleaners.
- **Hire a cleaning person one day a week, if you can.** If you can't, keep things simple. Put the knickknacks away for now, to simplify dusting. Lower your standards and catch up on the weekend. Remember that this stage won't last forever!

Chapter 14

Balancing Breastfeeding and the Rest of Your Life

In This Chapter

- Coping with siblings' responses to breastfeeding
- Nursing in the real world
- Traveling and breastfeeding

Breastfeeding isn't done in a vacuum, as a separate activity from the rest of your life. Isolated breastfeeding may work for a month or two after the baby's born, but sooner or later you need to breastfeed around your other children, your relatives, and sometimes the butcher, the baker, and the candlestick maker. You may need to breastfeed in planes, trains, automobiles, and turnpike rest stops!

In this chapter, we suggest ways to deal with normal curiosity about breastfeeding in everyone from your 2-year-old to your bowling team. We also explain how to succeed at breastfeeding when you're on the go.

Helping Older Children Adjust

If you have older children, they may react to your plans to breastfeed with anything from "Ohhh, gross!" to a demand to nurse as well. Approach breastfeeding as a family project from the beginning. Talk to everyone in the family about the fact that you're going to breastfeed, and try to get reactions ahead of time.

REMEMBER

If your kids are older than 10, they may be horribly embarrassed that you're pregnant to begin with and may refuse to even look at your chest after you say the word *breastfeeding*. If this is your first time breastfeeding, you may wonder if dealing with your older child's issues as well as your own insecurities is worth the trouble. Rest assured, it is.

Nursery school negativity

Children go out into the world with the values they learn at home. While breastfeeding may be business as usual at home, some children find themselves in the nursery school equivalent of the principal's office for pretending to breastfeed their dolls!

While you may feel frustration if your older child encounters negative attitudes toward breastfeeding outside your home, try to remember that not everyone sees things in the same way. Treat this as an opportunity to teach your older child a lesson about respecting a variety of opinions.

When you bring home the new baby, your older child, whether 2 years old or 12, has to adjust to not being the only kid on the block anymore. Breastfeeding may add fuel to the fire. If you already have more than one child at home, your situation may be a bit easier; kids with siblings tend to accept another baby into the home with good grace. And if they're already used to breastfeeding as the preferred method of feeding, so much the better!

REMEMBER

Kids of all ages are naturally curious. If you portray breastfeeding as the normal way to feed your baby, your older child is less likely to be obsessed with it. You may find him looking curiously, saying "What are they, mom?" or "What are you doing?" He may worry that the baby is hurting you, especially if he's aware that you were in the hospital and he equates the hospital with being sick. Encourage him to ask questions, and show him by your actions that breastfeeding is normal, not something to be ashamed of.

Nursing with a toddler in tow

When you picture breastfeeding with a toddler around, you may have horrible visions of your 3-year-old hanging out the second-story window while you race upstairs, baby hanging off one breast, to grab him. Watching a toddler and nursing a new baby requires preparation so you can avoid this scenario. (And you thought your Girl Scout days were over!)

REMEMBER

Even the best-adjusted child feels a small pang of jealousy over the loss of attention that results from a new baby's arrival. In most cases, this leads to child number one doing whatever he can to attract your attention. None of the things he does to attract your attention are likely to be good things, either! Be prepared for wall painting, window breaking, and general naughtiness. But we're here with suggestions for how to nurse child number two while keeping number one from self destructing.

First, prepare your toddler as much as possible for breastfeeding before the baby arrives. Many books and videos can give him an idea of what he's in for with the new baby. If he understands what's happening, it lessens the anxiety or feeling of competition with the new baby. *I'm a Big Brother/I'm a Big Sister* by Joanna Cole and *We Have a Baby* by Cathryn Falwell deal well with the topic of breastfeeding and new babies, as do many other books.

The best way to keep your toddler out of troublesome situations while you nurse is to head them off before they occur. The following suggestions can help you do just that:

- **Set up a room with your toddler's needs, as well as yours, in mind.** Would you be better off nursing in a room away from the hustle and bustle of the house, one where you can put a gate across the door to keep your toddler confined? Or would it be more conducive to nurse in the family room where he's used to playing, and where he can occasionally watch a video?

  Keep in mind that you'll be nursing frequently in the first few months, and shoving your toddler in front of the TV every time may not be such a good idea! Make sure that you have items such as books, puzzles, and snacks readily available.

- **Plan activities that you and your toddler can do together while you nurse.** Multi-tasking is the hallmark of motherhood. This translates into being capable of nursing the baby and reading to your toddler — or playing a game — at the same time. With breastfeeding, you have a free hand, which benefits your toddler. Reading to him or doing a puzzle can help him feel special even when you're busy with the baby.

  Use TV and videos sparingly; try to make nursing time a special time for your toddler. And don't forget how far a hug and kiss will go!

- **Create a *surprise box* and keep it next to your nursing chair or sofa.** Stock it with things like stickers, books, pictures (especially ones of the older child as a baby), and water color paints. Or put some costume jewelry or beads in it. Sometimes things other than toys are more interesting and hold a toddler's attention longer than the latest gadgets from Toys 'R' Us!

- **Enlist your toddler's help.** It's amazing how much real help you can get out of a toddler, and he or she feels like an important big brother or sister by doing so. Make sure that items such as burp cloths or baby wipes are within your toddler's reach. Ask him to get the burp cloth for you, and watch his face light up. Everyone wants to feel needed, even someone who's only 3 feet high.
- **Plan times where you and your older child can do something together, alone.** Enlist your partner's help to make this happen on a regular basis, so your toddler knows that he's still as special to you as ever!

Your older child needs to accept a new baby at his own pace. He shouldn't be forced into his new role as oldest child through anger or embarrassment. It could take some time to adjust, and some children even regress during this time. Be firm but patient. Recognize his feelings, even if you don't understand them. Eventually he'll come to realize that he isn't being pushed off the family ladder, but rather being elevated to a higher rung.

Dealing with a child's embarrassment

If you have children old enough to associate breasts with sexuality, they may feel embarrassed about your breastfeeding. It doesn't matter to them if you're nursing privately in your home in front of grandma or in the middle of Grand Central Station. Dealing with older children can be as challenging to you as a 2-year-old running around when you're trying to nurse. Try to identify this difficulty and deal with it early so that the simple act of feeding your baby isn't emotionally traumatic for anyone!

An embarrassed child is easy to recognize when you know the signs. Does he bolt from the room when you go to put the baby on the breast? Does he pretend not to know you when you nurse in public, even when you're doing it discreetly? Try to be sensitive to his emotions. Although breastfeeding is the best way to feed your new baby, a child doesn't understand this. He sees his mom "baring all," and it makes him uncomfortable.

Until your older child is comfortable with breastfeeding, try to nurse in a private area. Attempt to expose him to the process little by little, letting him see that no harm comes from nursing his sibling. Encourage him to talk with you or your partner about his embarrassment.

Appeasing a sibling who wants to nurse

Be forewarned: When your older child sees you nursing the baby, he may decide that he wants to breastfeed, too! Don't panic if this occurs. Your child may accept a simple response like "That's the baby's milk. Would you like a drink of juice for you?"

If your child persists in his requests to nurse, a taste of hand-expressed milk may cure him. He probably won't develop a taste for breast milk on a regular basis, unless he stopped nursing very recently.

With a young child — 2 or 3 years old — who insists on nursing, you can offer the breast if you're comfortable doing so. Try not to criticize him for wanting to nurse; your disapproval will only make matters worse. Kids are very perceptive; yours will sense your awkwardness and anxiety and may start demanding to nurse every time he wants immediate attention. If you do allow him to nurse, chances are good that he won't return to his breastfeeding days. First, he may not remember how to nurse! Second, he'll probably find it way too much work for a drink of milk.

However, if you recently stopped nursing your older child, you may find him wanting to return to it, at least temporarily. If you choose, you can nurse a toddler and a new baby at the same time; see Chapter 16 for more on tandem nursing.

Letting your child imitate nursing

Even if your toddler doesn't want to revisit his breastfeeding days, you may find him trying to nurse his favorite doll. If he doesn't have a doll, consider getting one for him. Children are great imitators, and pretending to breastfeed a doll is perfectly normal and healthy behavior.

Be aware that you can probably expect some shocked reactions from friends, family members, or even preschool teachers who see him doing this. Be sure to inform his teachers that he's been very interested in your breastfeeding the new baby; if they're prepared, they may be less likely to draw negative attention to his behavior.

The reactions of your child's peers may be more of a problem, especially if they've never seen their moms nursing. Make sure your toddler knows that not all babies are breastfed and that his friends may not understand what he's doing.

Try not to make your child's breastfeeding rerun a big deal. More than likely, he sees the attention that you give the baby and thinks, "Hey, I want a little piece of this action, too!" This may be his way of revisiting his babyhood.

Breastfeeding All Over Town

Sooner or later, you've got to go to the mall. Or a friend's house. Or any number of other places that don't afford you the same level of privacy you get in your own family room.

Breastfeeding in public places is truly a personal decision. Don't feel silly if you're uncomfortable nursing your baby in the middle of your local mall; we'd bet that most new moms feel the same way. Let's face it: Up to this point in your life, you probably didn't lift your blouse or unhook your bra too often while hundreds of people walked pass.

Even though it may feel funny at first, know that nursing in public is perfectly okay; it's not illegal or immoral in any way! Consider this: If a mom can offer her baby a bottle on a bench in the mall, you can feed your baby there, too. (See Chapter 15 for more on legal issues and breastfeeding.) And with a little practice, you can find ways to make yourself and your baby comfortable with the entire process.

Feeling at ease with public breastfeeding is one part emotional and one part physical. At least half the battle is getting over the "Everyone's watching me" feeling. But unless you look like a Playboy Bunny, chances are few people will be staring at you. Honestly, most passersby won't even know you're nursing.

In the following sections, we show you how to make nursing in public a positive experience rather than a cause for stress.

Setting the stage for public nursing

When nursing in public, the time you spend preparing is time well spent. Learning to nurse in public while keeping things private is like setting sail on uncharted waters. Experiment at home before you make your public debut. Try getting your baby to latch on discreetly while watching yourself in the mirror. Do you see anything that you wouldn't want anyone else to see? Test your skills in front of your family; see if you can breastfeed in front of them without feeling like you're on center stage.

When you're ready to go public, try to shut out your environment as you prepare your baby to nurse. Turn your back on the hustle and bustle of whatever area you're in, and focus on getting the baby settled in. After he's on the breast, you can turn back.

TIP

Wear clothes that are conducive to a quick-change act. You want tops that make the breast easily accessible, such as those we discuss in Chapter 5. Bring the baby close to you and then lift your top up enough to get the baby lined up to latch on. This sounds simple, but some practice sessions may be helpful before "meeting your public"!

You may find it less revealing to lift your shirt in the center, then pull it over toward the side on which the baby is going to nurse. The baby's body covers any exposed skin on your abdomen, and the extra fabric drapes down over your side to cover exposed skin there.

WARNING!

Many women feel most comfortable covering the baby with a blanket when they nurse, because it provides the most privacy. But be forewarned: Many a mom has been surprised by a well meaning (and nosy) passerby who pulled the blanket away because she wanted to see the baby!

Carol's public debut

I have never been known for finesse in my life. As a kid, I always had scars on my knees because I could fall over a piece of paper. When it came to breastfeeding in public, I definitely struggled.

My first times nursing in public, I discreetly tried to get the baby to latch onto my breast. I remember feeling like the world was looking as I manipulated the baby with one hand and lifted my blouse with the other — while both of them went in the wrong direction! What a disaster.

I knew that I had to do this, so I forged ahead. Initially, I found that I was more comfortable not trying this magic trick in front of people. I would go to a private place (such as a bedroom or restroom), put the baby on the breast, and then go back to wherever I was. Another trick was turning my body away, getting the baby to latch on, and then turning back. Both of these techniques worked well in the beginning, until I got my feet wet!

Generally, after your baby is firmly latched on, he's not likely to come up for air until his tummy if satisfied. Switching to the second breast, for some reason, just isn't as nerve-wracking.

Try not to call attention to your nursing baby. If someone approaches you while you're nursing, make eye contact. If your partner or a friend is with you, encourage them to provide a buffer zone for you and your baby.

Finding a prime nursing spot

Breastfeeding shouldn't make you break out in a cold sweat! If you're not relaxed, the stress can affect your let-down. But depending on your destination, you may have a tough time locating an area that affords you the comfort and privacy you'd like while you're nursing. The tips in this section can help you optimize your options.

Advance planning

TIP

Before you take your first outing, scope out possible breastfeeding stations. Send out a scout, such as your partner or another family member. Or let your fingers do the walking by telephoning your destination and asking what facilities are available for breastfeeding moms. Also ask your local lactation consultant (see Chapter 4) for her lists of breastfeeding-friendly facilities.

Many public places, such as malls, department stores, and churches, have rooms set up specifically for nursing moms. If at all possible, avoid restrooms, which usually aren't the nicest places to nurse. (When was the last time you ate your lunch in the bathroom? Why should your baby have to do this?)

In your car

No matter where you go, if the weather permits, you can retreat to your car to nurse. The atmosphere is fairly private and quiet, which is conducive to your baby nursing well. As a matter of fact, if you have other children, you may find yourself retreating to the car for peace and quiet on a regular basis, even when you're not going anywhere!

On a shopping spree

Some malls have nice restrooms with chairs. If the ladies' restroom doesn't have a place to sit down, look for a family restroom; many malls offer these facilities, which are specifically designed to make parents' lives a little easier.

If your mall restroom doesn't offer a place to sit and nurse, you may have to go to an upscale department store to find a nice dressing room. They often have a chair or bench to sit on, and even if they don't, you can sit on the floor!

TIP

If you have a Nordstrom in town, count yourself as fortunate. This department store chain goes out of its way to set up comfortable lounges that are perfect for nursing.

At the game

Moms with older children sometimes find themselves attending lots of football or baseball games or other sporting events. If this describes your life, be sure to travel with a folding chair in your trunk. While it's possible to breastfeed on a bench with parents all around you yelling "Go team!", you may find it much easier to set up your folding chair at the back of the bleachers so you can nurse in relative privacy.

In a friend's home

Nursing at other people's houses is great as long as the other people are comfortable with it. Before you put the baby to breast while sitting at the dining room table, ask your host if there's a quiet area you can use for nursing. This way, if your host is comfortable with your nursing anywhere you'd like, she can say so. And if she isn't, she won't feel awkward about directing you to a more private area.

Appreciating the convenience

The convenience of breastfeeding is probably one of the reasons you chose to breastfeed in the first place. Before a bottle-feeding mom can leave home, she has to pack bottles, canned or powder formula, and possibly bottled water. When she gets where she's going, she has to find a place to mix the formula and warm up the bottle, perhaps by running hot water in a bathroom.

Now, look at a mom going out with her breastfed baby. She grabs her diaper bag, stocked with things such as wipes and diapers, and off she goes. When she gets to her destination, the only thing she needs is a seat!

Breastfeeding certainly makes nursing on the go easier. But being able to nurse in public depends on your breast attitude. What is *breast attitude*? It's being able to say, "Yes, I've chosen to breastfeed, and I'm okay to nurse my baby when he needs to be fed, even if I'm out of the house."

Choosing not to breastfeed in public

If you know that breastfeeding in public is just not for you at this time, you need to prepare for public appearances in other ways.

Pump extra milk and freeze it so you can offer your baby a bottle of pumped milk when you're out. Doing so may be less stressful in the beginning than public breastfeeding. However, try to limit offering bottles to your baby until breastfeeding is well-established. Occasional bottles shouldn't cause problems, but offering a bottle on a regular basis could produce nipple confusion (see Chapter 5).

Deferring public breastfeeding is another option in the first few months. Plan short trips where you can get in, get out, and get home in time for the next feeding.

Vacationing with Your Baby

Although you may picture your family vacations beginning with everyone singing "We're Off on the Road to Morocco" as you dance down the road, reality is usually much different. Vacations are supposed to be enjoyable, but when you have small children, they're about as much work as they are fun. A little advance planning helps decrease the work and increase the fun.

Traveling with a nursing baby is easier than traveling with a bottle-fed baby in some ways and more difficult in others. You don't have to pack as much when you breastfeed, and you never have to worry about where you'll find clean water to mix a bottle. On the other hand, you wouldn't hesitate to put a bottle in a baby's mouth in public, but breastfeeding in the Basilica may give you pause.

Make traveling as easy as possible by wearing nursing-friendly clothing, and bring a supply of blankets to throw over yourself. (If you're like us, you'll need more than one blanket, because you're sure to drop food on them as you try to eat and nurse at the same time!)

Traveling by car

Not long ago, a woman was arrested for breastfeeding while driving her car. Not while *riding* in the car, mind you, but while actually *driving*. She was also talking on a cell phone at the same time. A trucker reported her to the police, which makes us wonder about the strange things truckers must see on the highway.

We're going to assume that you know that driving your car and holding your unbuckled baby between you and the steering wheel is a real no-no. However, you *can* breastfeed in the car, as long as you're not the driver. It takes a bit of maneuvering, but it can be done.

You need to be in the seat next to your baby, which means you need to be in the back seat. Already you can see why you can't be the driver, right? This works only if your baby is in a rear-facing carrier, unless you have really large and flexible breasts. You should be belted in but have enough play in the belt to lean forward to get your breast to the baby (see Figure 14-1). Obviously, you'll have a much easier time nursing on the side closest to the baby.

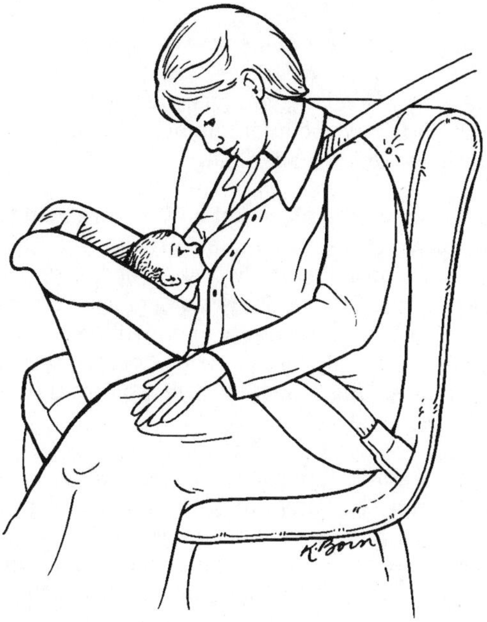

Figure 14-1: Nursing the baby while traveling in the car.

REMEMBER

Nursing in the car should be a stopgap, emergency measure to tide over a screaming infant until you can get to a rest stop. A few years ago a mother and baby were killed in an accident when the family was pulling out of a fast food restaurant and mom was nursing the baby in the back seat. She wasn't wearing a seat belt, and the baby was not in his car seat. It took only a second, and they weren't on a high-speed road. Don't take a chance. Nurse the baby out of her seat only when your car is pulled over.

TIP

When you do get to a rest stop, you may want to feed your baby in the car rather than going inside to nurse. Many rest stops are jammed full of people and have no chairs in the restrooms (or anywhere else, for that matter, except maybe the food areas). Not a restful atmosphere, in any case. You can find better places to eat while traveling than rest stops; keep reading for ideas.

Eating out in restaurants

Your coauthor Sharon's grandson has eaten in more nice restaurants than many adults. When our own kids were young, we often took them out to dinner at places whose cuisine far surpassed the local hamburger joint. We enjoyed eating out and wanted them to enjoy it, too. Don't be afraid to take your baby out to eat with you; just employ some common sense courtesy to those around you if she starts to fuss.

Some restaurants — such as chains known for their home cooking and some mom-and-pop operations — are kid-friendly. If you stick with the chains while traveling, you miss out on some great local gems. (However, you may also avoid being poisoned at a dive the locals all know to avoid! It's a dilemma.)

Wherever you go, scope the place out a bit before being seated, to see where you can breastfeed most unobtrusively. A table in the center of the room is probably the worst choice, especially if the chairs don't have arms. Booths are good because you can put an infant seat next to you to lean your arm on while you hold the baby, and booths are usually less centrally located than tables. Booths also are high enough to shield you a bit from the view of people sitting behind and in front of you.

WARNING!

Sit out of the line of traffic if possible, not only to nurse unobtrusively but also to keep the baby out of harm's way. Waitresses carrying trays loaded with food have been known to drop them. Never put an infant seat on the floor if you can avoid it; my brother tripped on one back in his busboy days and nearly knocked the baby out of it.

TIP

Most infant seats fit on standard restaurant wooden high chairs that are turned upside down; the grooves in the seat fit over the wooden rungs. So bring the infant seat in with you for use after nursing.

Some restaurants have chairs in the restroom that you can use for nursing; if they also have a changing table, that's an added bonus.

Coffee, tea, or valium: Flying with a baby

No matter how enticing the ads or the slogans about the friendly skies are, if you've flown recently, you know the truth: Flying these days is a hassle, and flying with a baby can be a nightmare. You can do it, but you'll be less likely to need sedatives at the end of the trip if you do some advance planning. Consider the following:

- **When making your reservations, pay attention to your layover times if you can't get a direct flight.** If a direct flight is available, take it, even if it costs a little more.

  To get yourself and the baby from one end of the airport to the other takes time, especially if you need to make a pit stop to feed or change her. Don't count on your connecting flight departing from the same part of the airport where you arrive, or even the same part of the county! Many airport flights require taking a shuttle to your connecting terminal, and you have to walk a mile first to get to the shuttle. Give yourself at least an hour and a half between flights if possible.
- **If you're a member of an airline's special club, or if you're in the military, use the members-only lounge between flights.** These lounges often are not crowded and have much better chairs than you find in the cattle hold . . . I mean, the waiting area.
- **If you want to nurse in a quiet spot, don't choose the waiting area or the bathroom.** Very few airport bathrooms have chairs. If you can't get into a lounge, go to a sit-down restaurant, assuming you can get a seat. You'll have a much easier time nursing there than in a waiting area.

Booking the best seats

Several schools of thought exist regarding the best place to sit if you're bringing baby on board. Lots of people like the bulkhead seats, which have much more leg room. Some also have a place to hang a bassinet, if your baby is tiny. (The airline supplies the hanging bassinet; don't bring your own.)

Bulkhead seats do have some disadvantages, though:

- **The tray tables come out of your armrests rather than pulling down from a seat in front of you.** While you don't have to worry about someone in front of you reclining for a long winter's nap and tilting your Coke until it's uncomfortably close, these folding trays are really awkward to use.
- **Airlines tend to load seats from front to back.** Therefore, if you didn't pay for a special seat for the baby, you're less likely to have the middle seat remain free.
- **The bulkhead area is usually a high-traffic area.** The bathrooms are often nearby, which can be handy for cleanup but means that lots of people will walk by your seat, and every one of them will look at you and the baby. If you have a hard time nursing in public, this kind of attention can be difficult.

Sitting in the back of the plane can be better than sitting in the bulkhead area because any empty seats will likely be located in the back. As a result, your chances of getting an extra seat for the baby are much higher.

Always choose the window seat over the aisle if you want to nurse without having the flight attendants run their carts into you and everyone gawking at you. Yes, it's harder to get out to the bathroom, but given the state of airplane bathrooms, how often do you want to go in there anyway?

Keeping your car seat with you

If you purchase a seat on the plane for your baby, be sure to bring his car seat to use during the flight. You may see catalogs that advertise vests for "lap children" to wear to keep them tethered to you during turbulence or during a crash. However, these vests are not approved for use on U.S. flights; you won't be allowed to use them at all for takeoff and landing, and you may not be allowed to use them in flight either. The best protection for your baby is an approved car seat!

Even if you haven't purchased a separate seat for your baby, always keep your car seat and stroller with you as you move through the airport, rather than checking them as luggage. When you arrive at the flight gate, ask an attendant to tag the seat and stroller so you can leave them on the jetway as you board the plane. That way, they'll be available as soon as you get off the plane, because they're loaded separately from the other luggage and retrieved right away.

If you haven't paid for a separate seat for your baby, also ask the attendant at the flight gate whether your flight is completely sold out or whether any empty seats remain. When seats are available, an attendant may be willing to help you secure a seat for your baby. In that case, take your car seat with you when you board rather than leaving it on the jetway.

Nursing in flight

Babies often feel pressure in their ears during takeoff and landing; that's why you're more likely to hear screaming at the beginning and end of your flight than when you're cruising at 30,000 feet. Breastfeeding during takeoff and landing reduces the pressure on your baby's ears, which should reduce the noise level on board.

If you're on a full flight, nursing discreetly in your seat may be difficult. Make sure you have your blankets with you to use as cover-ups, and pray that you're sitting next to someone who understands that breastfeeding is not an illegal activity!

Not long ago, a businessman made a huge fuss when the woman next to him on a flight not only breastfed her baby but also — horror of horrors — changed the baby's diaper in front of him! One can only hope that he someday marries a militant breastfeeder and has to eat humble pie a thousand times over for his anti-baby attitude. After this incident, Continental Airlines confirmed that breastfeeding on an airplane is not an illegal activity; neither is changing a diaper. (See Chapter 15 for more on legal issues and breastfeeding.)

Breastfeeding at your favorite vacation spots

Walt Disney World and Disneyland, being the kid-friendly places they are, have lots of places to breastfeed. You may want to nurse inside a dark ride such as "It's a Small World" or while watching the movie in the French pavilion in Epcot, although your baby may be distracted by the music and the colorful sights, if she's old enough to notice such things.

If breastfeeding inside rides doesn't appeal to you, quiet spots are tucked away throughout both parks. If you want to have a really marvelous experience, go to the Baby Care Centers where you can rock and nurse away from all the hubbub.

TIP

When you're looking for baby facilities in other amusement parks, look in the kiddie sections. Even if you don't find a "nursing moms only" spot, you'll probably be more comfortable nursing there than in front of the Screaming Meemie roller coaster line that's loaded with teens.

When visiting museums, look for the least popular exhibits and hope to spot a chair or bench in a quiet area. If the whole place is packed to the gills, look for the exhibits geared to young children. The parents in the area are less likely to stare if you end up nursing in the middle of the commotion; they'll be too busy trying to keep their own offspring from climbing on the dinosaurs!

REMEMBER

Be sure to keep your fluid intake up if you're at the zoo or any other outdoor attraction. You can easily get dehydrated on a hot day. Your best bet for a quiet nursing spot may be inside a sit-down restaurant.

Nursing at the beach is easy as long as you bring a chair and an umbrella along for shade. You can even tilt the umbrella to keep some prying eyes off you, although breastfeeding attire is probably among the most modest seen at the beach these days!

Chapter 15

Upholding Your Legal Right to Breastfeed

In This Chapter

- Looking at state laws that affect breastfeeding
- Keeping your child safe (and legal) in the car
- Requesting exemption from jury duty
- Nursing after a divorce or separation
- Exercising your rights at work

When it comes to breastfeeding, the law is on your side. Despite protests by people who don't want women to breastfeed in public, breastfeeding is legal everywhere mothers and babies are allowed in most states. This doesn't mean you can demand to breastfeed in the private quarters of the White House; if you and your baby can *legally* visit an area, you can also legally nurse there. In fact, breastfeeding is specifically exempt from public nudity laws in 13 states.

As a breastfeeding mom, you also have certain rights relating to child visitation in divorce cases, and you may be exempt from some civic duties, such as jury duty. In this chapter, we discuss the laws that affect breastfeeding and how those laws affect you.

Legislating Breastfeeding

Yes, laws exist for just about everything, including breastfeeding. More than half the states in the United States have enacted laws specifically encouraging breastfeeding as having benefits for both mothers and babies. Some states have passed laws saying that women hospitalized after childbirth must have access to breast-feeding counselors before being discharged.

Should breastfeeding be regulated by the government? A better question may be, "Why is government involved in a personal, natural maternal function?" Breastfeeding laws exist mostly to protect the rights of moms who have been told that breastfeeding on a plane, in a restaurant, or in a park is not allowed.

Of course, if this civilized world of ours considered breastfeeding to be a normal biologic function, such laws wouldn't be necessary. The fact that they are necessary shows how far we need to progress before breastfeeding is truly accepted as the best possible method for feeding young children.

Some states have gone beyond the obvious (that women should be allowed to breastfeed in public) and have passed laws related to other aspects of breastfeeding. Two states, California and Texas, have legislation related to milk banks (see Chapter 9) and the processing and distribution of human milk. Maryland exempts breastfeeding equipment, such as pumps, from sales tax. Louisiana prohibits daycare facilities from discriminating against breastfed babies. And Maine has made the age and breastfeeding status of a child an issue to be considered when assigning parental custody.

But as you're trying to quiet your screaming baby at the mall, you're probably most interested in laws governing nursing in public. So we'll start there.

Letting It All Hang Out in Public (Legally)

Do you find yourself glancing around furtively when you breastfeed in public, wondering whether you could be arrested or asked to stop nursing? Women are sometimes asked to stop nursing in public places; one recent case (which we discuss in Chapter 14) involved a woman on an airplane whose seatmate complained about her breastfeeding and then changing the baby's diaper. You may find it hard to believe that you could be confronted this way in this day and age, but it happens — especially in places where the law may not be completely clear (like on airplanes!).

The rules about breastfeeding in public can be summarized in one sentence: If you're in a place where you can comfortably bottle feed a baby, you have the right to breastfeed there, too.

Public breastfeeding has never been considered illegal in any state, because laws regarding indecent exposure do not pertain to a breastfeeding mother. However, breastfeeding in a *private* place, such as a restaurant, may not be a protected right in some states. This is why breastfeeding legislation is so important. As we write this book, 33 states have enacted legislation related to breastfeeding. Also, in September 1999, Congress passed a law that allows public breastfeeding on federal property.

State legislation targets key breastfeeding issues, such as breastfeeding in public places, breastfeeding and employment, breastfeeding and jury duty, and breastfeeding as it pertains to social assistance. To find out if your state has enacted pro-breastfeeding legislation, check the Web site `www.ncsl.org/programs/health/breast50.htm`. It identifies each state's breastfeeding legislation.

If you're confronted with a request to stop breastfeeding because you are making other people uncomfortable, you may have one of two normal human reactions: fight or flight. (Remember that from high school biology?) You'll either be totally mortified and quietly take your baby off the breast (flight), or you'll find yourself ready to raise quite a ruckus (fight)! Either response is perfectly normal. However, before you choose to fight, make sure that your state's legislation backs you up. Not all states have enacted specific laws that address issues such as nursing on private property. Know your rights, and don't hesitate to quote your state's laws when necessary.

Following Child Restraint Laws

As we mention in Chapter 14, a woman recently made national headlines when she was arrested for breastfeeding while driving. She and her husband argued that breastfeeding and driving at the same time was legal because their home state of Michigan exempts breastfeeding infants from child restraint laws. Two other states, Idaho and Tennessee, currently have laws exempting nursing children from seat belt laws. These are the only states that exempt nursing infants from being restrained at all times in an approved seat when the car is moving.

A little common sense should tell you that driving and breastfeeding at the same time is not what these states had in mind with these exemptions. No one should hold a child between themselves and the steering wheel while driving; even a minor accident could crush the baby. But what if you're the passenger, not the driver? Is it okay to take your child out of his car seat to breastfeed?

Rarely, if ever, is there a reason to ride in a moving vehicle and breastfeed at the same time. You can almost always pull over to the side of the road.

As we demonstrate in Chapter 14, you can breastfeed your baby while both of you are restrained if you sit in the back seat next to a rear-facing car seat. However, this is recommended only in an emergency situation, say when you're lost in a very bad neighborhood and don't dare pull over.

Asking for Exemption from Jury Duty

As with anything in life, just because you *can* do something doesn't necessarily mean that you *should.* As we mention earlier in this chapter, you can legally breastfeed in a federal building, including in a courtroom. However, doing so probably wouldn't help a jury's ability to concentrate on testimony during a trial.

A few states have enacted legislation specifically exempting breastfeeding mothers from jury duty, but most haven't. If you live in a state that doesn't specifically exempt you from jury duty, that doesn't mean you are required to serve. Many states excuse you from jury duty if you are the primary caretaker of a child younger than 6, regardless of whether you are breastfeeding or bottle feeding.

A *general hardship* exemption may be in order if you work part-time and can't pay for a childcare provider for a case that would require full-time attendance. Also, if you've never been separated from your child for extended periods of time, you may be able to apply for an exemption.

So you get summoned for jury duty — what do you do?

1. **Check the papers you received for a list of reasons to be excused from jury duty.** Many states provide check-off boxes stating reasons why you may be excused from jury duty. If that's the case, simply check the box and send the form back.

2. **If your paperwork doesn't include a list of exemptions, call the court and explain that you're a full-time mom who is breastfeeding.** Some states require written documentation verifying that you are a stay-at-home mom.

If you request exemption, your jury duty will likely be postponed until your status as a breastfeeding mom changes. Don't be surprised if you receive numerous notifications over the course of your childbearing years!

Some states require that you appear in person to explain why you can't attend jury duty. Try showing up with baby in tow; the judge won't likely sign you up for his courtroom.

The final decision to excuse you may ultimately be the judge's choice. It could be time-related, such as "When your child is 3 years old, you have to fulfill your duty." The judge can also say that because breastfeeding is recommended for the first year of life, you're excused only for that period of time. The judge usually has a fair amount of discretion within his power, ranging from totally excusing you to mandating that you attend. However, most courts will work with your circumstances.

If you find yourself hitting obstacles, try contacting your local La Leche League representative or lactation consultant. They usually have up-to-date local information regarding legal issues.

Balancing Nursing and Visitation Rights

We all know that adult relationships don't always work out. If you have an infant or toddler who is still breastfeeding when you and your partner separate, you may end up playing a complicated tug of ward with your ex-partner over breastfeeding and visitation rights.

Assuming that you have primary custody of your baby, the key issue is that you don't want your ex's visitation times to interfere with breastfeeding. The court will probably consider how much time you're away from your child each day. For example, if you work fivc days a week for eight hours a day, the court may feel that an eight-hour visitation on the weekend is okay, because you and your child are separated for that period each day during the week. However, if you breastfeed your baby every two hours every day, your partner's visits may be limited to a few hours.

Many states limit overnight stays with dad until your child is 18 months to 2 years old. If you are still breastfeeding at night after this time, bring it up to your lawyer. Some judges are quick to suggest weaning your child at this age in order to allow your child time with his dad. Even if overnight visits begin before you wean, you should be able to maintain your milk supply by pumping, because a child this age probably won't be breastfeeding that often.

WARNING! Most judges and lawyers deal with breastfeeding on a case-to-case basis, because everyone's situation is so different. Some lawyers have attempted to show that breastfeeding into and beyond the toddler years is child abuse and that custody should be given to the father based on "inappropriate" mothering. If you find yourself in this situation, go to court armed to the teeth with evidence on the benefits of prolonged nursing.

In the end, you may need to weigh your child's relationship with his father against continued breastfeeding. If your child is close to weaning, you may choose to wean him now so he can see his father more often. If your baby is small, you'll probably have a much harder time deciding how to continue breastfeeding and still have your baby stay close to his dad.

Of course, your feelings about your ex are a determining factor in your feelings about visitation. Keep in mind, though, that the court can grant visitation against your wishes; it may be better to give a little and work out an agreement without getting the courts involved.

Knowing Your Rights in the Workplace

We live in a legislative world — rules and regulations exist for almost everything, and they're always changing. Yet, for the most part, the important issue of breastfeeding at work is lacking official regulation.

Legislation is necessary to protect breastfeeding mothers from discriminating employers, and also to make sure employers who say they are pro-breastfeeding and family-friendly really are when the time comes for you to nurse or pump.

Doing your homework

Usually, by the time you are ready to return to work, your breastfeeding is well-established. (We discuss returning to work in detail in Chapter 13.) However, you may not be prepared for all the difficulties that breastfeeding and work can bring. And, unfortunately, most employers are too busy to think about how beneficial a breastfeeding mother can be to them and how they can help you succeed.

TIP

You must prepare yourself for the return to the work environment. Find out what state legislation is in place to support your continued breastfeeding while working. A good review of breastfeeding legislation all across the United States can be found at the Web site `www.lalecheleague.org/Law/summary`.

Approximately ten states have enacted some breastfeeding legislation to encourage employers to assist returning breastfeeding mothers. Some states mandate that moms be given the time to breastfeed or pump; others require that a private area for breastfeeding be provided. Some states offer legal recourse against employers who don't comply.

REMEMBER

Most state legislation is aimed at clarifying a working mother's right to continue her nursing experience by:

- Establishing that it is discriminatory to keep moms from breastfeeding or expressing milk during a break;
- Requiring employers to provide sufficient break time to express milk or nurse in a clean and private place; or
- Providing specific laws that give mothers an avenue to challenge violations of their rights.

Educating your employer

Because few states have work-related breastfeeding legislation in place, working with your employer in a non-confrontational way is probably your best avenue for getting what you need. Explain the advantages of your returning to work as a breastfeeding mom; we're sure you're a great employee, and your boss doesn't want to lose you!

TIP

Most bosses only want to hear how your situation can help them; they may not care about your personal reasons for breastfeeding. Arm yourself with a list reminding your boss what a treasure you are, and offer the following arguments:

- Breastfed babies receive immunities from their mothers' milk, which makes them less prone to illness.
- A healthier baby translates to less time off for the mom due to baby illness.
- If you take breaks to do something for your baby, you will be a happier, more productive employee. You've won't feel as if you've abandoned breastfeeding because you returned to work.

If your employer gives you a hard time, remind him nicely that the law prohibits discriminating against a breastfeeding woman, no matter which state you live in. What does this mean? If the employer allows cigarette breaks, he must allow pumping breaks, as long as they don't exceed the allotted time period.

Be flexible when you return to work; things aren't always going to be peaches and cream. At times, you may find it impossible to take a break to nurse or pump, no matter how supportive your boss is.

Keep in mind that most employers do want satisfied employees. They are willing to work with mothers as long as the company's needs are being met. Try to prepare for difficulties by anticipating potential problems and finding solutions to overcome them. If you can do this, everyone wins: The employer gets the work done, you earn your salary, and (best of all) your baby still is being breastfed!

Chapter 16

Breastfeeding and Your Next Pregnancy

In This Chapter

- Avoiding pregnancy until you're ready
- Planning your next pregnancy
- Nursing during pregnancy
- Breastfeeding two at a time

You may already know that you want another baby — but not immediately after the first one is born. In this chapter, we talk about the effects of breastfeeding on your menstrual cycle and discuss safe methods of avoiding pregnancy while you're breastfeeding.

We also discuss nursing number one while pregnant with number two, as well as how pregnancy affects your milk production. Last but not least, we look at nursing two babies of different ages at the same time so you can ensure the needs of both children are met.

Being Smart about Birth Control

Perhaps you've heard two conflicting pieces of advice regarding breastfeeding and getting pregnant:

- You don't have to worry about birth control while you're breastfeeding, because you can't get pregnant.
- You must use birth control while you nurse, because breastfeeding doesn't protect you from pregnancy.

Both are a little bit correct.

Breastfeeding is 98 to 99 percent effective as birth control — as effective as birth control pills — but only under certain conditions. To achieve this high degree of protection against pregnancy while breastfeeding, you must:

- Breastfeed exclusively — that means no formula, no water, no solid food, and little or no pacifier use.
- Wait no longer than four hours between feedings during the day, and six hours at night.
- Not have started having periods after delivery. (Having periods means you may be ovulating.)

You can ovulate even if your periods haven't started again, especially if you're supplementing or not nursing regularly.

To understand why breastfeeding protects against pregnancy, we take you back to Biology 101. Today's topic is female reproduction, and there will be a quiz at the end, so pay attention!

Revisiting your reproductive cycle

The reproductive cycle — yawn. We understand. Your coauthor Sharon found this to be the most boring subject of all my nursing classes, and now my career centers around it. Knowing the reproductive cycle is crucial for my profession, and you'll find it equally important if you'd prefer not to have two babies ten months apart!

We all know the basics: You can't get pregnant unless you *ovulate,* which means you develop and release a mature egg. But how, exactly, does this happen?

Every month, a hormone called Gonadotropin Releasing Hormone (GnRH) instructs your pituitary gland to release two other hormones: Follicle Stimulating Hormone (FSH) and Leutenizing Hormone (LH). When this happens, your ovaries start to develop a number of *follicles* (small cavities) that each contain an egg. One follicle becomes dominant and produces an estrogen called *estradiol,* which causes the level of FSH in your body to drop. When the follicle is developed enough, your LH levels rise and direct the follicle to rupture so the egg inside is released.

Breastfeeding disrupts the normal rhythm of these hormones. GnRH, which is normally released in a pulsating fashion, is released irregularly when you breastfeed. As a result, FSH and LH don't receive the signals from the pituitary gland that normally cause follicles to grow. Even if a follicle does start to grow, it doesn't receive the cue to release the egg if the LH signal is disrupted.

Science isn't quite clear on why the baby's suckling triggers this contraceptive effect, but the end result is that exclusive nursing offers a high level of protection against another pregnancy. This probably occurs because your body needs a chance to recover and nourish one child before moving on to the next.

Most women who breastfeed don't start having periods for 4 to 24 months after delivery, while moms who don't breastfeed may start ovulating again as soon as 1 to 2 months after delivery. Another great benefit of breastfeeding!

Want to know even more about your reproductive cycle? Your coauthor Sharon is also the coauthor of *Fertility For Dummies* (Wiley) — we encourage you to check it out!

Using nursing for birth control

Breastfeeding is a very effective method of birth control under the right conditions. In fact, breastfeeding prevents more pregnancies worldwide than any other method of birth control! But to optimize your protection, you've got to be diligent about avoiding supplemental sucking of any kind, including pacifiers. And if you resume having periods, you need to assume you're ovulating and use another method of birth control.

As we discuss in Chapter 10, by the time your baby is 6 months old, he requires supplementation with solid food. As soon as you start feeding him solid food, the effectiveness of breastfeeding as birth control decreases. At that time, you need to start using another method of birth control. You can continue to use breastfeeding for birth control if you combine it with natural family planning, which we discuss next.

Considering other methods

Maybe exclusive breastfeeding is out of the question for you, or your baby is nearing the 6-month-old mark, and you're not ready for another pregnancy. You want to use a contraceptive method that is safest for the baby as well as for you. You've got lots of choices.

Natural family planning

If you want to sound really scientific, tell people you're using *LAM* (lactation amenorrhea method) with *NFP* (natural family planning) for birth control. This combination may sound high tech, but it's actually the least invasive of all birth control methods (besides abstinence, which we assume you're not interested in using).

Natural family planning, sometimes called *fertility awareness,* is based on avoiding intercourse around the four to five days that you're releasing an egg, because you can't get pregnant without an egg. NFP requires you to be aware of what's happening to your body; you need to be willing to check your cervical mucus, the position of your cervix, and your temperature daily. You may also want to purchase a fertility monitor or ovulation predictor kits to make sure you're avoiding the days around ovulation. Used consistently, NFP alone is more than 90 percent effective in preventing pregnancy. For normal people, who sometimes make mistakes, the rate of effectiveness is around 75 percent.

Right before ovulation, you notice an increase in cervical mucus, which becomes clear, slippery, and stretchy. Your cervix becomes softer and easier to locate, because it moves forward a bit in the vagina. Your temperature may drop slightly just before ovulation and will rise after ovulation, due to the effects of progesterone released from the leftover follicle (called the *corpus luteum*).

After you've ovulated, you can't get pregnant until you have a period, and the reproductive cycle begins again. So if you take NFP a step further and have sex only during the *luteal phase,* the two-week period after you ovulate and before your period starts, your chances of getting pregnant are only about 1 percent. But this form of birth control requires avoiding sex for long periods, which may not work for you — or for your partner!

NFP has a high satisfaction rate because it doesn't involve taking any drugs that could be passed on to the baby through breast milk. However, it does require dedication — and strong willpower!

Several books are available that offer in-depth instructions on NFP. Two that we suggest considering are:

- *Taking Charge of Your Fertility* (Quill) by Toni Weschsler. This book discusses how to get pregnant, as well as how to avoid it.
- *The Art of Natural Family Planning* (Couple to Couple League) by John and Sheila Kippley. This book has very strong religious and moral overtones that some may find offensive.

Barrier methods

Keeping your partner's sperm away from your egg prevents pregnancy. You can block sperm from entering your cervix by using condoms, cervical caps, or a diaphragm. All are completely safe for use while you're breastfeeding, although they have other drawbacks. For more specifics about each method, check out *Sex For Dummies,* 2nd Edition, by Dr. Ruth Westheimer.

Condoms decrease sensation (which your partner may not be crazy about) and can cause vaginal irritation (which you may not be crazy about), especially because breastfeeding can reduce your body's production of cervical mucus. Your partner needs to have a condom in place before any penetration takes place. The effectiveness rate of condoms, when used correctly, is around 90 percent.

Diaphragms and cervical caps should be used with a spermicidal jelly to be between 80 and 90+ percent effective; again, the higher numbers belong to people who use these methods perfectly. You need to be refitted for a diaphragm after delivery, because you may need a different size.

Hormonal birth control

Birth control pills, taken correctly, prevent pregnancy around 99 percent of the time. The downside to the pill, besides the chance that you may forget to take it on a busy day, is that it contains hormones that may decrease your milk supply.

TIP

Some pills combine synthetic estrogen and progesterone; others contain only progesterone. The progesterone-only pills are less likely to impact your milk supply. You should wait six weeks after delivery before starting the pill, just to make sure your milk supply is well established. The American Academy of Pediatrics says birth control pills are safe to use while breastfeeding, as long as you're aware of the possible decrease in milk supply.

Birth control patches, such as OrthoEvra, are worn for a week at a time, so the risk of forgetting your birth control is less than if you take the pill. If the patch causes a problem, such as severe headaches or mood swings, it can be easily removed.

WARNING!

The patch is 99 percent effective, unless you weigh over 198 pounds. Women who weigh more than this may have an increased risk of pregnancy.

Injectable hormones, such as Depo Provera (given every three months) or Lunelle (given once a month), are also considered safe for use with breastfeeding. However, if you experience a drop in your milk supply, it takes a long time for the drug to leave your system. By the time the drug is gone, your milk supply may be diminished considerably. For this reason, you're better off taking a daily pill rather than using injectables while you're breastfeeding.

Some intrauterine devices (IUDs) contain progesterone, and others do not. IUDs are also considered safe to use while you're breastfeeding. You shouldn't insert an IUD until you've had a checkup six weeks after delivery.

Permanent methods of birth control

If you decide to have a tubal ligation after delivery, that procedure may be done a few days after you give birth or, if you have a cesarean section, at the time of delivery.

If you have a tubal ligation while you're breastfeeding, check out Chapter 9 for tips on nursing while you undergo surgery. The temporary disruption in breastfeeding shouldn't cause any problems, although you may have to keep those kicking feet away from your incision for a few days.

Deciding to Have Another Baby

If your first baby has been just a bundle of joy, you may feel ready to jump right back on the pregnancy train. However, if your little one has been more like a freight train, you may feel like you don't want another baby until this one is in college!

REMEMBER

Sometimes the feeling of needing to have another baby right away is related to breastfeeding. Many women experience mild depression when their babies start to decrease the amount of nursing time. Be sure that you and your partner discuss your reasons for wanting another baby so soon — you want to make the right decision not only for yourselves, but also for the child you already have.

Preparing for your next pregnancy

If you decide that you're ready to give Junior a sibling, and you're still breastfeeding, you need to counteract Mother Nature a bit. As we discuss earlier in the chapter, exclusive breastfeeding can give your body a natural break from pregnancy. So what can you do to encourage your menstrual cycle to resume?

TIP

- **Eliminate feedings.** Start by eliminating the night feeding.
- **Increase the time between feedings.** Going six hours between some feedings will probably restart your reproductive engines. Supplementing one feeding a day with formula will give you a six-hour stretch each day without nursing.
- **Lessen the duration of each feeding.** Gradually decrease a feeding by a few minutes over a period of time until you've eliminated the entire feeding.

Usually, if you decrease the total amount of time that your baby nurses on the breast, you trigger a return of your menses and (hopefully) your fertility. This tends to occur naturally after the baby is about 6 months old, when he starts eating solid food. Keep in mind that even when your period returns, it doesn't necessarily mean that pregnancy is right around the corner.

When your period returns, you may notice a decrease in your milk supply. That's because your level of *prolactin,* the hormone that helps you produce milk, may decrease. This could translate into a baby who develops a disinterest in breastfeeding. However, most moms don't experience a significant enough decrease to trigger the baby to wean himself. Many a mother is still nursing her first baby when she finds out that she's pregnant with number two.

Some babies are sensitive to hormonal changes; yours may be disinterested in nursing for a few days when you have your period. He should resume his normal nursing patterns after a few days.

Nursing while you're pregnant

If you're having a great nursing experience when you find out that you're pregnant again, you may wonder what nursing while you're pregnant entails — or if it's even possible. If you wish to continue to nurse while you're pregnant, you absolutely can do so.

Following are some things to consider if you aren't sure whether to continue breastfeeding:

- You may hear that breastfeeding causes uterine contractions that could put you into labor. Nipple stimulation does cause contractions, but they aren't strong enough to start labor in early pregnancy. The American Academy of Pediatrics endorses breastfeeding during a healthy pregnancy. These are the guys who'd be charged with taking care of a premature baby — why would they endorse breastfeeding if it were dangerous?

  However, if you have a history of preterm labor or miscarriages, you should notify your obstetrician about your plans to continue to nurse. She can advise you of the risks, and she may suggest that you reconsider your decision.

- You don't have to "eat for three" if you nurse while you're pregnant. You do, however, need to be very aware of your nutritional intake because, as we discuss in Chapter 7, your eating habits can impact your milk supply. If your baby is under a year old, you want to be sure that he is getting enough nutrition to gain weight. Usually a child older than 1 year does fine because most of his nutritional needs are met by solid food.

- You may hear that your milk changes during pregnancy and tastes terrible to your baby. Well, you'll just have to ask Junior about this! Somewhere between four and eight months of pregnancy, your milk does start changing from mature milk back to *colostrum,* the first type of milk that you gave your baby. The colostrum usually tastes a little different than mature milk, so you may find your baby not as interested in this new menu item and starting the process of weaning.
- Your milk supply will likely diminish during the second trimester. Although breastfeeding is a supply-and-demand process, the hormonal changes you experience during pregnancy can override this. Even with frequent nursing, your supply is probably going to remain low. As a result, your child may begin to wean. If this happens, don't feel guilty; know that what's happening is natural.

REMEMBER

Some kids develop a fickle personality, weaning and then returning to the breast either at the end of the pregnancy (when your milk supply increases) or after the new baby is born. Just be open to your baby's suggestions, and you'll both do fine.

Anticipating questions

As with many aspects of pregnancy and child-rearing, people in general — and particularly those in your family — often feel the need to share unsolicited advice and opinions. If you decide to nurse while you're pregnant, someone is bound to suspect that you've gone a little mad. Talk with your doctor before making your decision; if you have your doctor's full support, you'll have an easier time answering questions and ignoring criticism.

REMEMBER

You aren't hurting your unborn baby if you continue to nurse; no evidence exists that breastfeeding decreases the nutrients available to either child, as long as you eat a proper diet. If you consume enough calories to satisfy your hunger, you're probably eating enough for you and your babies.

Expecting physical changes

"Oh, my aching nipples!" You may find yourself *uddering* (sorry, we couldn't help ourselves!) these words when you become pregnant and continue to nurse. During pregnancy, just like when you're menstruating, your nipples become more sensitive. When you breastfeed, this sensitivity can become downright uncomfortable.

TIP

Try to relieve the discomfort with cold compresses, or nurse your child in a more comfortable position. The length of this discomfort varies from person to person. Some mothers experience it only during early pregnancy because of the hormone changes, while others feel it throughout most of the pregnancy.

Some mothers find that breastfeeding affects morning sickness. The stimulation and let-down of milk increases nausea for some, while others find that the nausea becomes worse after they wean.

If you experience nausea, first try the typical morning sickness treatments, such as eating small meals throughout the day and sucking on lemon drop candies. (For more suggestions, see *Pregnancy For Dummies,* 2nd Edition.) Try changing your position while you breastfeed to reduce nausea. For example, try lying down and avoid a position where your child is lying on your stomach.

Breastfeeding may help you enjoy the last days alone with your "old baby" before your "new baby" comes along. Or it may become physically uncomfortable for you. Your child may lose interest as your supply drops and wean himself. Whatever the circumstances, enjoy this special time together.

Tackling Tandem Nursing

If the phrase *tandem nursing* makes you think of yourself as a restaurant with a line of hungry customers forming in front of you, you're almost right. *Tandem nursing* describes nursing two or more children (who are not twins) at the same time. You don't have to literally nurse both at the exact same time, of course — you can nurse them one after the other or at different times of the day.

Perhaps you plan to nurse your 2-year-old and your new baby at the same time, or perhaps you fall into it more or less by accident because your oldest doesn't wean by the time the next baby arrives. You may be a closet tandem nurser, just like some women are closet toddler nursers (see Chapter 10). In fact, you can be a closet tandem and toddler nurser at the same time!

If you make it through pregnancy without your older baby weaning herself, you almost certainly will have enough milk to nurse her and your new baby at the same time. Keep the following guidelines for tandem nursing in mind:

- **Make sure the new baby is getting enough.** Nurse the newborn before your older child, to be sure your newborn gets a good amount of milk. Keep an eye on the new baby's weight, especially if your older child steps up her nursing after the baby's born (which may happen because she needs reassurance and/or because you have such a bountiful milk supply!).
- **Keep yourself healthy.** You need to eat well to nurse two children, and you may be more exhausted after delivery of number two than you were after having number one.

- **Keep an eye on your own emotional state.** Many moms find themselves getting annoyed at the older nursing child's demands, even if they were happily nursing her right up to the day of the baby's birth. Your hormones and protectiveness of the new baby may cause some resentment; the helplessness of the new baby may also have you feeling annoyed at your demanding older child.

  REMEMBER

  If you find yourself feeling really annoyed, you may need to think hard about whether you want to continue nursing both children. Many moms find they can tandem nurse if they limit their older child's nursing by setting a timer, counting to ten, or allowing "a few sips." You're not doing your older child any favors if you resent letting him nurse and hate every minute.

Some moms have nursed several children for several years, even adding a third to the tandem string! If this works for you, great. If it doesn't, don't feel guilty. Parenthood is full of things to feel guilty about; weaning your 2- or 3-year-old shouldn't be one of them!

Part V
The Part of Tens

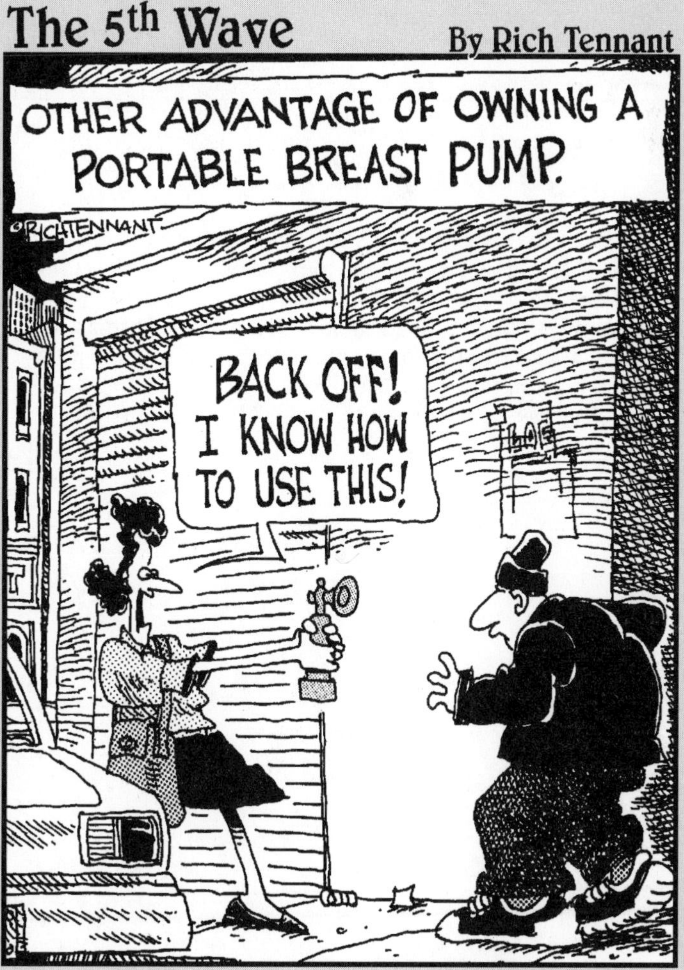

In this part . . .

Want to buy some fun stuff, like bumper stickers and T-shirts that announce to the world your views about breastfeeding? Are you hearing all sorts of old wives' tales about breastfeeding that are giving you nightmares? Or do you just want to know where to find more breastfeeding information, so you can chat the long night away with other sleep-deprived new moms? Look no further.

Chapter 17

(Almost) Ten Little Things That Make Breastfeeding More Fun

In This Chapter

- Taking yourself less seriously!
- Wearing hot bras and cool T-shirts
- Watching fun (or at least instructional) videos
- Journaling your experiences
- Choosing classy accessories

Breastfeeding can be beneficial and rewarding — and it can also be fun! In this chapter, we show you where to find interesting stuff to add a little spice to your breastfeeding experience. Some items, such as bumper stickers and T-shirts, advertise your commitment. Others, such as cool nursing bras, are just for your benefit (and perhaps your partner's!). Ready to have fun? Us, too!

Bumper Stickers

You see them everywhere — bumper stickers proclaiming everything from political views to personal habits. They're a great way to make a proclamation on whatever subject you choose.

If you choose to tell the guy behind you that you're pro-nursing, you can find bumper stickers to help you do it. Some are modest; some are militant. The following Web sites offer breastfeeding bumper stickers, and some sites let you create your own:

- `www.mammasmilk.com/resources.htm`
- `http://bflrc.com/products/stickers.htm`

- www.winter-branch.com/LLL-bumper-sticker.html
- www.bumperstatements.com/make.ihtml
- www.cafeshops.com/cp/store.aspx?s=bfingadvocacy
- www.healthed.cc/bumper_stickers.htm

TIP: The Web site "Breastfeeding Resources: Advocacy" can be found at http://bf.marie.org/resources/advocacy.html. This site lists many other sites where you can find breastfeeding promotion materials.

Cool Nursing Bras

Looking for some leopard print nursing bras? How about floral or polka dots? You've got it! Bravado makes nursing bras not only in leopard print, but also in black and, of course, basic white. But why stick to basics when you can have stuff that really makes you "feel like a woman"? Check out the Web site www.bravadodesigns.com.

REMEMBER: The nice thing about the Internet is that you don't have to leave your house to buy a new bra when your old one is in tatters; just type in "nursing bra" and order the undergarment of your dreams for delivery right to your door! Okay, so maybe even Bravado's aren't exactly the bras of your dreams, but they're better than plain white until you can get back into Victoria's Secret, aren't they?

Videos on Breastfeeding

This is your coauthor Carol speaking: As I look back at the years when my kids were growing up, I think "How did that time go so fast?" However, as I was going through a typical day it seemed that it would never end. I never had time to relax, and I rarely had time to read about how to improve my parenting skills.

One resource available today that I wish I'd had is instructional videos about parenting and breastfeeding. No matter how hectic your day is, you can probably convince yourself to take a few minutes to sit down, have a cup of tea, and unwind by watching a video. If not, then take advantage of nursing sessions by watching a video as you breastfeed.

Although we certainly hope this book becomes your breastfeeding Bible, we also know that videos can offer you a type of instruction you simply can't get from a book. Following are some Web sites where you can find helpful and informative videos:

- www.eaglevideo.com/versions.htm
- www.motherstuff.com. Visit the section on "Breastfeeding," and go to the subsection on "Videos."
- yahoo.com/Business_and_Economy/Shopping_and_Services. From the "Shopping and Services" page, click on "Health." On that page, click on "Reproduction." If you choose the "Birth" or "Pregnancy" categories, you find a wealth of resources, including Web sites where you can purchase videos and other breastfeeding supplies.
- www.breastfeeding.com. If you click on "Video Clips" from the home page, you find dozens of short videos you can download directly from the site onto your computer.

Pro-Nursing Shirts

Are you looking at your expanded chest and wondering if you should rent it out as a billboard? Why not be a billboard for breastfeeding instead? The Internet is full of Web sites that sell T-shirts both for you and your baby that proclaim nursing's benefits.

In addition to the sites listed in the "Bumper Stickers" section of this chapter, check out the following for T-shirts:

- www.justduckybabies.com. This Web site has embroidered T-shirts, which may hold up under frequent washings better than silk screened.
- www.cafeshops.com/ottogear/83421. Cafeshops.com has links to many great breastfeeding sites. We love OttoGear's T-shirt for moms that says "moo," with an accompanying baby shirt that says "baby moo"!
- www.dianadesigns.com. For some really elegant shirt designs, check out this site.

A Baby Journal

Baby journals are a far cry from the marble composition books you may have kept a diary in as a child. You can purchase great journals both in retail stores and online. Whether you choose a traditional baby book, use a plain notebook you buy at the drugstore, or make your own and decorate the cover with ribbons and bows, a journal is your trip back to your child's babyhood. You probably want to buy one before your baby is born, so you can have it handy in the hospital in case you get a few minutes to jot down your experiences.

TIP

Make the time to write all the important milestones down, because this information will be incredibly handy 10 or 20 years from now. You wouldn't believe how many times we've been asked, "When did your child start to walk?" or "How old was he when he started talking?" Recently your coauthor Sharon asked Carol about her breastfeeding experiences, and Carol couldn't remember how long she breastfed each child!

Journals can also serve purposes other than helping you remember your child's development. For example, your coauthor Carol had a daughter with major health problems. My husband kept a journal of our daughter's months with us, and doing so seemed to help him achieve a catharsis after all the difficulties. A journal helps you reflect on times both good and bad.

REMEMBER

A journal can also be a great tool for looking back at breastfeeding difficulties and how you handled them. This resource can come in handy when you have a second child and run into the same problem. Your journal then becomes a personal reference book!

Following is a sampling of baby journals online, but don't forget to check your local bookstores, which probably have beautiful personal journals in stock:

- `www.humblebumbles.com/products/babyjournal`. This site features a product called *Humble Bumbles Baby Journal: A Keepsake Journal for Baby's First Three Years.*
- `www.amazon.com`. From Amazon's home page, search for the book titled *Goodnight Moon Baby Journal.* Remember that one from your childhood? It's one of our personal favorites, and now my grandson loves it, too. One Amazon review says this is a great journal for busy moms — do you fit into that category?
- `www.babysstory.com`. You may want to keep up with the times by using an online baby book where you can record your baby's firsts up to age 6.

A Classy Diaper Bag

A diaper bag that does what you want can be a lifesaver. Lucky for you, it won't need to be filled up with bottles, formula, and a portable microwave for warming bottles! Okay, maybe we're stretching it a little, but a diaper bag needs to carry a lot of stuff. If you don't have all your necessities organized in a tidy bag, your trip to grandma's house can turn into a full-blown disaster.

If you didn't receive a diaper bag at your baby shower (and even if you did!), make sure you get one that meets your needs in the color of your choice. Get a bag that has a place for everything: diapers, wipes, diaper cream, a changing pad, medications, snacks, spare outfits, your wallet, and so on. An organized bag really helps when your hands are full, and you need to find something fast.

Trial and error can help you find the right bag, and you may find that you prefer to have more than one. Don't feel stuck using a bag you received as a present if it doesn't work for you. You can always find another use for it, for example as a tote for your baby's toys.

As long as it's functional, make sure you get something you really like, because your diaper bag is your handbag for a few years. (Does Gucci make a diaper bag?) If you care about how something looks — and who doesn't? — look around. Keep your receipt for the return in case the bag isn't as functional as you thought.

REMEMBER

Your diaper bag doesn't have to scream *baby!* Lots of moms use a generic type of bag with lots of pockets, such as a backpack. Make sure the bag is made from a substantial fabric like canvas or heavy vinyl and is washable.

Videos to Watch While Breastfeeding

TIP

If you spend hours in the nursing chair worrying about the long-term effects of soap opera dialogue on your baby, we have a suggestion. The Baby Einstein series of videos combines great music with beautiful graphics that entertain you and the baby at the same time. If you're harboring hopes of a future concert pianist, play *Baby Beethoven* or *Baby Mozart.* If your child looks more like a future scientist to you today, put on *Baby Newton.* Raising an artiste? Expose him to *Baby Van Gogh.* A marine biologist? *Baby Neptune.*

These videos are calming and enjoyable at the same time; you may find yourself watching them even when your kids aren't around! (We won't tell anyone.) Check out `www.babyeinstein.com` for a complete list of products.

Scrapbooks

Scrapbooking is a blast! This is one of your coauthor Sharon's current obsessions, and I wish I'd started when my kids were little. Chronicling your family's history in pictures is fun to do now and will provide you and your family with years of entertainment down the road. You can taking nursing pictures that are discreet, so that your (now) baby won't be horribly embarrassed by them when he's 15. And wait until you see how funny those outfits you're wearing look in 15 years!

All large craft stores have huge scrapbooking sections; don't get carried away buying supplies until you have a feel for what you want to do. You may have a page or two for every month of your baby's life, or you may do an events-oriented book: first bath, first smile, first step. The kind of book you do may change as you become more experienced at scrapbooking.

You need an album, preferably one that you can add to when you run out of pages. A good pair of scissors and a straight-edge ruler will get you started cropping pictures. Don't forget to write a little on every page so you remember the stories that go with the pictures in years to come.

TIP

Lots of stores have scrapbooking classes, and this is a great way to meet other moms so you can have connections for play dates in a few years.

Check out Creative Memories (`www.creativememories.com`), which offers lots of ideas to keep your scrapbooking quick and easy, especially when the duties of motherhood keep you running.

Chapter 18

Ten Resources for Breastfeeding

In This Chapter

- Catching up on your reading
- Relying on lactation consultants, doctors, and nurses
- Asking help from support groups, friends, and family

Whether you're an experienced breastfeeder or a first-timer, you're bound to have questions (even after you memorize every word of this book!). It helps to know where to look for answers.

In this chapter, we list some classic breastfeeding books, show you where to find online support groups, and tell you how to get in touch with a lactation consultant. We also give you ideas for setting up your own support group, getting help from your doctor or the nurses at your local hospital, and much more.

Reading Breastfeeding Books

As much as we'd like to believe that this book is the only one you'll ever need, we encourage you to check out other titles as well. Following are some classics that are widely available:

- *The Womanly Art of Breastfeeding* (Plume). This classic is La Leche League's official breastfeeding book.
- *Breastfeeding, Pure and Simple* (La Leche League International). This resource covers breastfeeding basics.
- *The Nursing Mother's Companion* (The Harvard Common Press). This book addresses just about every aspect of breastfeeding thoroughly.
- *The Complete Book of Breastfeeding* (Bantam Books). This thorough book was written by a pediatrician and a nursing mom.

TIP: If you're looking for some humor and good information at the same time, check out *So That's What They're For!* (Adams Media Corporation). Written by a lactation consultant and nursing mom, this book gives lots of facts in a humorous way.

The following are also recommended by nursing moms:

- *The Breastfeeding Book: Everything You Need to Know About Nursing Your Child From Birth Through Weaning* (Little, Brown and Co.)
- *The Ultimate Breastfeeding Book of Answers* (Prima Publishing)
- *Nursing Mother, Working Mother: The Essential Guide for Breastfeeding and Staying Close to Your Baby After You Return to Work* (Harvard Common Press)

Perusing Parenting Magazines

Parenting magazines often have very helpful articles on breastfeeding, as well as many other parenting issues. Your public library most likely carries magazines such as *Parent and Child, Parenting, American Baby, Child,* and *ePregnancy* (which is actually a hard-copy magazine, as well as an online publication); browse through them and see which might be worth ordering.

TIP: Arrange a magazine swap with a friend to keep your costs down; you order one magazine while she gets another. Or, if you organize your own breastfeeding group, build up a great library with each of you ordering one magazine and sharing with the others.

Surfing the Web

You can find everything from personal stories to articles from medical journals online. The Internet is also a great place to find breast pumps and other paraphernalia that your local stores may not carry. Better yet, you can compare prices easily and have the stuff sent right to your front door — a godsend for the first few hectic weeks of your baby's life when a trip to Wal-Mart takes more planning than the Normandy invasion.

Chatting Online

Sharon speaking here: One night, when one of my sons was facing an unusual problem, I searched the Internet for parent groups dealing with what was currently consuming my thoughts. Guess what? I found one! (More than one, in fact.)

Countless bulletin boards and chat rooms exist where you can discuss anything in anonymity, if you choose. If you don't mind sharing your identity, doing so can open up possibilities for more personal contact with your online buddies: I've been involved in online groups where members actually met for dinner.

TIP

Yahoo!, AOL, and MSN all have multiple bulletin board and chat groups on breastfeeding. So do `www.babycenter.com`, `www.ivillage.com`, and La Leche League (`www.lalecheleague.org`). If one is too strident or too laid back for you, find another.

Meeting a Lactation Consultant

As we discuss in Chapter 4, a good lactation consultant can save you hours of worry and confusion, especially if you're having difficulty breastfeeding. Look for a certified consultant; call the hospital you plan to deliver at and ask if it has a consultant on staff. Or check your phone book or the Internet.

Some consultants are associated with hospitals, and you'll see them for free after delivery. Others practice independently and charge a fee; your insurance may help cover the cost.

Picking Helpful Doctors

REMEMBER

Also in Chapter 4, we explain the importance of finding a good obstetrician and pediatrician. These doctors can make or break your breastfeeding success both in the hospital and in the months after delivery. Don't assume that every doctor will automatically support your decision to breastfeed — you may be disappointed.

As unbelievable as it seems, most doctors receive little or no formal training related to breastfeeding. A doctor who has taken classes to increase her knowledge of breastfeeding is worth her weight in gold.

Talking to the Hospital Nurses

Like doctors, many nurses receive very little training in breastfeeding. But some maternity nurses and labor and delivery nurses (like us!) take courses related to breastfeeding, read a lot of literature, and pay close attention to their patients' experiences. A good nurse can make your first breastfeeding days a pleasure. If you've been assigned Nurse Bottlefeed, ask your doctor if any of the nurses on your floor are especially good with breastfeeding mothers.

Utilizing Support Groups

If you live in an area with an established support group, such as La Leche League, and the group's general philosophy fits yours, you're in luck! Visit occasionally, or become a once-a-week regular. Undoubtedly you'll make friends with some special moms and babies — then you'll have all the ingredients for a play group!

No support groups in your area? Maybe you should start one. Stick a notice up on the supermarket bulletin board, talk to other moms at your 3-year-old's nursery school, or put a notice in the church bulletin. Even consider running an ad in your local paper.

Try to make sure your members have the same general breastfeeding philosophies, because you don't want to spend every meeting arguing with each other! If you write an ad, word it in a way that reveals your general philosophy. If you mention La Leche, people will get the idea. If you say "laid back," they'll understand that, too.

Listening to Friends and Family

People you know can be a great breastfeeding resource — or they can be real saboteurs. Choose carefully the people you want to talk with about breastfeeding. Some of your older neighbors and relatives may have breastfed their children — let them know you're nursing, and ask them for suggestions.

Attending Birthing Class

Most hospitals offer a birthing class for expectant parents; this may be a one- or two-day seminar, or it may be an eight-week class. If at all possible, go. Most childbirth instructors are also breastfeeding advocates. They can give you lots of information in class and serve as a resource after the baby is born. If you like your instructor and she seems to know her stuff, hang on to her card so you can get in touch with her after the baby's born.

Chapter 19

Ten Breastfeeding Wives' Tales

In This Chapter

- Clearing up misconceptions
- Separating truth from fiction

Our friends and family have good intentions — really. But if they actually listened to some of their own suggestions, even they might question them. When it comes to breastfeeding, the people who have never done it are likely to have the most opinions, and those people may be your nearest and dearest, like your mother.

Don't get fooled into believing every tale you're told about breastfeeding; start now to develop a filter to keep out some of the nonsense you may hear. This chapter — full of supposed "Tales from the Dark Side of Nursing" — can help.

Size Is Everything

Here's what you may hear: "Your breasts are way too small, you'll never make enough milk." Or, conversely, "Your breasts are too big, you'll smother the baby."

Many women have nursed their babies successfully with a size A cup bra. Your coauthor Sharon is related to one such person, who was nearly in tears because she couldn't find any nursing bras made in a 32A. (She was a successful breastfeeder for a year, by the way.) And besides, in the period right after delivery (when your breasts are engorged), even a double A becomes fairly well endowed!

There is no truth at all to the idea that the size of your breasts impacts your ability to produce adequate milk, or that big breasts are weapons of destruction. No one has ever smothered a baby with her breasts during nursing — we promise.

Blondes Don't Have More Fun

Here's what you may hear: "Being a redhead or a blonde makes you more susceptible to nipple pain." Blondes and redheads, because they are usually fair-skinned, are often told that they'll regret trying to breastfeed because their skin is too sensitive to nurse.

This is simply not the case. If you experience nipple discomfort, your hair color is not to blame. Instead, consider the possibility that your baby isn't latching on correctly or that you're holding her in an uncomfortable position (see Chapter 6).

Heavy Breasts Mean More Milk

Here's what you may hear: "You can tell how much milk is in your breasts by how much they weigh." The last time we checked our breasts, they didn't have a weight gauge on them!

Many people will tell you this and really mean it. But what they're talking about is the engorgement that occurs within the first couple days after birth, when you experience an increased flow of blood to the breasts, and they're definitely heavier.

When engorgement subsides after a day or two, your breasts will feel and look like they weigh about 10 pounds less than they did a few days before. This has nothing to do with the amount of milk in them; your breasts are just settling down to the job of making milk.

You Can't Eat Anything Good

Here's what you may hear: "When you nurse, you have to stay away from milk and desserts and coffee and spicy foods and. . . ." If you really tried to avoid all the foods people say not to eat when nursing, you'd find yourself feeling a little deprived at the dinner table. That's not what nursing is about.

Many foods do pass through the breast milk to the baby, just as many drugs do. But you don't need to stick to a fruit and rice diet when you're nursing; just pay attention to what you eat if the baby's not a happy camper. Your coauthor Carol once ate hot dogs, sauerkraut, and baked beans for dinner. I hope I enjoyed that meal, because the baby didn't, and I paid dearly for the next 24 hours! I lived and learned. You just have to do the same.

A Crying Baby Must Be Hungry

Here's what you may hear: "Your baby cries a lot. I don't think he's getting enough milk." Many new moms hear this, especially from people who don't understand breastfeeding. Or babies.

Babies cry for many reasons. And most of the time, hunger isn't the prime suspect. Rest assured that if you're nursing every few hours for 15 to 30 minutes each time, and if your pediatrician is comfortable with your baby's weight gain, your baby is getting plenty of milk.

Keep Your Partner's Hands Off

Here's what you may hear: "Your partner needs to know that those breasts are off-limits in your lovemaking." This is definitely not true, at least from a medical perspective. Only you and your partner can determine what's comfortable and what's not. It's your bedroom — you make the rules.

Rest assured that your baby's food supply will not decrease if you get your breasts involved in lovemaking. However, keep in mind that *oxytocin* — the hormone that releases milk — doesn't turn off during lovemaking. Your breasts may spray milk during a climax. (This takes a "milk bath" to the next level!) We talk more about sex and breastfeeding in Chapter 11.

Sour Moms Make Sour Milk

Here's what you may hear: "If you're angry or upset, you'll sour your milk." Sheer nonsense. Unless you're practicing to be a Stepford Wife, you're going to become angry and upset at some point while you're nursing. If the baby seems to get upset after a tense feeding, it may be because she's picked up your tension, not because you've curdled your milk.

Nursing Leads to Sagging

Here's what you may hear: "Breastfeeding makes your breasts sag." Unfortunately, breasts sag all by themselves as you age. Whether you breastfeed or not makes no difference — even women who never get pregnant must eventually face the reality of sagging.

Public Nursing Is Criminal

Here's what you may hear: "Don't even think about nursing in public, or you'll get arrested." If this were true, half the breastfeeding women in the United States would have been arrested by now! Women have been breastfeeding in public places for years. Some states have instituted laws that specifically exclude breastfeeding from public nudity laws. See Chapter 15 for more information about your legal rights related to breastfeeding.

Breastfeeding Is Birth Control

Here's what you may hear: "You can't get pregnant while you're breastfeeding." Many women have learned, to their shock, that this isn't necessarily true. While breastfeeding may delay your first ovulation after delivery, it doesn't delay it forever, and the degree of protection against another pregnancy is directly related to how you're breastfeeding.

The best way to protect against another pregnancy is to breastfeed exclusively at least every four hours around the clock, without using any supplements or pacifiers. Doing so can be a very effective method of birth control, as effective as using birth control pills.

REMEMBER

You can ovulate even if your periods haven't started again, especially if you're supplementing or not nursing regularly. Don't assume you're safe from using birth control because your periods haven't resumed yet! For much more information about birth control and breastfeeding, see Chapter 16.

Index

• A •

• C •

• D •

• E •

• F •

• M •

• N •

• O •

• P •

• T •

• U •

• V •

• W •

• Y •

• Z •

FOR DUMMIES®

A world of resources to help you grow

TRAVEL

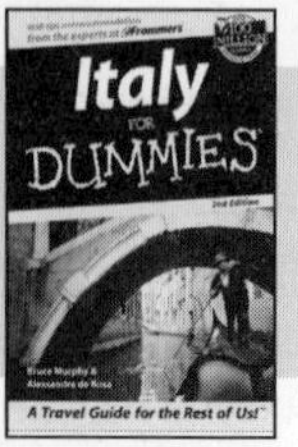

0-7645-5453-0

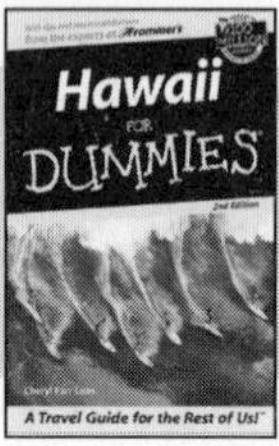

0-7645-5438-7

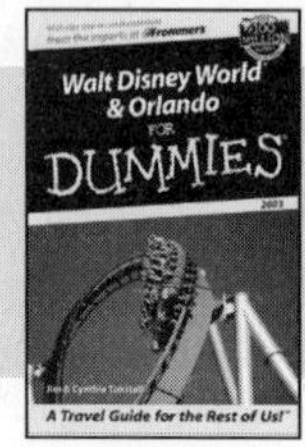

0-7645-5444-1

Also available:

America's National Parks For Dummies (0-7645-6204-5)

Caribbean For Dummies (0-7645-5445-X)

Cruise Vacations For Dummies 2003 (0-7645-5459-X)

Europe For Dummies (0-7645-5456-5)

Ireland For Dummies (0-7645-6199-5)

France For Dummies (0-7645-6292-4)

Las Vegas For Dummies (0-7645-5448-4)

London For Dummies (0-7645-5416-6)

Mexico's Beach Resorts For Dummies (0-7645-6262-2)

Paris For Dummies (0-7645-5494-8)

RV Vacations For Dummies (0-7645-5443-3)

EDUCATION & TEST PREPARATION

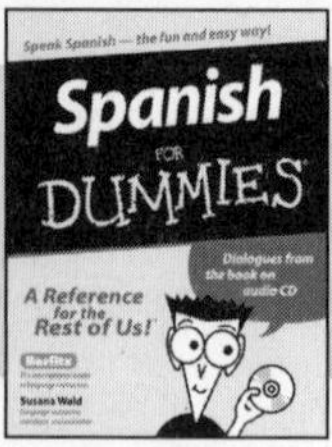

0-7645-5194-9

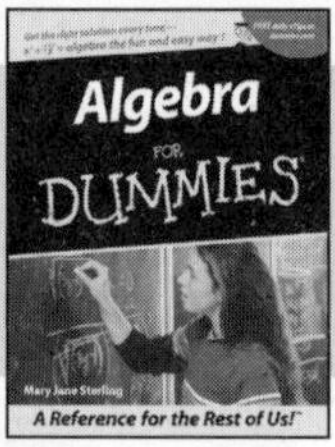

0-7645-5325-9

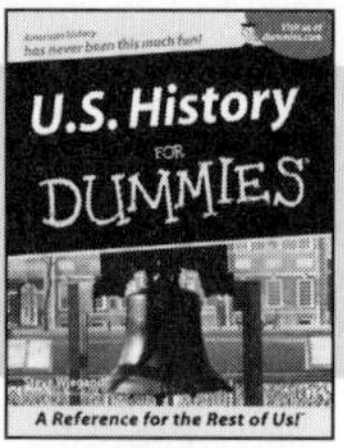

0-7645-5249-X

Also available:

The ACT For Dummies (0-7645-5210-4)

Chemistry For Dummies (0-7645-5430-1)

English Grammar For Dummies (0-7645-5322-4)

French For Dummies (0-7645-5193-0)

GMAT For Dummies (0-7645-5251-1)

Inglés Para Dummies (0-7645-5427-1)

Italian For Dummies (0-7645-5196-5)

Research Papers For Dummies (0-7645-5426-3)

SAT I For Dummies (0-7645-5472-7)

U.S. History For Dummies (0-7645-5249-X)

World History For Dummies (0-7645-5242-2)

HEALTH, SELF-HELP & SPIRITUALITY

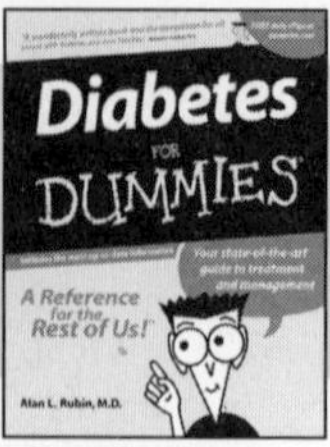

0-7645-5154-X

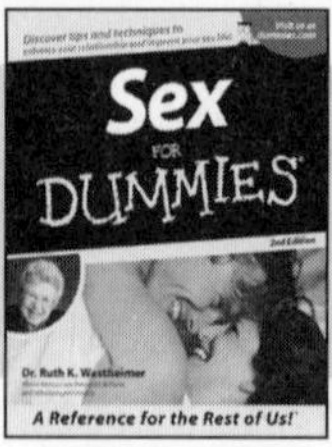

0-7645-5302-X

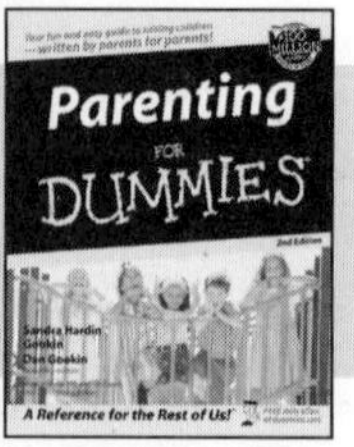

0-7645-5418-2

Also available:

The Bible For Dummies (0-7645-5296-1)

Controlling Cholesterol For Dummies (0-7645-5440-9)

Dating For Dummies (0-7645-5072-1)

Dieting For Dummies (0-7645-5126-4)

High Blood Pressure For Dummies (0-7645-5424-7)

Judaism For Dummies (0-7645-5299-6)

Menopause For Dummies (0-7645-5458-1)

Nutrition For Dummies (0-7645-5180-9)

Potty Training For Dummies (0-7645-5417-4)

Pregnancy For Dummies (0-7645-5074-8)

Rekindling Romance For Dummies (0-7645-5303-8)

Religion For Dummies (0-7645-5264-3)

Available wherever books are sold. Go to www.dummies.com or call 1-877-762-2974 to order direct

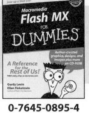

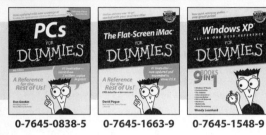

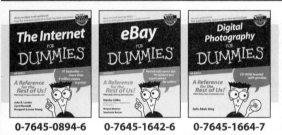

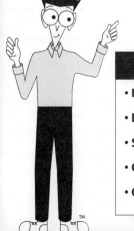

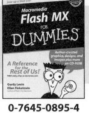

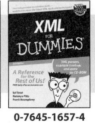

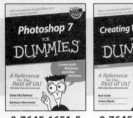

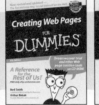

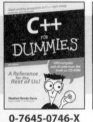

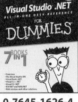

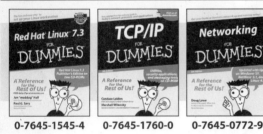

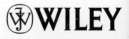